Liver Pathology

Editor

JOHN HART

SURGICAL PATHOLOGY CLINICS

www.surgpath.theclinics.com

Consulting Editor
JASON L. HORNICK

June 2018 • Volume 11 • Number 2

ELSEVIER

1600 John F. Kennedy Boulevard • Suite 1800 • Philadelphia, Pennsylvania, 19103-2899

http://www.theclinics.com

SURGICAL PATHOLOGY CLINICS Volume 11, Number 2
June 2018 ISSN 1875-9181, ISBN-13: 978-0-323-58420-3

Editor: Stacy Eastman
Developmental Editor: Donald Mumford

Surgical Pathology Clinics (ISSN 1875-9181) is published quarterly by Elsevier Inc., 360 Park Avenue South, New York, NY 10010. Months of issue are March, June, September, and December. Business and Editorial Office: Elsevier Inc., 1600 John F. Kennedy Blvd., Ste. 1800, Philadelphia, PA 19103-2899. Accounting and Circulation Offices: Elsevier Inc., 3251 Riverport Lane, Maryland Heights, MO 63043. Periodicals postage paid at New York, NY and at additional mailing offices. Subscription prices are $206.00 per year (US individuals), $279.00 per year (US institutions), $100.00 per year (US students/residents), $258.00 per year (Canadian individuals), $318.00 per year (Canadian Institutions), $258.00 per year (foreign individuals), $318.00 per year (foreign institutions), and $120.00 per year (international & Canadian students/residents). Foreign air speed delivery is included in all *Clinics'* subscription prices. All prices are subject to change without notice. **POSTMASTER:** Send address changes to *Surgical Pathology Clinics*, Elsevier, 3251 Riverport Lane, Maryland Heights, MO 63043. **Customer Service: 1-800-654-2452 (US). From outside the United States, call 1-314-447-8871. Fax: 1-314-447-8029. E-mail: JournalsCustomerServiceusa@elsevier.com (for print support) and JournalsOnlineSupport-usa@elsevier.com (for online support).**

Reprints. For copies of 100 or more, of articles in this publication, please contact the Commercial Reprints Department, Elsevier Inc., 360 Park Avenue South, New York, NY 10010-1710. Tel. 212-633-3874; Fax: 212-633-3820; E-mail: reprints@elsevier.com.

Surgical Pathology Clinics of North America is covered in *MEDLINE/PubMed (Index Medicus)*.

Contributors

CONSULTING EDITOR

JASON L. HORNICK, MD, PhD
Director of Surgical Pathology and
Immunohistochemistry, Brigham and Women's
Hospital, Professor of Pathology, Harvard
Medical School, Boston, Massachusetts, USA

EDITOR

JOHN HART, MD
Professor and Chief of GI and Hepatic
Pathology, The University of Chicago
Medicine, Chicago, Illinois, USA

AUTHORS

JOSEPH AHN, MD, MS, MBA, FAASLD
Associate Professor of Medicine, Director of
Clinical Hepatology, Oregon Health & Science
University, Portland, Oregon, USA

**VENANCIO AVANCINI FERREIRA ALVES,
MD, PhD**
Professor, Department of Pathology, Director,
Surgical Pathology, University of Sao Paulo
School of Medicine, Sao Paulo, Brazil

EUN-YOUNG KAREN CHOI, MD
Assistant Professor, Department of Pathology,
University of Michigan, University of Michigan
Hospitals, Ann Arbor, Michigan, USA

WON-TAK CHOI, MD, PhD
Assistant Professor, Department of Pathology,
University of California, San Francisco,
San Francisco, California, USA

**ANDREW D. CLOUSTON, MBBS, PhD,
FRCPA**
Professor, Faculty of Medicine, The University
of Queensland, Brisbane, Queensland, Australia

RYAN M. GILL, MD, PhD
Associate Professor, Department of Pathology,
University of California, San Francisco,
San Francisco, California, USA

RAUL S. GONZALEZ, MD
Assistant Professor, Department of Pathology
and Laboratory Medicine, University of
Rochester Medical Center, Rochester,
New York, USA

RONDELL P. GRAHAM, MBBS
Divisions of Anatomic Pathology and of
Laboratory Genetics and Genomics,
Mayo Clinic, Rochester, Minnesota, USA

CYNTHIA D. GUY, MD
Duke University, DUHS, Durham,
North Carolina, USA

DAVID E. KLEINER, MD, PhD
Senior Research Physician, Chief,
Post-Mortem Section, Laboratory of
Pathology, National Cancer Institute,
Bethesda, Maryland, USA

ANNE KOEHNE DE GONZALEZ, MD
Assistant Professor, Department of Pathology
and Cell Biology, Columbia University,
New York, New York, USA

JAMIE KOO, MD
Assistant Professor, Department of Pathology
and Laboratory Medicine, Cedars-Sinai
Medical Center, Los Angeles, California, USA

ALYSSA M. KRASINSKAS, MD
Professor, Department of Pathology and
Laboratory Medicine, Director of
Gastrointestinal and Liver Pathology
Fellowship, Emory University, Atlanta,
Georgia, USA

STEPHEN M. LAGANA, MD
Assistant Professor, Department of Pathology
and Cell Biology, Columbia University,
New York, New York, USA

LAURA W. LAMPS, MD
Godfrey D. Stobbe Professor of
Gastrointestinal Pathology, Department of
Pathology, University of Michigan, University of
Michigan Hospitals, Ann Arbor, Michigan, USA

MEREDITH E. PITTMAN, MD, MSCI
Assistant Professor, Department of Pathology
and Laboratory Medicine, Weill Cornell
Medicine, New York, New York, USA

MICHAEL H. SCHILD, DO
Duke University, DUHS, Durham,
North Carolina, USA

MICHAEL TORBENSON, MD
Professor of Laboratory Medicine and
Pathology, Mayo Clinic, Rochester,
Minnesota, USA

HANLIN L. WANG, MD, PhD
Professor, Department of Pathology and
Laboratory Medicine, David Geffen School of
Medicine at UCLA, Los Angeles, California,
USA

KAY WASHINGTON, MD, PhD
Professor, Department of Pathology,
Microbiology, and Immunology, Vanderbilt
University Medical Center, Nashville,
Tennessee, USA

MARIA WESTERHOFF, MD
Associate Professor of Pathology, University of
Michigan, Ann Arbor, Michigan, USA

RHONDA K. YANTISS, MD
Professor and Chief of Gastrointestinal
Pathology, Department of Pathology and
Laboratory Medicine, Weill Cornell Medicine,
New York, New York, USA

Contents

Hepatic granulomas are encountered in approximately 2% to 10% of liver biopsies. There are many potential infectious and noninfectious causes; granulomas can be generally classified by their morphology, which may be helpful in refining the differential diagnosis. This article provides a review of hepatic granulomas, with an emphasis on infectious causes.

From the standpoint of the surgical pathologist "hepatitis" is defined as the set of histologic patterns of lesions found in livers infected by hepatotropic viruses or by nonhepatotrophic viruses leading to liver inflammation in the context of systemic infection or due to an autoimmune disease, drug, or toxin involving the liver. This article is centered on the histologic patterns of injury in acute viral hepatitis, encompassing the hepatotropic viruses A, B, C, D, and E and the "icteric hemorrhagic fevers" (dengue, hantavirus, yellow fever). A brief mention of viruses causing hepatitis in immunosuppressed patients also is presented.

Nonalcoholic fatty liver disease (NAFLD) is a major health concern, and the prevalence continues to increase in many industrialized and developing countries around the world. NAFLD affects adults and children. NAFLD-related cirrhosis is expected to become the top indication for liver transplant in the near future, and the incidence of NAFLD-related hepatocellular carcinoma is also increasing. Nonalcoholic steatohepatitis is the more severe form of NAFLD. The pathogenesis of NALFD/nonalcoholic steatohepatitis is complex, and new concepts continue to evolve. The diagnosis and categorization of nonalcoholic steatohepatitis currently rests on hepatopathologists. Accurate morphologic interpretation is important for therapeutic, prognostic, and investigational purposes.

The hepatitis C virus (HCV) is the most common blood-borne infection in the United States and is the most common cause of end-stage liver disease requiring liver transplant. Over the last 10 years, direct acting antiviral therapies have revolutionized HCV treatment, increasing the cure rates from less than 50% to more than 90% in those who reach access to care. This article is an overview for pathologists and clinicians covering the histologic findings of HCV as well as direct acting antiviral therapy.

Drug-induced liver injury (DILI) is constantly changing as new drugs are approved and as new herbals and dietary supplements (HDS) reach the market. The pathologist plays a key role in the evaluation of DILI by classifying and interpreting the histologic findings considering patients' medical history and drug exposure. The liver biopsy findings may suggest alternative explanations of the injury and additional testing that should be performed to exclude non-DILI causes. Recent reports of iatrogenic liver injury are reviewed with attention to immunomodulatory and antineoplastic agents, as well as reports of injury associated with HDS use.

The inherited diseases causing conjugated hyperbilirubinemia are diverse, with variability in clinical severity, histologic appearance, and time of onset. The liver biopsy appearances can also vary depending on whether the initial presentation is in the neonatal period or later. Although many of the disorders have specific histologic features in fully developed and classic cases, biopsies taken early in the disease course may be nonspecific, showing either cholestatic hepatitis or an obstructive pattern of injury requiring close correlation with the laboratory and clinical findings to reach the correct diagnosis. In addition, increased understanding of the range of hepatic changes occurring in mild deficiencies of bile canalicular transporter proteins suggests that these disorders, particularly ABCB4 deficiency, may be more common than previously recognized; improved awareness should prompt further investigation.

Primary biliary cholangitis and autoimmune hepatitis are common autoimmune diseases of the liver. Both have typical clinical presentations, including certain autoantibodies on serologic testing. Histologic features are also often typical: primary biliary cholangitis shows bile duct destruction (sometimes with granulomas), and autoimmune hepatitis shows prominent portal and lobular lymphoplasmacytic inflammation. Both have a wide differential diagnosis, including one another; they may also simultaneously occur within the same patient. Careful use of clinical and histologic criteria may be necessary for diagnosis. First-line therapy is immunosuppression for autoimmune hepatitis and ursodeoxycholic acid for primary biliary cholangitis. Both diseases may progress to cirrhosis.

Rapid advances in molecular and anatomic pathology have greatly improved our understanding of hepatocellular adenomas. Principal among them is a clinically relevant, histology-based classification that identifies hepatic adenomas at greatest risk for malignant transformation. This new classification system has led to general consensus on the major subtypes of hepatic adenomas. However, controversy remains regarding how to incorporate less common types of hepatic adenomas into the classification system and how to incorporate adenoma subtyping into clinical care. This article provides an in-depth review of how adenomas are classified, with a focus on the current rationale, the consensus, and controversies.

definition of humoral (antibody-mediated) rejection has been greatly expanded in recent years. The histopathologic assessment of allograft biopsies continues to serve an important role in the diagnosis of rejection and to facilitate patient management. The diagnosis of both acute and chronic antibody-mediated rejection requires integration of the results of donor-specific antigen testing and C4d immunostaining, as well exclusion of other potential causes of graft dysfunction. Chronic antibody-mediated rejection should also be included in the differential diagnosis for unexplained allograft fibrosis.

Meredith E. Pittman and Rhonda K. Yantiss

Intraoperative consultation requires skills in gross examination and histologic diagnosis, as well as an ability to perform rapid interpretations under time constraints. This article provides surgical pathologists with a framework for dealing with hepatic specimens in the frozen section area by covering common clinical scenarios and histologic findings. Differential diagnoses are considered in relation to primary hepatic neoplasia and metastatic diseases. Benign mimics of malignancy and other pitfalls in frozen section diagnosis of lesional tissue are covered. Finally, assessment of donor liver biopsy for organ transplant evaluation is discussed.

SURGICAL PATHOLOGY CLINICS

RELATED INTEREST

Clinics in Liver Disease, May 2015 (Vol. 19, No. 2)
Hepatocellular Carcinoma in Adults and Children
Adrian Reuben, *Editor*

THE CLINICS ARE AVAILABLE ONLINE!
Access your subscription at:
www.theclinics.com

Preface

Hepatic Pathology: Evolving Concepts in Diagnosis and Pathogenesis for Medical Diseases and Tumors

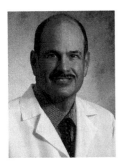

John Hart, MD

Editor

Percutaneous and transjugular liver biopsy tests have been utilized for over 50 years for the evaluation of medical liver disease and for the diagnosis of hepatic mass lesions. The increasing use of noninvasive methods for assessing liver fibrosis, coupled with the expanding utilization of direct-acting antiviral medications for the treatment of chronic HCV hepatitis, has clearly led to a recent decrease in the volume of liver biopsies. Nevertheless, histologic assessment of a liver biopsy specimen remains the gold standard for diagnosis of most medical liver diseases and mass lesions. Moreover, there have been exciting recent developments in our understanding of the molecular pathogenesis of many hereditary, metabolic, autoimmune, and neoplastic disorders that have made pathologic assessment of liver tissue samples more informative and clinically relevant than ever before.

In this issue, recent developments in the pathology of a variety of medical liver diseases and tumors are reviewed. There has been a significant expansion of the clinically important bacterial, fungal, parasitic, and viral infections of the liver that must be considered in an era of ever-increasing global travel. The enormous differential diagnosis of granulomas and acute hepatitis now faced by the surgical pathologist requires a systematic approach for liver biopsy diagnosis. While chronic HCV hepatitis is no longer the leading indication for liver transplantation in the United States, having been supplanted by nonalcoholic steatohepatitis, there are still intriguing histologic features present in the biopsies of patients who have achieved sustained virologic response after treatment with a direct-acting antiviral agent. At the same time, our understanding of the pathogenesis of nonalcoholic steatohepatitis increases yearly in parallel with the increasing number of liver biopsies performed to assess this disorder. The pathologic features of steatohepatitis are being delineated in ever greater detail, making histologic assessment more valuable for clinical management decision making.

One of the increasingly common and important indications for liver biopsy is the assessment for possible drug-induced liver injury. As biologic agents are utilized more frequently to treat advanced malignancies, clinically significant hepatic toxicity has become a critical limiting factor in their use. The number of new medications of all types is seemingly rising every year, resulting in an ever-expanding spectrum of histologic features of drug-induced injury. At the same time, progress in identifying the key molecular events responsible for several of the common and rare hereditary and autoimmune disorders of the liver has led to a better delineation of the key histologic features necessary for their diagnosis. Hereditary cholestatic conditions due to defects in canalicular

Surgical Pathology 11 (2018) xi–xii
https://doi.org/10.1016/j.path.2018.04.001
1875-9181/18/© 2018 Published by Elsevier Inc.

transporter proteins in particular are being increasingly recognized and diagnosed based on a combination of key histologic features and molecular testing performed on liver biopsy samples. Meanwhile, as our knowledge of the clinical and molecular features of autoimmune hepatitis and primary biliary cholangitis becomes more refined, the histologic spectrum of features is also becoming more detailed and clinically relevant.

Liver biopsy has always been a mainstay in the diagnosis of hepatic mass lesions, whether primary or metastatic. Tissue acquisition is even more important now as next-generation sequencing is utilized routinely to also identify mutations that can be targeted for therapeutic intervention. Our increasing knowledge of the molecular pathogenic mechanisms of hepatocellular adenoma development has led to the creation and refinement of a new classification scheme that is utilized for management decision making. New diagnostic and prognostic immunohistologic and molecular techniques are also being developed and applied in the diagnosis of hepatocellular carcinoma, fibrolamellar carcinoma, cholangiocarcinoma, and primary liver tumors with progenitor cell phenotypes. The diagnosis of lymphoproliferative disorders involving the liver also increasingly relies on the carefully considered application of an expanding selection of immunohistologic and molecular diagnostic assays.

Every practicing surgical pathologist must be prepared for frozen section consultations on liver specimens, for diagnosis of primary and metastatic tumors as well as many medical liver diseases. Donor liver biopsy frozen section evaluation is also a critical component of the decision-making process for organ suitability for transplantation and is often performed in the middle of the night

without backup from colleagues. As the donor pool is expanded to meet the demand for organs, the spectrum of histologic abnormalities that needs to be evaluated in donor liver biopsies is also rising. The pathologic evaluation of posttransplant liver biopsies, after a long and dynamic period of progressive gain in experience and accumulated knowledge, has now seemingly settled into a mature field of well-defined pathologic entities. Nevertheless, as new immunosuppressive regimens are instituted and as long-term allograft survival increases, there is still an evolving understanding of the pathologic features of allograft rejection and tolerance.

This issue of *Surgical Pathology Clinics* is devoted to the most recent developments in each of these areas of hepatic pathology. The intent is for the reader to use this text as a resource for the most up-to-date information available for each of the 14 topics covered, with numerous high-quality and carefully curated photographs to illustrate the key features described in the text. I am grateful to all of the expert liver pathologists who have accepted the invitation to contribute. They have undertaken to provide the reader with a concise and well thought-out approach to the most common and problematic issues in hepatic pathology, and I believe they have met the challenge exceptionally well.

John Hart, MD
Department of Pathology
University of Chicago Medicine
MC 6101, 5841 South Maryland Avenue
Chicago, IL 60637, USA

E-mail address:
John.hart@uchospitals.edu

Granulomas in the Liver, with a Focus on Infectious Causes

Eun-Young Karen Choi, MD*, Laura W. Lamps, MD

KEYWORDS

• Liver • Granuloma • Infection • Granulomatous inflammation

Key points

- Granulomas in the liver can be generally classified by morphology, which can be helpful in suggesting the cause.
- There are many possible causes of hepatic granulomas, including infectious and noninfectious diseases. Clinical history and other laboratory tests are often helpful in the evaluation of hepatic granulomas.
- A cause of hepatic granulomas cannot be identified for some cases, even following extensive clinical and histologic workup; in some cases, hepatic granulomas are incidental and have no clinical significance.

ABSTRACT

Hepatic granulomas are encountered in approximately 2% to 10% of liver biopsies. There are many potential infectious and noninfectious causes; granulomas can be generally classified by their morphology, which may be helpful in refining the differential diagnosis. This article provides a review of hepatic granulomas with an emphasis on infectious causes.

GENERAL CONSIDERATIONS

Hepatic granulomas have been reported in 2% to 10% of biopsies[1-4] and may be localized to the liver or be a part of a systemic disease. They have been associated with both infectious and noninfectious causes, but in some cases, a cause cannot be identified even after extensive histologic, clinical, and laboratory workup.

Granulomas in the liver can also be an incidental finding with no clinical significance or only a minor component of a pathologic process. The histologic features of hepatic granulomas, however, may be suggestive of a cause that can guide further evaluation of patients. This article discusses the causes of hepatic granulomas as they relate to histologic patterns, with an emphasis on infectious diseases.

Granulomas can be roughly classified by their morphology (**Table 1**). *Aggregates of foamy histiocytes* (**Fig. 1**A) are usually infectious in cause and most often occur in immunocompromised patients. Examples include *Mycobacterium avium-intracellulare* (MAI), *Mycobacterium leprae* (leprosy), *Tropheryma whipplei* (Whipple disease), and *Rhodococcus equi* infections.

Epithelioid granulomas are discrete, well-formed collections of epithelioid histiocytes with well-defined borders. Non-necrotizing

---

Disclosure Statement: The authors have nothing to disclose.
Department of Pathology, University of Michigan, University of Michigan, 5231B Medical Science I, 1301 Catherine Street, SPC 5602, Ann Arbor, MI 48109, USA
* Corresponding author.
E-mail address: ekchoi@med.umich.edu

Surgical Pathology 11 (2018) 231–250
https://doi.org/10.1016/j.path.2018.02.008
1875-9181/18/

Table 1
Classification of hepatic granulomatous processes by morphology

Granuloma Morphology	Possible Causes
Aggregates of foamy macrophages	Usually infectious: *Rhodococcus equi,* MAI in immunocompromised patients, lepromatous leprosy, Whipple disease

Epithelioid granulomas with or without necrosis	Infectious
	    Tuberculosis (usually with caseating necrosis), MAI in immunocompetent patients, brucellosis, tuberculoid leprosy, syphilis, rarely Whipple disease and viral infections
	Noninfectious
	    Sarcoidosis, drug reaction, foreign body reaction, common variable immunodeficiency, autoimmune diseases, primary biliary cholangitis, neoplasm-associated, chronic granulomatous disease

Fibrin-ring granulomas	Infectious
	    Q fever, typhoid fever, Epstein-Barr virus, cytomegalovirus, toxoplasmosis, leishmaniasis
	Noninfectious
	    Drug reaction, lupus, metastases

Granulomatous inflammation associated with prominent suppurative inflammation	Usually infectious: tularemia, listeriosis, melioidosis

Granulomatous inflammation with central stellate microabscess	Infectious
	    Cat-scratch disease, *Nocardia*, tularemia, *Candida*, actinomycosis, other fungi
	Noninfectious
	    Chronic granulomatous disease

Lipogranulomas	Mineral oil, fatty liver disease, hepatitis C
Microgranulomas	Nonspecific reaction to liver injury

Abbreviation: MAI, mycobacterium avium-intracellulare complex.

epithelioid granulomas can be seen in many conditions (**Fig. 1**B), and the differential is broad. Epithelioid granulomas with caseating necrosis (**Fig. 1**C), however, are highly suggestive of an infectious cause (eg, *Mycobacterium tuberculosis*); these are often randomly distributed throughout the liver with destruction of surrounding architecture.

Fibrin-ring granulomas are composed of epithelioid macrophages with a central fat vacuole surrounded by a ring of fibrin (**Fig. 1**D). They are classically associated with Q fever but have been associated with many infectious causes, including cytomegalovirus, Epstein-Barr virus (EBV), leishmaniasis, and toxoplasmosis,[5] as well as noninfectious causes, such as adverse drug reactions.[5,6]

Granulomatous inflammation, composed of poorly formed granulomas with indistinct borders, is often intermixed with other types of inflammatory cells (**Fig. 1**E). When accompanied by prominent suppurative inflammation, the findings raise suspicion for infectious causes, such as tularemia, listeriosis, and melioidosis. Granulomatous inflammation with associated hepatocellular or bile duct injury raises the possibility of an adverse drug reaction.

Granulomatous inflammation with a central stellate microabscess is usually infectious as well, and examples include *Bartonella* (cat-scratch disease) (**Fig. 1**F) and *Candida* infections and, more rarely, *Nocardia,* tularemia, and actinomycosis.

Lipogranulomas are small collections of macrophages and lipid droplets (**Fig. 1**G). They have been linked to mineral oils in foods and have also been associated with fatty liver disease and hepatitis C virus infection. Lipogranulomas may have associated fibrosis, but they are not thought to

Fig. 1. Types of granulomas by morphology. (*A*) Aggregate of histiocytes with foamy, pale cytoplasm. (*B*) Epithelioid granuloma. The granuloma is non-necrotizing, has discrete well-defined borders, and is composed of epithelioid macrophages mixed with other inflammatory cells. (*C*) Epithelioid granuloma with caseating necrosis.

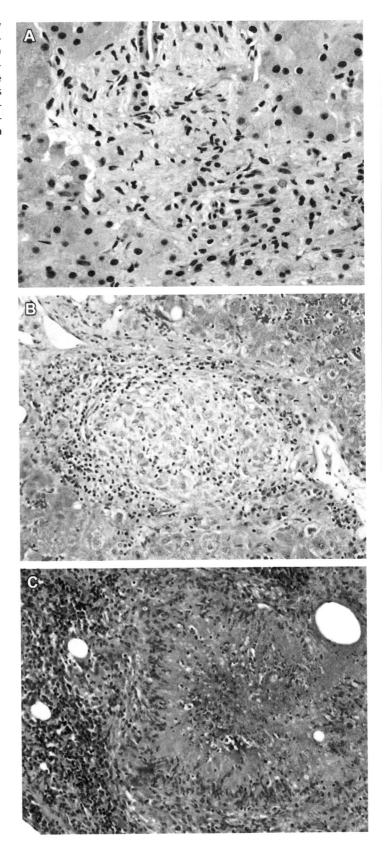

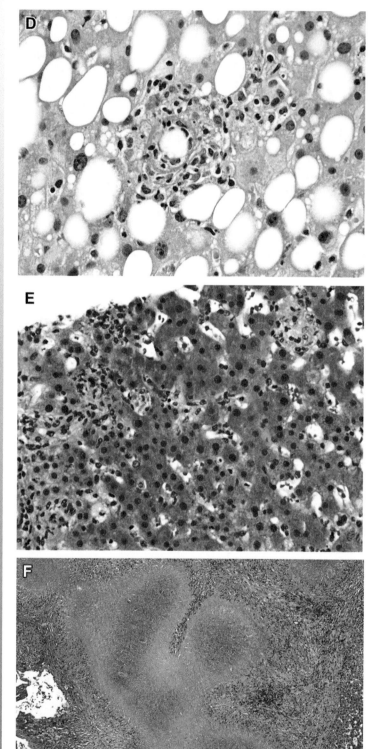

Fig. 1. (continued). (*D*) Fibrin-ring granuloma. A central lipid vacuole is surrounded by a ring of fibrin and epithelioid macrophages. (*E*) Granulomatous inflammation. This type of granuloma is composed of small collections of macrophages with indistinct borders and often intermixed with other types of inflammatory cells. (*F*) Granulomatous inflammation with a central stellate microabscess.

Fig. 1. (*continued*). (*G*) Lipogranuloma composed of lipid droplets, macrophages, and lymphocytes. (*H*) Microgranuloma composed of a few macrophages and other inflammatory cells (hematoxylin-eosin, original magnification ×400 [*A, D, G, H*]; original magnification ×200 [*B, C, E*]; original magnification ×40 [*F*]).

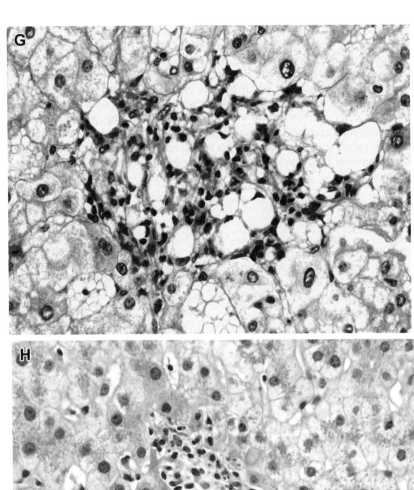

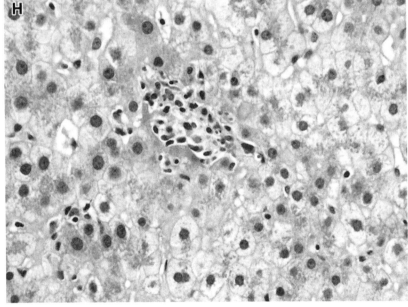

contribute to the progression of fibrosis in chronic liver diseases. Lipogranulomas are commonly encountered and are generally not clinically significant.

Microgranulomas are small clusters of histiocytes (about 3–7) that are often mixed with other inflammatory cells and hepatocellular apoptotic debris (**Fig.** 1H). This pattern is nonspecific, can be seen following many forms of cellular injury,

and is often associated with an adverse drug reaction.

In addition to the morphology of the granulomas, other histologic features, such as accompanying inflammatory cell infiltrate, location in the liver parenchyma, and presence of identifiable organisms or foreign material, may be helpful in suggesting a cause. Clinical information, such as patients' past medical history, immune status, drug and toxin exposure, recreational drug use, contact with animals, and history of recent travels, may also provide clues regarding the cause of hepatic granulomas. Other tests, such as special stains, cultures, and molecular assays, may be needed for further evaluation as well. Ultimately, determination of the likely cause of a granulomatous process in the liver is often made clinically, but the findings in the liver biopsy can potentially help narrow down the differential diagnosis.

INFECTIOUS CAUSES OF HEPATIC GRANULOMAS

There are many infectious causes of hepatic granulomas, including bacterial, fungal, parasitic, and viral infections. Select examples of infectious causes associated with granulomatous reactions are discussed.

BACTERIAL INFECTIONS

Granulomas can be seen in many mycobacterial infections, including M tuberculosis, M leprae, and MAI infections. M tuberculosis is the causative agent of tuberculosis. The liver is involved in most cases of hematogenous dissemination (miliary tuberculosis), and hepatic tuberculosis is also common in association with pulmonary tuberculosis and in localized extrapulmonary tuberculosis.[7,8] Signs and symptoms may include fever, abdominal pain, hepatomegaly, and serum liver enzyme elevations, most commonly alkaline phosphatase and gamma-glutamyl transferase elevations.[7,9] Microscopically, the granulomas are epithelioid, often with caseating necrosis and giant cells. Acid-fast stains (eg, Ziehl-Neelsen) are needed to visualize the bacilli; but they have low sensitivity, and microbial culture and polymerase chain reaction (PCR) are useful adjuncts.[10]

M leprae is the etiologic agent of leprosy (Hanson disease). It is a slow-growing, obligate intracellular pathogen that primarily affects skin and peripheral nerves. Liver infection occurs in approximately 20% cases of tuberculoid leprosy and more than 60% cases of lepromatous leprosy.[11–13] The granulomas of lepromatous leprosy are typically composed of aggregates of foamy macrophages containing numerous acid-fast bacilli (lepra cells) scattered in the lobules and portal tracts. The granulomas of tuberculoid leprosy are often discrete, non-necrotizing epithelioid granulomas with associated giant cells and few detectable organisms (Fig. 2). The bacilli can be highlighted by acid-fast stains (eg, Fite stain), and PCR testing is also available.[14] Risk factors for infection include close contact with patients who have leprosy and, in the southern United

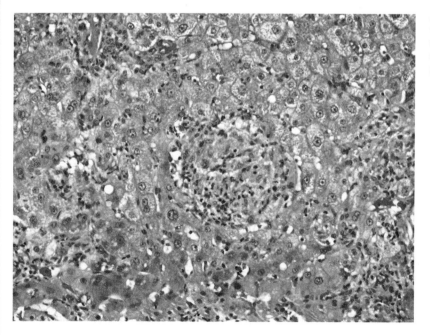

Fig. 2. A discrete epithelioid granuloma in tuberculoid leprosy (hematoxylin-eosin, original magnification ×200).

States, exposure to the 9-banded armadillo, in which *M leprae* is enzootic.[15]

MAI complex infections are most commonly encountered in patients with AIDS. The liver can be involved in disseminated disease.[16,17] In immunosuppressed patients, the granulomas are typically composed of foamy macrophages in the lobules and portal tracts (**Fig. 3**A) with numerous acid-fast organisms identifiable by the acid-fast stain (**Fig. 3**B). Epithelioid granulomas with rare bacilli may be present, particularly in immunocompetent patients. Culture and PCR can be very helpful in establishing a diagnosis.

Whipple disease is caused by *T whipplei*, a Gram-positive bacillus. The disease predominantly affects middle-aged white men; common symptoms include weight loss, chronic diarrhea,

Fig. 3. (*A*) Collections of foamy macrophages in MAI infection (hematoxylin-eosin, original magnification ×100). (*B*) Numerous acid-fast bacilli in foamy macrophages highlighted by a Ziehl-Neelsen stain (Ziehl-Neelsen, original magnification ×300).

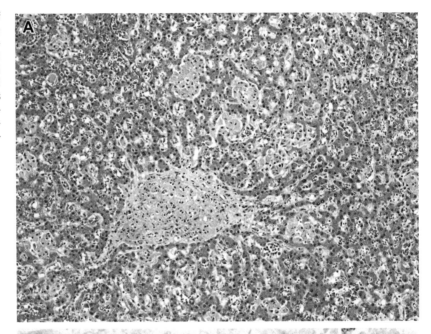

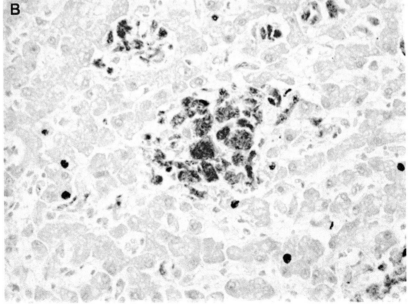

abdominal pain, and joint symptoms.[18,19] Hepatic involvement is not commonly reported, but it can be seen in multi-organ disease. Histologically, there may be aggregates of foamy macrophages in the portal tracts or sinusoidal Kupffer cells that have granular periodic acid-Schiff (PAS)–diastase positivity, and bluish gray intracytoplasmic material in macrophages may be visible on the hematoxylin-eosin stain.[20–23] Epithelioid noncaseating granulomas in the liver, described by some as sarcoidlike and lacking PAS positive material, have been reported in patients with Whipple disease.[20,24,25] The bacteria are negative for acid-fast stains (eg, Ziehl-Neelsen), which can help distinguish *T whipplei* from *M avium-intracellulare*. PCR can be a

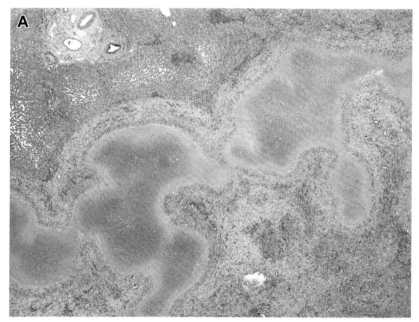

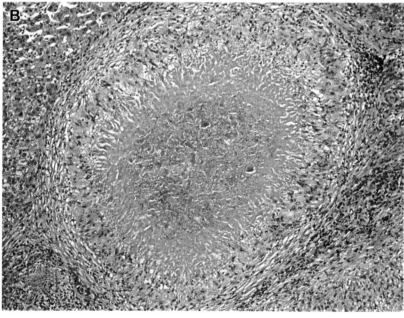

Fig. 4. (*A, B*) Characteristic lesion of cat-scratch disease with a central stellate microabscess surrounded by palisading histiocytes and an outer rim of fibrosis (hematoxylin-eosin, original magnification ×20 [*A*] and original magnification ×100 [*B*]).

helpful diagnostic aid.[18] The organisms can also be identified by immunohistochemistry[26] and electron microscopy.

Bartonella henselae is the etiologic agent of most cases of cat-scratch disease. Affected individuals are usually immunocompetent and present with localized disease of the skin and regional lymph nodes near the site of inoculation. The liver and other visceral organs can be involved in a small number of cases; the characteristic skin papule and peripheral lymphadenopathy at the primary inoculation site are often absent in this subset of patients, who may instead present with fever, abdominal pain, weight loss, multiple liver lesions, and abdominal lymphadenopathy.[27,28] The hallmark granulomatous lesion of cat-scratch disease has a distinctive zonal morphology with a central stellate microabscess, surrounding palisaded granulomatous inflammation, and an outer rim of fibrosis[27] (Fig. 4). Temporal heterogeneity may be seen within the same specimen with morphologies ranging from the characteristic stellate microabscess to older lesions with only fibrosis and central granulation tissue. Clinical history of exposure to cats, liver impregnation stains (eg, Warthin-Starry and Steiner stains), immunohistochemistry, molecular methods (eg, PCR), and serologic tests can aid in the diagnosis.

Brucellosis is a zoonotic infection caused by Brucella melitensis, Brucella abortus, Brucella suis, and Brucella canis, which are intracellular gram-negative coccobacilli transmitted from infected farm animals (eg, sheep, goats, cattle, buffalo) or ingestion of contaminated food products.[29] Symptoms include fever, malaise, headache, and arthralgias; and hepatosplenomegaly and lymphadenopathy may be present.[29] Liver involvement is common. Microscopically, nonspecific reactive hepatitis is the most common finding; granulomatous inflammation may also be present.[30–32] The granulomas are often noncaseating and epithelioid, sometimes admixed with lymphocytes and accompanied by giant cells or they may be small and poorly formed.[30–34] (Fig. 5). The bacteria are rarely identified by special stains. Cultures can be performed, but Brucella is difficult grow. Clinical history of potential exposures and serologic assays are helpful in establishing a diagnosis.

Coxiella burnetii is the infectious agent of Q fever. Fibrin-ring granulomas are classically associated with Q fever, but the granuloma morphology is often intermediate between fibrin-ring and epithelioid granulomas.[35,36] Serologic testing and PCR can be helpful diagnostic aids.

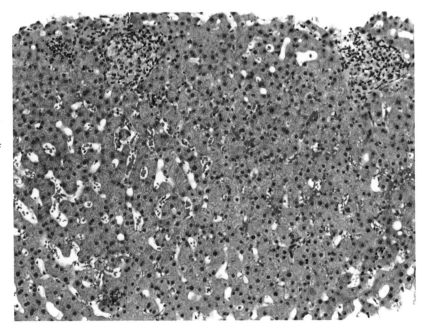

Fig. 5. This liver biopsy from a patient with brucellosis shows small epithelioid granulomas with admixed lymphocytes in a background of patchy lobular inflammation and reactive hepatocellular changes (hematoxylin-eosin, original magnification ×100). (Courtesy of Dr John Hart, Chicago, IL).

Francisella tularensis is the etiologic agent of tularemia, a rare but potentially fatal disease that is endemic to many parts of North America.[37] *F tularensis* is highly infectious, and modes of transmission to humans include direct contact with infected animals (eg, rodents and rabbits) and arthropod bites.[37] Patients with disseminated disease often have hepatic involvement, and signs may include hepatomegaly and elevated transaminases.[38,39] Microscopically, there are typically suppurative microabscesses with occasional surrounding macrophages, which may become more granulomatous with time[39] (**Fig. 6**). There may also be well-delineated areas of cortical necrosis in periportal lymph nodes.[39] Special stains rarely identify organisms; serologic tests, PCR, and microbiologic culture may aid in the diagnosis.

FUNGAL INFECTIONS

Fungal infections of the liver are usually seen in the context of disseminated disease in immunocompromised patients. When the liver is involved, patients may have hepatomegaly, abdominal pain, and elevated transaminases and bilirubin. Fungi can sometimes be seen on hematoxylin-eosin–stained sections; but special stains, such as Grocott methenamine silver (GMS) and PAS stains, remain valuable diagnostic aids. Although the morphology of the fungus in tissue sections can suggest the correct classification, microbiologic testing (eg, cultures or molecular testing) are more accurate and reliable for speciation, which has important implications for therapy.

Candida hepatitis often features granulomas with suppurative inflammation surrounded by palisading histiocytes and lymphocytes, which may resemble the lesions of cat-scratch disease.[40] The granulomas can be of various sizes, and some may have central caseating necrosis (**Fig. 7**A). Giant cells may be present. GMS (**Fig. 7**B) and PAS histochemical stains can be used to highlight the fungi.

Hepatic histoplasmosis often demonstrates portal lymphohistiocytic inflammation and sinusoidal Kupffer cell hyperplasia with organisms present in both the portal and sinusoidal macrophages (**Fig. 8**).[41] Discrete granulomas and giant cells are uncommon.

Cryptococcus produces variable histologic findings depending on the immune status of the host, ranging from mixed suppurative and necrotizing granulomatous inflammation in immunocompetent patients to virtually no inflammatory cell reaction in immunocompromised patients (**Fig. 9**A).[42,43] Purely granulomatous inflammation can occur as well.

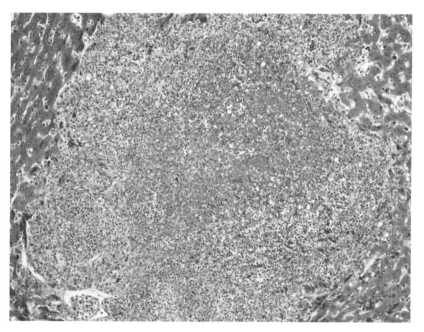

Fig. 6. A case of tularemia with central suppurative microabscess and surrounding granulomatous inflammation (hematoxylin-eosin, original magnification ×100).

A

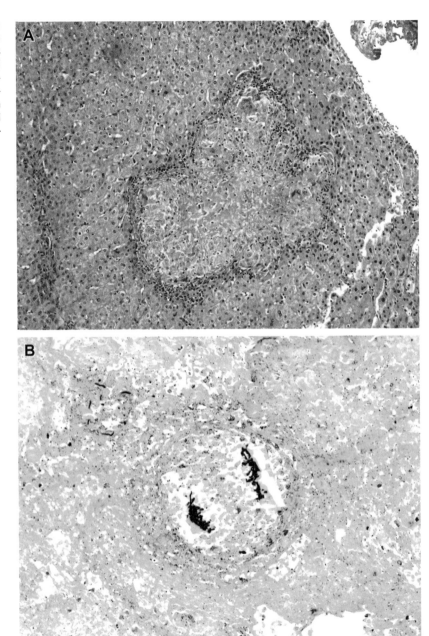

Fig. 7. (*A*) Granuloma with central necrosis in a case of hepatic candidiasis with a few multinucleated giant cells (hematoxylin-eosin, original magnification ×100). (*B*) GMS stain highlights the fungi (GMS, original magnification ×100).

Mucicarmine histochemical stain highlights the capsule of *Cryptococcus* (**Fig.** 9B), but some strains are capsule deficient and will either lack mucicarmine staining or only have focal staining. In such cases, Fontana-Masson or GMS stains (**Fig.** 9C) may be helpful in visualizing the organisms.

PARASITIC INFECTIONS

Schistosoma mansoni, *Schistosoma japonicum*, and *Schistosoma mekongi* are responsible for most human hepatobiliary infections. They have a preference for mesenteric and portal veins, where they copulate and produce thousands of

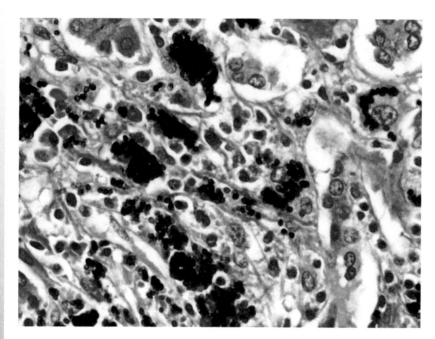

Fig. 8. Portal lymphohistiocytic reaction to hepatic histoplasmosis. Methenamine silver highlights *Histoplasma* in macrophages (methenamine silver and hematoxylin-eosin stain, original magnification ×600).

eggs, many of which remain in patients and incite an inflammatory response that leads to fibrosis and obstructive hepatobiliary disease. Patients may present with signs of portal hypertension, such as variceal bleeding. Grossly, the liver may be enlarged and nodular, with a pattern of fibrosis known as pipestem or Symmers fibrosis. Histologically, there is typically a granulomatous response to the parasite eggs, leading to progressive, dense fibrosis of portal tracts. Parasite eggs are often more difficult to find as the disease progresses, and many will ultimately calcify (**Fig. 10**). Schistosome pigment produced by adult worms during hemoglobin catabolism can be seen as brown pigment in granulomas and Kupffer cells.[44] Identification of the eggs in tissue, urine, feces, serology, and PCR tests are helpful for diagnosis.

Visceral leishmaniasis (kala-azar) most often affects patients with AIDS. Microscopically, there are usually hypertrophic Kupffer cells containing parasites, which can aggregate and form loose granulomas. Fibrin-ring and epithelioid granulomas have also been described.[45,46]

Enterobius vermicularis (pinworm) is a common human parasite. The parasite can rarely produce a hepatic granuloma consisting of a hyalinized nodule and peripheral inflammation, and central necrosis with remnants of the worms and eggs can be seen.[47]

VIRAL INFECTIONS

Granulomas occur infrequently in viral infections. The classic morphology of EBV hepatitis is a diffuse sinusoidal infiltrate of lymphocytes arranged in single files; but there may also be small clusters of Kupffer cells, discrete noncaseating granulomas, or fibrin-ring granulomas.[48] Cytomegalovirus liver infections may similarly have fibrin-ring and epithelioid granulomas (**Fig. 11**),[49,50] and epithelioid granulomas can also occur in chronic hepatitis B[51] and C infections.[52,53]

NONINFECTIOUS CAUSES OF HEPATIC GRANULOMAS

There are many possible noninfectious causes of hepatic granulomas. The following is a limited discussion of some of the more important noninfectious causes to consider in the differential diagnosis.

Liver involvement is very common in sarcoidosis, and the hepatic granulomas are morphologically similar to those in other anatomic sites. There are typically multiple non-

Fig. 9. (*A*) *Cryptococcus* infection in a patient with AIDS with little inflammatory cell response (hematoxylin-eosin, original magnification ×600). (*B*) Mucicarmine stains the capsule (mucicarmine, original magnification ×600). (*C*) Grocott methenamine silver stain is particularly helpful in cases of mucin deficient strains of *Cryptococcus* (GMS, original magnification ×600) and highlights the variation in size that is typical of *Cryptococcus*.

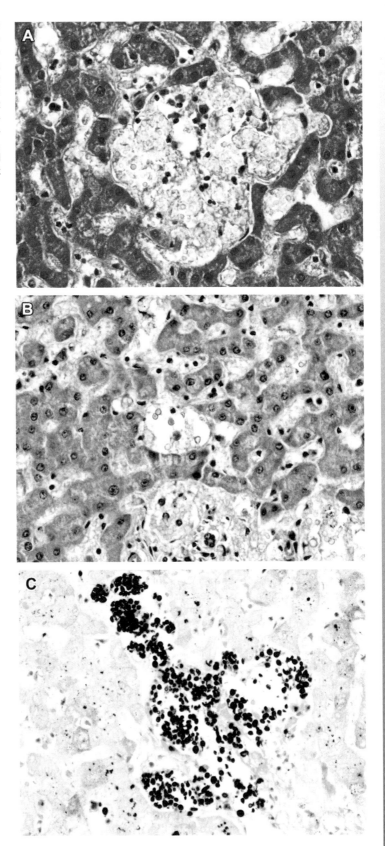

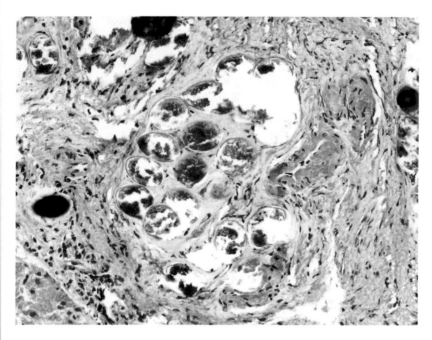

Fig. 10. Chronic schistosomiasis with dense portal fibrosis and calcification of Schistosoma eggs (hematoxylin-eosin, original magnification ×200).

necrotizing granulomas, which are often confluent, sclerotic (**Fig. 12A, B**), portal, or periportal in distribution and sometimes associated with lymphocytes and giant cells. Inclusions (eg, asteroid bodies and Schaumann bodies) and fibrinoid necrosis can be seen (**Fig. 12C**), but true caseating necrosis should be absent. Patients may develop cirrhosis, portal hypertension, or a chronic cholestatic process with progressive bile duct destruction that resembles primary biliary cholangitis (PBC).[54]

Granulomas may be seen in chronic cholestatic liver diseases, most often PBC. The florid duct lesions of PBC and antimitochondiral antibody (AMA)-negative PBC are classically small, poorly formed epithelioid granulomas that are associated with bile duct damage and often accompanied by dense lymphoid aggregates (**Fig. 13**). Although quite uncommon, non-necrotizing epithelioid granulomas have been reported in primary sclerosing cholangitis.[3,55]

Adverse drug reactions should always be considered in the differential diagnosis of hepatic granulomatous inflammation. The morphologic findings are variable, but necrosis in granulomas is rare. There are usually other accompanying findings, such as hepatocellular injury, a mixed inflammatory cell infiltrate, and/or cholestatic changes. Some of the common

drugs associated with a granulomatous inflammation are listed in **Box 1**.[3,5,56] Fibrin-ring granulomas have been reported in some drug reactions, including allopurinol and the checkpoint inhibitors ipilimumab and nivolumab[6] (**Fig. 14**).

Common variable immunodeficiency (CVID) is a heterogeneous primary immunodeficiency

Box 1
Common drugs associated with hepatic granulomas
Allopurinol
Amiodarone
Cephalexin
Diazepam
Isoniazid
Nitrofurantoin
Penicillins
Phenytoin
Propylthiouracil
Quinidine
Sulfa drugs

Fig. 11. (*A*) Cytomegalovirus (CMV) hepatitis with a rare epithelioid granuloma. (*B*) A cell with CMV viral inclusions in the center of photomicrograph is surrounded by neutrophils (mini-microabscess) and lymphohistiocytic inflammation (hematoxylin-eosin, original magnification ×400 [*A, B*]).

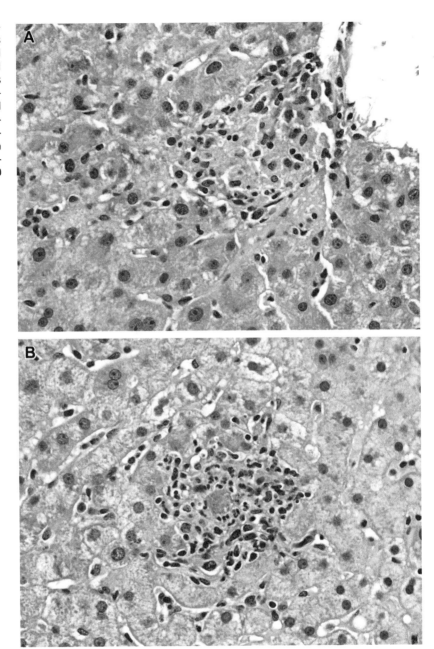

disorder in which there is impaired B-cell differentiation with hypogammaglobinemia. Defects in T cells and antigen-presenting cells are also thought to be contributing factors, though the pathogenesis is poorly understood.[57] Patients can present with elevated liver tests, which may prompt a liver biopsy. The cause, clinical presentation, and histologic findings of liver involvement in CVID are quite variable. The liver may be involved by infections, autoimmunity, primary malignancies, and drug/toxic exposures; signs may include elevated alkaline phosphatase, hepatomegaly, and splenomegaly.[57] Patients with CVID can have granulomatous disease, which often involves the liver[58,59] and typically consists of small,

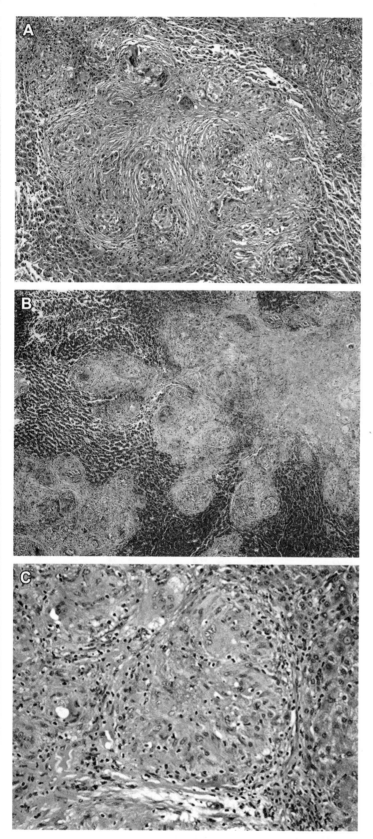

Fig. 12. Sarcoidosis. (*A*) Typical epithelioid, noncaseating, confluent, sclerosing, granulomas (hematoxylin-eosin, original magnification ×100). (*B*) Trichrome stain highlights extensive fibrosis associated with the granulomas (trichrome, original magnification ×40). (*C*) Granulomas with fibrinoid necrosis can be seen in sarcoidosis (hematoxylin-eosin, original magnification ×200).

Fig. 13. Florid duct lesion in PBC. A granuloma is associated with duct destruction and dense portal inflammation (hematoxylin-eosin, original magnification ×200).

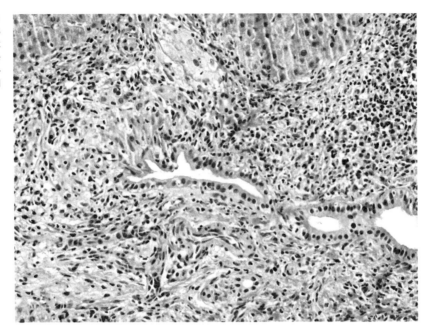

epithelioid, non-necrotizing granulomas located in the lobules and portal tracts[60,61] (**Fig. 15**). The absence of plasma cells may be a clue to the diagnosis, and there may be accompanying lymphocytic portal and lobular inflammation.[58,60]

Granulomas can be found associated with tumors. These tumors include hepatocellular carcinoma (**Fig. 16**), Hodgkin and non-Hodgkin lymphomas, hepatocellular adenomas, and metastases. Other noninfectious causes of liver granulomas include foreign body reaction (eg, talc from intravenous drug use), vascular diseases (eg, polyarteritis nodosa), and chronic gastrointestinal diseases, such as idiopathic eosinophilic enteritis.

Fig. 14. Adverse drug reaction with multiple fibrin-ring granulomas in a patient with metastatic melanoma being treated with ipilimumab and nivolumab (hematoxylin-eosin, original magnification ×200).

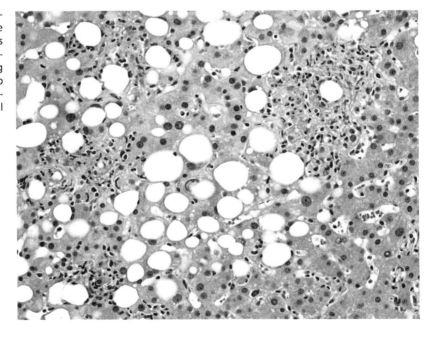

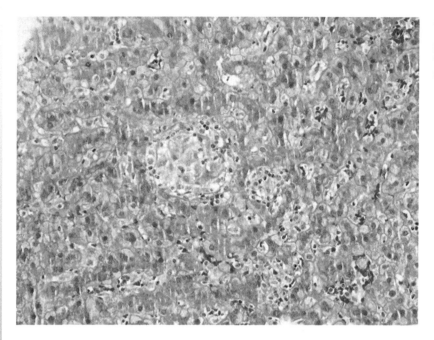

Fig. 15. A small epithelioid granuloma in a patient with CVID (hematoxylin-eosin, original magnification ×200).

In summary, hepatic granulomas can be of infectious or noninfectious cause. When an infectious cause is suspected, special stains performed on liver biopsies can be helpful; but the absence of organisms does not exclude the possibility of infection. Ancillary laboratory tests and correlation with clinical history and findings are often necessary as part of the workup.

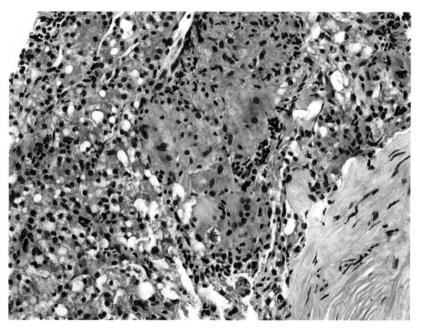

Fig. 16. An epithelioid granuloma with multinucleated giant cells within a hepatocellular carcinoma. An asteroid body is seen in one of the giant cells (hematoxylin-eosin, original magnification ×200).

REFERENCES

1. Harrington PT, Gutierrez JJ, Ramirez-Ronda CH, et al. Granulomatous hepatitis. Rev Infect Dis 1982; 4(3):638–55.
2. Lagana SM, Moreira RK, Lefkowitch JH. Hepatic granulomas: pathogenesis and differential diagnosis. Clin Liver Dis 2010;14(4):605–17.
3. Gaya DR, Thorburn D, Oien KA, et al. Hepatic granulomas: a 10 year single centre experience. J Clin Pathol 2003;56(11):850–3.
4. Lamps LW. Hepatic granulomas, with an emphasis on infectious causes. Adv Anat Pathol 2008;15(6): 309–18.
5. Marazuela M, Moreno A, Yebra M, et al. Hepatic fibrin-ring granulomas: a clinicopathologic study of 23 patients. Hum Pathol 1991;22(6):607–13.
6. Everett J, Srivastava A, Misdraji J. Fibrin-ring granulomas in checkpoint inhibitor-induced hepatitis. Am J Surg Pathol 2017;41(1):134–7.
7. Hickey AJ, Gounder L, Moosa MY, et al. A systematic review of hepatic tuberculosis with considerations in human immunodeficiency virus co-infection. BMC Infect Dis 2015;15:209.
8. Oliva A, Duarte B, Jonasson O, et al. The nodular form of local hepatic tuberculosis. A review. J Clin Gastroenterol 1990;12(2):166–73.
9. Essop AR, Posen JA, Hodkinson JH, et al. Tuberculosis hepatitis: a clinical review of 96 cases. Q J Med 1984;53(212):465–77.
10. Luo RF, Scahill MD, Banaei N. Comparison of single-copy and multicopy real-time PCR targets for detection of Mycobacterium tuberculosis in paraffin-embedded tissue. J Clin Microbiol 2010; 48(7):2569–70.
11. Karat AB, Job CK, Rao PS. Liver in leprosy: histological and biochemical findings. Br Med J 1971; 1(5744):307–10.
12. Chen TS, Drutz DJ, Whelan GE. Hepatic granulomas in leprosy. Their relation to bacteremia. Arch Pathol Lab Med 1976;100(4):182–5.
13. Sehgal VN, Tyagi SP, Kumar S, et al. Microscopic pathology of the liver in leprosy patients. Int J Dermatol 1972;11(3):168–72.
14. Gillis T, Vissa V, Matsuoka M, et al. Characterisation of short tandem repeats for genotyping Mycobacterium leprae. Lepr Rev 2009;80(3):250–60.
15. Sharma R, Singh P, Loughry WJ, et al. Zoonotic leprosy in the Southeastern United States. Emerg Infect Dis 2015;21(12):2127–34.
16. Farhi DC, Mason UG 3rd, Horsburgh CR Jr. Pathologic findings in disseminated Mycobacterium avium-intracellulare infection. A report of 11 cases. Am J Clin Pathol 1986;85(1):67–72.
17. Klatt EC, Jensen DF, Meyer PR. Pathology of Mycobacterium avium-intracellulare infection in acquired immunodeficiency syndrome. Hum Pathol 1987; 18(7):709–14.
18. Dolmans RA, Boel CH, Lacle MM, et al. Clinical manifestations, treatment, and diagnosis of tropheryma whipplei infections. Clin Microbiol Rev 2017;30(2): 529–55.
19. Bai JC, Mazure RM, Vazquez H, et al. Whipple's disease. Clin Gastroenterol Hepatol 2004;2(10):849–60.
20. Cho C, Linscheer WG, Hirschkorn MA, et al. Sarcoidlike granulomas as an early manifestation of Whipple's disease. Gastroenterology 1984;87(4): 941–7.
21. Enzinger FM, Helwig EB. Whipple's disease. Virchows Arch Pathol Anat Physiol Klin Med 1963;336:238–69.
22. Upton AC. Histochemical investigation of the mesenchymal lesions in Whipple's disease. Am J Clin Pathol 1952;22(8):755–64.
23. Burt AD, Ferrell LD, Hubscher SG, editors. MacSween's pathology of the liver. 7th edition. Philadelphia: Elsevier; 2018.
24. Torzillo PJ, Bignold L, Khan GA. Absence of PAS-positive macrophages in hepatic and lymph node granulomata in Whipple's disease. Aust N Z J Med 1982;12(1):73–5.
25. Caravati CM, Litch M, Weisiger BB, et al. Diagnosis of Whipple's disease by rectal biopsy with a report of three additional cases. Ann Intern Med 1963;58: 166–70.
26. Lepidi H, Fenollar F, Gerolami R, et al. Whipple's disease: immunospecific and quantitative immunohistochemical study of intestinal biopsy specimens. Hum Pathol 2003;34(6):589–96.
27. Lamps LW, Gray GF, Scott MA. The histologic spectrum of hepatic cat scratch disease. A series of six cases with confirmed Bartonella henselae infection. Am J Surg Pathol 1996;20(10): 1253–9.
28. Larsen CE, Patrick LE. Abdominal (liver, spleen) and bone manifestations of cat scratch disease. Pediatr Radiol 1992;22(5):353–5.
29. Pappas G, Akritidis N, Bosilkovski M, et al. Brucellosis. N Engl J Med 2005;352(22):2325–36.
30. Akritidis N, Tzivras M, Delladetsima I, et al. The liver in brucellosis. Clin Gastroenterol Hepatol 2007;5(9): 1109–12.
31. Young EJ, Hasanjani Roushan MR, Shafae S, et al. Liver histology of acute brucellosis caused by Brucella melitensis. Hum Pathol 2014;45(10): 2023–8.
32. Cervantes F, Bruguera M, Carbonell J, et al. Liver disease in brucellosis. A clinical and pathological study of 40 cases. Postgrad Med J 1982;58(680): 346–50.
33. Ablin J, Mevorach D, Eliakim R. Brucellosis and the gastrointestinal tract. The odd couple. J Clin Gastroenterol 1997;24(1):25–9.

34. Williams RK, Crossley K. Acute and chronic hepatic involvement of brucellosis. Gastroenterology 1982; 83(2):455–8.

35. Srigley JR, Vellend H, Palmer N, et al. Q-fever. The liver and bone marrow pathology. Am J Surg Pathol 1985;9(10):752–8.

36. Pellegrin M, Delsol G, Auvergnat JC, et al. Granulomatous hepatitis in Q fever. Hum Pathol 1980;11(1): 51–7.

37. Centers for Disease Control and Prevention (CDC). Tularemia - United States, 2001-2010. MMWR Morb Mortal Wkly Rep 2013;62(47):963–6.

38. Ortego TJ, Hutchins LF, Rice J, et al. Tularemic hepatitis presenting as obstructive jaundice. Gastroenterology 1986;91(2):461–3.

39. Lamps LW, Havens JM, Sjostedt A, et al. Histologic and molecular diagnosis of tularemia: a potential bioterrorism agent endemic to North America. Mod Pathol 2004;17(5):489–95.

40. Johnson TL, Barnett JL, Appelman HD, et al. Candida hepatitis. Histopathologic diagnosis. Am J Surg Pathol 1988;12(9):716–20.

41. Lamps LW, Molina CP, West AB, et al. The pathologic spectrum of gastrointestinal and hepatic histoplasmosis. Am J Clin Pathol 2000;113(1): 64–72.

42. Bonacini M, Nussbaum J, Ahluwalia C. Gastrointestinal, hepatic, and pancreatic involvement with Cryptococcus neoformans in AIDS. J Clin Gastroenterol 1990;12(3):295–7.

43. Washington K, Gottfried MR, Wilson ML. Gastrointestinal cryptococcosis. Mod Pathol 1991;4(6): 707–11.

44. Sano M, Ishii A. Experimental studies of schistosomal pigment from Schistosoma japonicum. Experientia 1979;35(4):472–3.

45. Moreno A, Marazuela M, Yebra M, et al. Hepatic fibrin-ring granulomas in visceral leishmaniasis. Gastroenterology 1988;95(4):1123–6.

46. Daneshbod K. Visceral leishmaniasis (kala-azar) in Iran: a pathologic and electron microscopic study. Am J Clin Pathol 1972;57(2):156–66.

47. Daly JJ, Baker GF. Pinworm granuloma of the liver. Am J Trop Med Hyg 1984;33(1):62–4.

48. Nenert M, Mavier P, Dubuc N, et al. Epstein-Barr virus infection and hepatic fibrin-ring granulomas. Hum Pathol 1988;19(5):608–10.

49. Clarke J, Craig RM, Saffro R, et al. Cytomegalovirus granulomatous hepatitis. Am J Med 1979;66(2):264–9.

50. Lobdell DH. 'Ring' granulomas in cytomegalovirus hepatitis. Arch Pathol Lab Med 1987;111(9): 881–2.

51. Tahan V, Ozaras R, Lacevic N, et al. Prevalence of hepatic granulomas in chronic hepatitis B. Dig Dis Sci 2004;49(10):1575–7.

52. Harada K, Minato H, Hiramatsu K, et al. Epithelioid cell granulomas in chronic hepatitis C: immunohistochemical character and histological marker of favourable response to interferon-alpha therapy. Histopathology 1998;33(3):216–21.

53. Ozaras R, Tahan V, Mert A, et al. The prevalence of hepatic granulomas in chronic hepatitis C. J Clin Gastroenterol 2004;38(5):449–52.

54. Devaney K, Goodman ZD, Epstein MS, et al. Hepatic sarcoidosis. Clinicopathologic features in 100 patients. Am J Surg Pathol 1993;17(12):1272–80.

55. Kleiner DE. Granulomas in the liver. Semin Diagn Pathol 2006;23(3–4):161–9.

56. Sartin JS, Walker RC. Granulomatous hepatitis: a retrospective review of 88 cases at the Mayo Clinic. Mayo Clin Proc 1991;66(9):914–8.

57. Song J, Lleo A, Yang GX, et al. Common variable immunodeficiency and liver involvement. Clin Rev Allergy Immunol 2017.

58. Ardeniz O, Cunningham-Rundles C. Granulomatous disease in common variable immunodeficiency. Clin Immunol 2009;133(2):198–207.

59. Morimoto Y, Routes JM. Granulomatous disease in common variable immunodeficiency. Curr Allergy Asthma Rep 2005;5(5):370–5.

60. Daniels JA, Torbenson M, Vivekanandan P, et al. Hepatitis in common variable immunodeficiency. Hum Pathol 2009;40(4):484–8.

61. Malamut G, Ziol M, Suarez F, et al. Nodular regenerative hyperplasia: the main liver disease in patients with primary hypogammaglobulinemia and hepatic abnormalities. J Hepatol 2008;48(1): 74–82.

Acute Viral Hepatitis: Beyond A, B, and C

Venancio Avancini Ferreira Alves, MD, PhD

KEYWORDS

- Acute viral hepatitis • Hepatotropic viruses • Icteric hemorrhagic fevers • Immunosuppression

Key points

- Acute hepatitis due to any of the hepatotrophic viruses produces a histologically similar generic lobular hepatitis pattern.
- The non-hepatotrophic viruses do not produce a lobular hepatitis pattern histologically, but instead exhibit distinctive histologic features.
- Viral hemorrhagic fevers can produce severe acute hepatitis with characteristic histologic features.

ABSTRACT

From the standpoint of the surgical pathologist "hepatitis" is defined as the set of histologic patterns of lesions found in livers infected by hepatotropic viruses, by non-hepatotrophic viruses leading to liver inflammation in the context of systemic infection, or due to an autoimmune disease, drug, or toxin involving the liver. This article is centered on the histologic patterns of injury in acute viral hepatitis, encompassing the hepatotropic viruses A, B, C, D, and E and the "icteric hemorrhagic fevers" (dengue, hantavirus, yellow fever). A brief mention of viruses causing hepatitis in immunosuppressed patients also is presented.

OVERVIEW

The epidemiology of viral hepatitis has substantially changed over the past decade due to progress in vaccine development and protocols for prevention, diagnosis, and treatment.[1–3] However, marked differences in incidence of each type of viral hepatitis still remain. In 2015, Gupta and colleagues[4] reported a series of 206 cases of acute viral hepatitis from India and determined that hepatitis E virus (HEV) infection was responsible in 95 cases, hepatitis A virus (HAV) in 36, hepatitis B virus (HBV) in 18, and concurrent infections of these viruses in an additional 27 cases. Hepatitis C virus (HCV) was detected in only 1 patient, whereas the other 29 cases were ascribed to CMV or EBV. In the United States, a summary of reports of acute hepatitis from the Centers for Disease Control and Prevention (CDC) for 2014 include 1239 cases of HAV and an increase to 1390 cases in 2015. A total of 2791 cases of acute HBV hepatitis was reported in in 2014 and an increase to 3370 in 2015. Newly reported acute HCV hepatitis cases totaled 2194 in 2014 with an increase to 2436 in 2015. The CDC also reported that cases of acute HCV infection increased more than 2.9-fold from 2010 through 2015, with an increased incidence each year during this period. Unfortunately no data regarding case numbers for acute HEV were reported, but elsewhere on the Web site, the CDC states that in the United States, HEV infection is believed to be uncommon, and when symptomatic hepatitis E does occur, it is usually in individuals who are from or have traveled to a country where hepatitis E is endemic.[5]

Acute liver failure may result from viral hepatitis. In 2015, the CDC reported 8 deaths in the United States ascribed to fulminant HAV infection.[5] Deaths due to acute hepatitis B infection were reported in 20 cases. In contrast, chronic HBV hepatitis was considered the cause of

Department of Pathology, Surgical Pathology, University of Sao Paulo School of Medicine, Sao Paulo, Brazil
E-mail address: venancio@uol.com.br

Surgical Pathology 11 (2018) 251–266
https://doi.org/10.1016/j.path.2018.02.014

death of 1715 patients. The CDC report did not mention death due to acute HCV hepatitis, but chronic HCV hepatitis was considered the cause of death of 19,629 patients.[5] Acute liver failure due to acute HEV infection is not mentioned by the CDC, but in other countries, acute liver failure occurs in 0.1% to 4.0% of infected patients, with a predilection for pregnant women, 30% of whom may develop acute liver failure.[6]

HISTOLOGIC FINDINGS IN ACUTE VIRAL HEPATITIS

The lobular inflammation and hepatocellular injury in acute hepatitis is much more striking than the portal tract changes, resulting in a low-power pattern that could be termed "lobular hepatitis" (**Fig. 1**). Variable numbers of swollen/ballooned hepatocytes are intermingled with more normal-appearing hepatocytes. Lymphocytes, histiocytes, and plasma cells appear as single cells or in small groups, even in early infection, surrounding the damaged hepatocytes or fragments of dead hepatocytes, a lesion known as lytic necrosis or spotty necrosis.[7] Scattered individual hepatocytes undergo apoptosis and are known as *acidophilic bodies* or *Councilman-Rocha Lima bodies*. Cellular remnants phagocytized by Kupffer cells may be highlighted by use of the periodic acid–Schiff–diastase (PAS/D) stain, which is extremely useful for the diagnosis of resolving acute hepatitis when the appearance in the hematoxylin-eosin (H&E) stain is nearly normal (**Fig. 2**). Portal tract findings are variable; there may be minimal edema and generally sparse to mild mononuclear cell infiltrates that are almost always less impressive than the parenchymal hepatocellular injury and inflammation. Bile duct injury is usually mild, although mild cholangitis has been reported in acute hepatitis E infection.[8] Mild cholestasis may be seen in acute hepatitis, with bile pigment found in the cytoplasm of hepatocytes or in biliary canaliculi. The presence of more significant cholestatic changes rarely may be seen in elderly patients, but also should raise the possibility of drug-induced injury or even bile duct obstruction.

In acute hepatitis, hepatocytes at the interface with the portal tract are usually not damaged, although in acute HAV hepatitis lymphocytes often spill over the limiting plate. Because portal fibrosis and neoangiogenesis are not features of acute hepatitis, when patterns of both acute and chronic hepatitis coexist, the pathologist must consider the possibility of an acute viral infection

as a second hepatic insult occurring in the setting of underlying chronic liver disease. An important example of such a scenario is hepatitis D virus (HDV) superinfection of livers chronically infected by HBV.[9]

In most cases of acute hepatitis, especially those due to hepatitis A and E, the loss of individual hepatocytes because of apoptosis and spotty necrosis do not disturb the underlying trabecular architecture, and once the viral infection resolves, usually within 2 to 4 months after infection, regeneration from neighboring hepatocytes leads to complete restoration of structure and function of the liver.

In some cases of acute viral hepatitis, groups of hepatocytes die, resulting in collapse of reticulin framework, known as *confluent necrosis*.[7,10] When confluent necrosis links central veins (terminal hepatic venules) to the neighboring ones, a "vascular bridge" ensues ("central-central bridging" or "central-portal bridging"). Almost 50 years ago, Boyer and Klatskin[11] suggested that confluent necrosis linking central veins to portal tracts might lead to a presinusoidal-postsinusoidal shunt, with a high risk of evolution to cirrhosis (**Fig. 3**). This hypothesis is still a matter of debate, and will require additional sophisticated morphologic and functional assessment in cohorts of affected patients.

Fulminant hepatitis is defined as acute liver failure occurring a few weeks after the onset of acute hepatitis. Viral hepatitis and drugs are reported as major causes of this rather infrequent but potentially severe condition. Confluent necrosis may become extensive, leading to *submassive* or even *massive necrosis* (**Fig. 4**). Because of the irregular distribution of necrosis, histologic features from needle liver biopsies may not predict clinical outcome in such instances[12]

Extensive necrosis may be mistaken as fibrosis; the distinction can be aided by silver impregnation stains, such as the Gomori silver stain. Confluent necrosis leads to approximation of reticulin fibers (collagen III fibers) due to parenchymal collapse, whereas chronic active fibrogenesis leads to deposition of both collagen III and collagen I fibers. Collagen III appears as narrow black fibrils (reticulin fibrils), whereas collagen I bands appear brown. Chronic fibrogenesis is accompanied by production of elastic fibers, visualized by the Shikata orcein, van Gieson, or Weigert stain, whereas acute collapse lacks elastic fibers.[13] These histologic and histochemical features are even more important in the assessment of biopsies demonstrating acute-on-chronic liver failure, to discriminate which lesions are ascribable to acute events

Fig. 1. Histologic features of lobular hepatitis. (*A*) Hepatocyte ballooning (H&E, original magnification ×40). (*B*) Hepatocyte apoptosis (H&E, original magnification ×100). (*C*) Spotty hepatocyte necrosis (H&E, original magnification ×100).

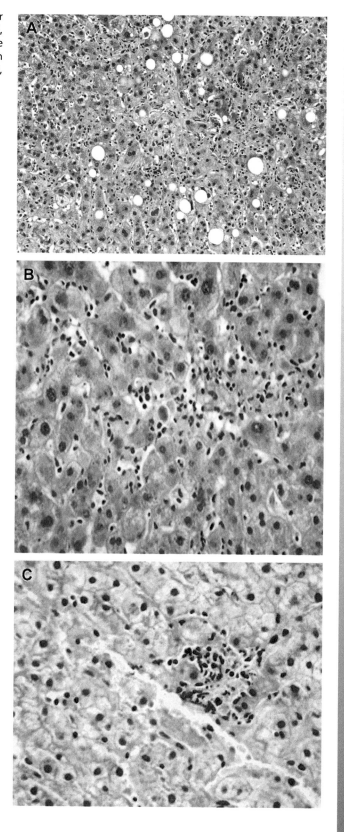

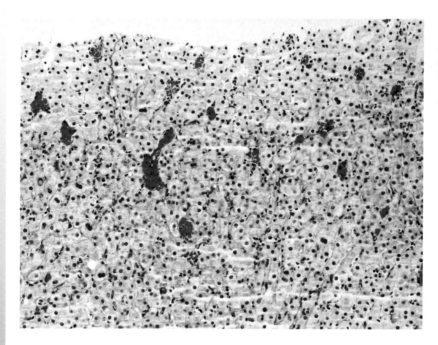

Fig. 2. Resolving acute hepatitis with numerous scattered Kupffer cells containing cellular debris highlighted by a PAS/D stain (PAS/D, original magnification ×40).

(mainly infections) superimposed on preexisting chronic liver disease, and such determination may be relevant for selection of patients who should be prioritized for liver transplantation[14] Liver regeneration in cases of confluent or submassive necrosis is based on activation of progenitor cells, leading to a "ductular reaction," a network of small tubular-canalicular structures reminiscent of biliary ductules (positive for CK19) embedded in variable amounts of collagen[15]

The fate of the liver microarchitecture after acute hepatitis depends on the etiologic agent and the patterns of necrosis and regeneration. Hepatic structure and function are usually completely restored in a few months in cases in which the extent of parenchymal damage is limited to

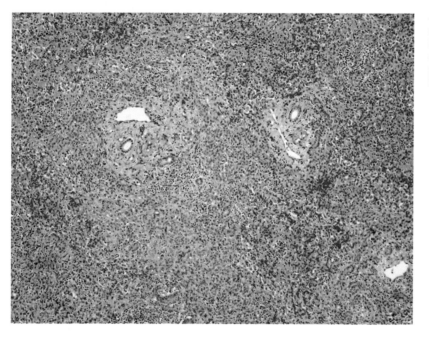

Fig. 3. Confluent necrosis in a case of acute HAV hepatitis. Note the approximation of the portal tracts (H&E, original magnification ×200).

Fig. 4. Submassive necrosis due to acute viral hepatitis.

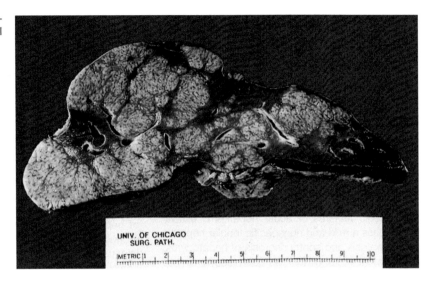

UNIV. OF CHICAGO
SURG. PATH.

apoptosis or spotty necrosis, whereas fibrosis development is more likely in cases with more extensive confluent or submassive/massive hepatocyte necrosis, even after resolution of the infection.

Histologic Clues to the Causative Virus in Acute Hepatitis

At present, etiologic diagnosis of acute hepatitis is based on serology, with sensitive tests detecting viral antigens in hepatitis B or antibodies to viral proteins in hepatitis A, C, D, and E infection. Molecular assays, most of them based on polymerase chain reaction (PCR), are also important for the diagnosis of ongoing infection by these viruses

and also for the causative agents in icteric hemorrhagic syndromes and viruses infecting immunocompromised patients. Although the histologic appearance is similar for all types of acute viral hepatitis, there are some distinctive features that are associated with specific viruses.

Hepatitis A

Lobular features are usually predominant, with spotty necrosis and many apoptotic bodies. However, in acute HAV hepatitis, the portal infiltrate also may be impressive, with plasma cells and lymphocytes frequently "spilling over" the limiting plate into the zone 1 hepatocytes (Fig. 5). Serologic testing is key for proper diagnosis, especially

Fig. 5. Acute HAV hepatitis exhibiting marked lobular hepatitis (H&E, original magnification ×40).

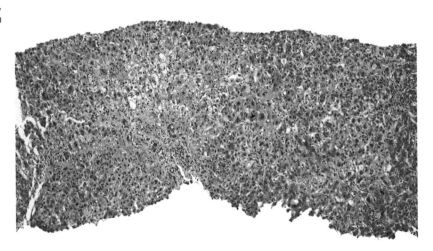

in cases with prolonged or relapsing disease, which may last for more than 6 months. Mild cholestasis may be seen in these cases.[16]

Hepatitis E

Hepatitis E infection is endemic in India, sub-Saharan Africa, and Mexico, where infection is waterborne, mostly due to genotypes 1 and 2. More recently, foodborne zoonotic disease or bloodborne infections have been reported in the United States, Germany, France, Japan, and England, with a predominance of genotypes 3 and 4, transmitted as a zoonosis mainly via contaminated meat.[17–20]

Histologic features of acute hepatitis E usually encompass a mild and nonspecific lobular hepatitis with apoptosis and spotty necrosis of hepatocytes. Bile pigment accumulation has been reported in hepatocytes and bile canaliculi and cellular debris may be found in hypertrophic Kupffer cells (Fig. 6). A rather striking finding in some cases is the presence of a mixed inflammatory cell infiltrate consisting of several polymorphonuclear cells and lymphocytes. In an 11-case series from France, marked lobular necroinflammatory activity was found in 9 patients and confluent necrosis in 5, leading to death in 3 patients.[17] Characteristic pathologic signs of acute hepatitis E included severe intralobular necrosis, neutrophilic inflammation, and acute cholangitis. Drebber and colleagues[8] found HEV RNA sequences by reverse-transcriptase PCR in 7 of 221 formalin-fixed paraffin-embedded liver biopsy samples with acute hepatitis of obscure etiology from Germany. The histologic appearance was a generic lobular hepatitis pattern with cholestatic features and in some cases confluent hepatocyte necrosis in zone 3.

Among major determinants of the severity of illness caused by HEV infection are viral factors, such as the HEV strain (genotype or subtype), viral load, and other coinfections. Genotype 3 and 4 strains are described as less pathogenic for humans than genotypes 1 and 2.[21] Host factors are also relevant: severe acute hepatitis, including cases of fulminant/submassive necrosis have been reported in pregnant patients, and immunosuppressed patients have developed chronic HEV infection progressing to cirrhosis.[21,22]

In a promising approach to the etiologic diagnosis of hepatitis E, Gupta and colleagues[23] produced monoclonal antibodies directed to recombinant HEV proteins codified at ORF2 and ORF3. An immunohistochemical assay tested on 30 liver biopsies collected postmortem from patients who died of acute liver failure caused by HEV infection yielded positive results in all paraffin-embedded samples from these 30 cases, whereas 15 controls (5 noninfected liver tissues, 5 HBV-infected and 5 HCV-infected liver tissues) were all negative. If these results are reproduced in larger studies, this immunohistochemical approach may prove a valuable tool for prospective and retrospective assessment of the extent of HEV hepatitis worldwide.

Hepatitis B

As opposed to chronic HBV hepatitis, in which ground-glass hepatocytes and sanded nuclei serve as important histologic clues for diagnosis, acute HBV hepatitis does not produce specific

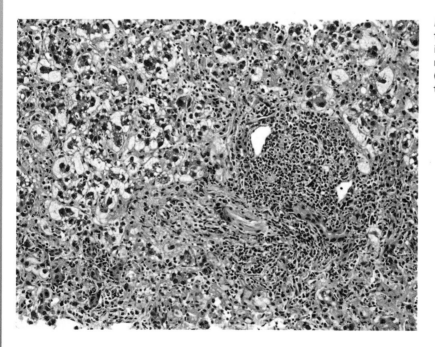

Fig. 6. Acute HEV hepatitis with moderate portal inflammation as well as marked lobular hepatitis (H&E, original magnification ×100).

histologic pattern features. Moreover, viral antigens cannot be detected at this stage of infection using immunohistologic stains due to ongoing immune clearance of the virus. The lack of immunohistochemical expression of hepatitis B surface antigen or hepatitis B core antigen in acute hepatitis B has been used to differentiate it from chronic disease in asymptomatic cases with minimal histologic changes at biopsy.[24]

Hepatitis C

Descriptions of the histologic findings in acute HCV hepatitis in immunocompetent patients usually includes mild lobular inflammation and relatively mild hepatocytic injury with less ballooning and fewer apoptotic bodies than is seen with other forms of acute viral hepatitis (**Fig. 7**).[25] In a series of 5 symptomatic cases from Johns Hopkins, 2 cases biopsied in the first 2 weeks demonstrated mild cholestasis and ductular reaction, raising possibility of early findings of biliary tract disease.[26] Two cases biopsied at 8 weeks showed mild to moderate lobular and portal lymphocytic inflammation without cholestasis. The patient biopsied at 18 weeks showed mild portal lymphocytic inflammation, minimal interface hepatitis, and moderate lobular lymphocytic inflammation, probably reflecting evolution to chronicity. Immunohistochemical detection of HCV antigens is not sensitive enough to be useful for routine diagnosis, although the expression of HCV core protein has been reported in one study to predict severe relapse in posttransplant recurrent hepatitis C.[27]

OTHER VIRUSES CAUSING ACUTE HEPATITIS

Hepatitis D (Delta) Virus

HDV, an incomplete replication-defective RNA virus that requires the molecular machinery of HBV to complete its life cycle, causes acute and chronic hepatitis by coinfection or superinfection with HBV.[28,29] Replication of HDV depends on the delta antigen, which binds to viral RNA in the nucleus of infected hepatocytes by a double rolling-circle mechanism. Similar to HBV, HDV is most often transmitted by contact with contaminated blood and body fluid.[30]

In the Amazon regions of South America and in Africa, superinfection of HBV carriers with HDV may lead to epidemic bouts of severe acute viral hepatitis, also known as "black vomiting fever." This disease is also known as Bangui fever in Africa, Santa Marta hepatitis in Colombia, and Labrea hepatitis in Brazil.[31–33] The disease may progress to hepatic failure and death within a few days or weeks, especially in children and young adults.[32] In Brazil, the clinical course of Labrea hepatitis may resemble fulminant yellow fever, with fever, jaundice, bloody vomiting ("black vomits"), and, finally, hepatic coma and death.[29,32]

Typically acute HDV/HBV hepatitis demonstrates submassive/massive hepatic necrosis (see **Fig. 6**). In addition, reports from Latin America and Africa have emphasized the presence of microvesicular steatosis and hepatocyte ballooning degeneration with the presence of large "spider/morula cells," and variable lymphocytic infiltrates (**Fig. 8**).[8,31,32] Histologic distinction from

Fig. 7. Acute HCV hepatitis with lobular disarray (H&E, original magnification ×20).

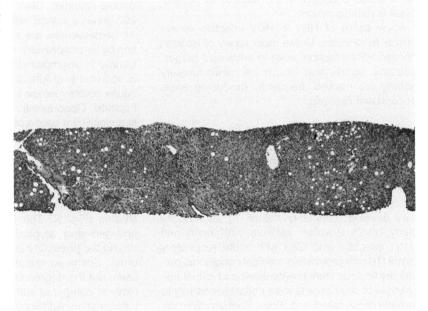

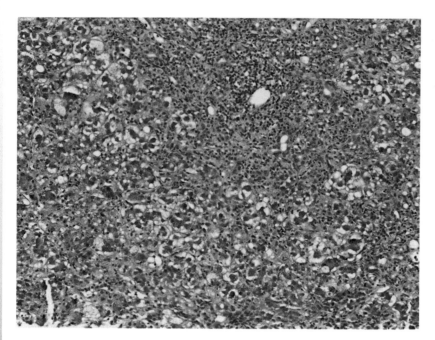

Fig. 8. Chronic HBV hepatitis with superinfection by Delta virus, showing marked lobular hepatitis (H&E, original magnification ×100).

hepatitis due to yellow fever is difficult. In a study comparing these 2 forms of fulminant hepatic failure from patients from the Amazon basin, the most discriminating findings in the HBV/HDV hepatitis cases were the presence of extensive, predominantly lytic hepatocytic necrosis, portal and hepatic vein phlebitis, and the presence of "morula cells" (large hepatocytes with large central nuclei and microvesicular steatosis) in a background of chronic liver disease.[8] When present, reactivity for hepatitis D antigen in the nucleus of hepatocytes is pathognomonic.[8,31]

Many cases of HBV + HDV infection evolve rapidly to cirrhosis. Unlike most cases of isolated chronic HBV infection, even in advanced stages, interface activity and lobular necroinflammatory activity are marked, frequently producing areas of confluent necrosis.[8,31,32]

Influenza: H1N1

Most patients with influenza, including those infected with the epidemic H1N1 virus, present with upper respiratory symptoms with a benign course, whereas those patients with comorbidities may develop respiratory failure. In an autopsy study of 21 Brazilian patients with confirmed H1N1 infection who died with acute respiratory failure (16 with preexisting medical conditions) pulmonary findings were predominant and pathologic changes in other organs were mainly secondary to multiple organ failure and shock. Sections from the

liver showed erythrophagocytosis and a few mononuclear inflammatory cells in the sinusoids in all patients, and variable degrees of shock-related centrilobular necrosis. Remarkably, the only pregnant patient in the series presented clinically with hepatic failure and sections demonstrated massive hepatic necrosis.[32]

Herpesviruses

Herpesviridae is a family of large, encapsulated, double-stranded DNA viruses encoding 100 to 200 genes encased within an icosahedral capsid. All herpesviruses are nuclear-replicating.[34] Infection by herpesviruses is highly prevalent worldwide. Usually asymptomatic, primary infection is acquired in childhood. Congenital infection may cause severe disease in multiple organs, including hepatitis. Opportunistic infection by herpesviruses is a significant cause of morbidity and mortality in immunocompromised individuals.

Epstein-Barr virus

Epstein-Barr virus (EBV)-related hepatitis is characterized by prominent lymphocytic infiltrates in the sinusoids as well as mild to moderate portal infiltrates (Fig. 9). The lymphoid cells are mildly enlarged and atypical appearing ("activated"), raising the possibility of a lymphoproliferative disorder. Scattered apoptotic hepatocytes may be seen, but the degree of hepatocellular damage is minimal compared with the degree of sinusoidal inflammation. Additionally, although the lymphoid

Fig. 9. EBV hepatitis exhibiting a distinctive sinusoidal in filtrate of activated lymphocytes (H&E, original magnification ×200).

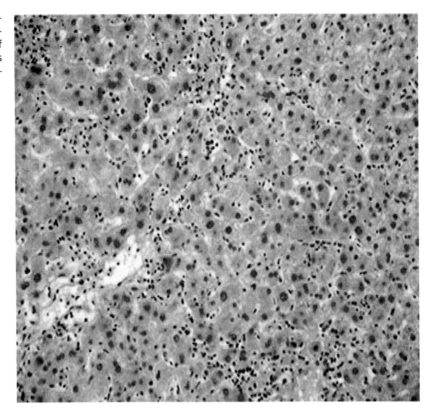

infiltrate may spill over from the portal tracts into the adjacent parenchyma, it does not destroy cells at the portal interface.[35,36] Although diagnosis relies primarily on serologic/molecular virological methods, immunohistochemistry for EBV viral capsid antigen or in situ hybridization (ISH) for EBV nucleic acids are also useful. ISH is much more sensitive, especially for detecting EBV-encoded RNA sequences, for which it is reported to be as sensitive as PCR.[36]

Cytomegalovirus

Congenital cytomegalovirus (CMV) is frequently asymptomatic, but may lead to premature birth, various neurologic manifestations, jaundice, and hepatosplenomegaly. In the post-neonatal period, primary CMV infection, especially in teenagers, presents as an infectious mononucleosis–like syndrome, sometimes with liver dysfunction, occasionally leading to fulminant hepatic failure.[37]

Histologically congenital CMV infection may lead to neonatal hepatitis, with portal and lobular inflammation, cholestasis, variable degrees of extramedullary hematopoiesis, and giant cell transformation of hepatocytes. A firm histologic diagnosis requires the identification of typical CMV inclusions in bile duct epithelium, hepatocytes, or endothelial cells. The infected cells demonstrate an enlarged nucleus with an inclusion that may be either eosinophilic or basophilic, surrounded by a clear halo leading to a characteristic "owl's eye" appearance. Variable numbers of basophilic granules can be present in the cytoplasm of the infected cells.

The histologic features of CMV hepatitis in immunocompetent patients are usually not pathognomonic because CMV inclusions are usually not found. Variable degrees of lymphocytic portal infiltrate may coexist with sinusoidal lymphocytes, similar to the histologic appearance of EBV hepatitis. Aggregates of macrophages sometimes form microgranulomas, whereas hepatocyte injury is generally not present, with the exception of rare apoptotic bodies. In immunosuppressed patients, CMV hepatitis may present as a rather mild lobular hepatitis or, less frequently, as a more severe form.[38] Microabscesses consisting of collections of neutrophils surrounding an infected hepatocyte containing a CMV inclusion is a typical finding. Immunohistochemistry (IHC) detects early-expression genes encoded protein in the nucleus of infected cells, whereas late-expression genes encode for proteins that may be found in the cytoplasm of infected cells. IHC has been considered slightly more sensitive than ISH for CMV (75.7% vs 67.6%), both claimed to be highly specific.[39]

Human herpesvirus-6

Acute infections due to human herpesvirus-6 (HHV-6) are frequently asymptomatic and resolve spontaneously. Rarely, especially in immunosuppressed patients, serious clinical manifestations involving the central nervous system, liver, gastrointestinal tract, lungs, and bone marrow occur.[40] In solid organ transplant recipients HHV-6 has been reported to rarely cause acute hepatitis, sometimes leading to fulminant hepatitis.

Herpes zoster

Although herpes zoster virus (HZV) almost never infects immunocompetent patients, submassive/massive hepatic necrosis may ensue in patients receiving high doses of steroids or with chemotherapy. In most of these cases, pathognomonic intranuclear herpetic inclusions are abundant. IHC for detection of early-expressed proteins is sensitive and specific for herpes groups. PCR detection of HZV DNA yields the most sensitive and type-specific diagnosis.[41]

Herpes simplex virus types 1 and 2

Although herpes simplex virus (HSV)-1 and HSV-2 most commonly infect immunosuppressed patients, acute hepatitis and even fulminant hepatic failure may be rarely found in immunocompetent individuals[42,43]

Histologically patchy areas of coagulative necrosis with sharp borders ("punched-out necrosis" and "punctate necrosis") are surrounded by hepatocytes with enlarged nuclei with "ground-glass" intranuclear viral inclusions; syncytial multinucleated cells are frequent (Fig. 10). Viral antigen can be demonstrated by immunohistochemistry.[44] Rare cases in pregnant patients or in neonates show diffuse, almost total hepatic necrosis with no viral inclusions and virtually no inflammatory response[45] Two types of viral inclusions, Cowdry A and B bodies, have been described in HSV infection. Cowdry A inclusions are small, round, and eosinophilic and are separated from the nuclear membrane by a halo. Cowdry B inclusions are large, ground-glass, eosinophilic, centrally located structures that push nuclear material to the rim of the nucleus. Type A bodies represent an early stage of nuclear infection, whereas type B bodies represent a later stage.

In a recent report of a case of an immunocompetent 67-year-old man with 1 week of fever and abdominal pain showed CT and MRI images compatible with liver abscesses, but with characteristic HSV histologic lesions stresses. Once again, the utility of liver biopsy for diagnosis was shown, using either immunohistochemical detection of viral antigens or of DNA sequences by in situ hybridization for HSV diagnosis.[46,47]

Adenovirus

Adenovirus is a nonenveloped, double-stranded DNA virus that causes respiratory tract infection in infancy and early childhood. Ronan and colleagues[48] collected and reviewed 89 cases of hepatitis due to adenovirus from the published literature, all occurring in immunosuppressed patients, with only 27% survival. Histologically, adenovirus hepatitis is characterized by random punched-out areas of hepatocyte necrosis (Fig. 11). Hepatocytes at the periphery of these necrotic areas usually contain nuclear viral inclusions. These are basophilic and slightly angulated and have a "ground-glass" appearance, making the nucleus look "smudgy." Cytoplasmic aggregates of basophilic material represent viral products. A variable but generally mild infiltrate of inflammatory cells accompany the infected hepatocytes and consist mostly of macrophages and lymphocytes. The centers of the necrotic areas may contain neutrophils or nuclear debris. Variable amounts of mononuclear portal inflammatory infiltrate and scattered granulomas may be seen. IHC with specific antibodies identifies viable infected cells at the periphery of the necrotic areas.[49]

Icteric Hemorrhagic Fevers

Systemic involvement by non-hepatotropic viruses can sometimes involve the liver. Patients present with high and prolonged fever, variable elevations of serum transaminase levels, and signs of multiorgan dysfunction.[50] Because these viruses tend to preferentially infect endothelial cells, the clinical picture often also includes evidence of vascular injury, including petechial rash, internal bleeding, and, in fatal cases, massive hemorrhage, shock, and disseminated intravascular coagulation.

Viral hemorrhagic fevers (VHFs) are due to enveloped RNA viruses from the families Flaviviridae, Arenaviridae, Filoviridae, and Bunyaviridae, which depend on animal reservoirs (arthropods, rodents, ruminants, and primates) and, so, they usually infect humans in regions where these animals live, mostly the Tropics. Human-to-human transmission or aerosol infections have occasionally been detected.[51]

Yellow fever

The major hepatic histologic manifestations are hemorrhagic hepatocyte necrosis and apoptosis, with a characteristic predominant midzonal (zone 2) accentuation (Fig. 12). The presence of non-necrotic rings of periportal and perivenular hepatocytes in zones 1 and 3 is useful for the morphologic

Fig. 10. HSV hepatitis. (*A*) Gross photograph showing extensive hepatocyte necrosis. (*B*) At low power a random area of hepatocyte necrosis is evident (H&E, original magnification ×40).

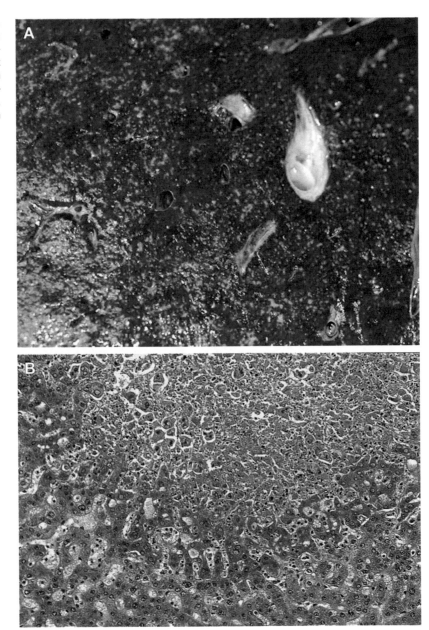

differential diagnosis with other causes of extensive hepatic necrosis. Numerous apoptotic bodies (Councilman-Rocha Lima bodies) are found amidst and at the borders of the necrotic areas. Macrovesicular and microvesicular steatosis also may be present.[52,53] Yellow fever viral antigen is exuberant in apoptotic cells as well as in hypertrophic Kupffer cells.[9] Molecular tests have been developed to allow distinction between infections caused by the wild-type virus versus the 17D vaccine strain, which is quite useful in patients with severe

hepatitis who have been recently vaccinated in Brazil and in the United States.[54,55]

Dengue virus

According to the World Health Organization, Dengue virus (transmitted primarily by the *Aedes aegypti* mosquito) has infected 100 million individuals worldwide, mostly residing in tropical and subtropical regions. The potentially severe hemorrhagic form of the disease has been diagnosed in 250,000 persons.[56] Multiple outbreaks of Dengue

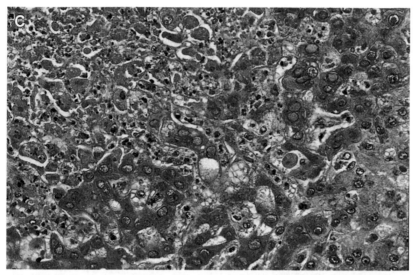

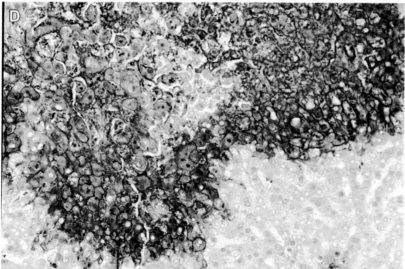

Fig. 10. (continued). (C) Viral intranuclear inclusions, including in multinucleated cells, are evident (H&E, original magnification ×100). (D) An immunostain for HSV antigen confirms the diagnosis (original magnification ×40).

infection in Latin America in the past decade has led to an endemic state in several countries. During the decade 2000 to 2010, Brazil identified 8,440,253 cases, 221,043 (2.6%) of which were classified as severe, and 3058 fatalities.[57] According to the CDC, the last reported dengue outbreak in the United States occurred in south Texas in 2005. A small dengue outbreak also occurred in Hawaii in 2001.[58]

Liver involvement varies from asymptomatic elevation of serum aminotransferases to severe hepatitis and occasionally acute liver failure.[56] Hepatocyte apoptosis leads to the presence of numerous Councilman-Rocha Lima Bodies in biopsies or at autopsy. Apoptosis may be the result of combined direct viral cytopathic effect, hypoxic mitochondrial dysfunction, the immune response, and accelerated endoplasmic reticular stress.[59] Necrosis of midzonal and centrilobular hepatocytes may result from the fact that the liver cells in these areas are more sensitive to the effects of anoxia or immune response or may be a preferential target zone of the dengue viruses.[59,60] Although not pathognomonic, more intense hepatocytic injury in zone 3 in dengue is useful for the differential diagnosis with yellow fever, which remarkably spares zone 3. Portal and lobular inflammation in dengue is usually sparse, composed mostly of lymphocytes and macrophages.

Fig. 11. Adenovirus hepatitis. There is a small focus of hepatocyte necrosis rimmed by hepatocytes with smudgy intranuclear inclusions typical of adenovirus (H&E, original magnification ×100).

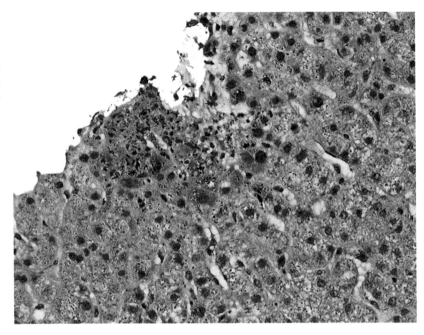

Other arboviruses: zika and chikungunya virus

Numerous cases of other arthropod-borne viruses causing acute hepatitis, specifically zika virus and chikungunya virus, have recently been reported from several Latin American countries and even from southern states of the United States. Up to now, the liver has not been shown a major target for these agents.[61,62]

Ebola and Marburg viruses

Person-to-person transmission led to very severe outbreaks in several African countries, where bats serve as major reservoirs[63] Clinical manifestations included high fever and massive hemorrhage, shock, and disseminated intravascular coagulation. Histopathology of the liver was similar to other VHFs causing acute hepatitis characterized by spotty to confluent hepatocellular necrosis with minimal inflammatory cell infiltrates.[63] Characteristic intracytoplasmic viral inclusions can be identified within hepatocytes of patients dying with Ebola infection and, less frequently, in those infected with Marburg viruses. The viral inclusions can be confirmed by IHC.[64] Mild to moderate microvesicular steatosis and Kupffer cell hypertrophy and hyperplasia are also found, but cholestasis has not been reported.[63] A small number of Ebola cases were diagnosed in Europe and the United States recently in patients who had traveled to West Africa.[64]

Hantavirus

These rodent-borne viruses are most prevalent in Asia but have also been detected in the United States and Europe.[65,66] Febrile illness is usually followed by renal failure, but in more recent outbreaks, multiorgan involvement with fever and pulmonary edema and hemorrhage have been described. In an autopsy study from Sao Paulo, Brazil,[67] a lobular hepatitis with lymphocytes and macrophages surrounding foci of necrotic hepatocytes was evident in patients who died due to severe acute edematous/hemorrhagic pulmonary disease. These patients had a history of contact with rodents, requiring consideration of bacterial infections such as leptospirosis. The correct diagnosis was confirmed by identification of Hanta viral antigens in endothelial cells and macrophages[67] by immunohistochemistry using an antibody developed by Zaki and colleagues.[65]

SUMMARY

A multidisciplinary approach for the proper diagnosis of acute viral hepatitis presently includes careful review of routine sections and the identification of viral antigen by IHC or finding viral nucleic acid sequences by in situ hybridization and/or PCR and next-generation sequencing methods. These results are then considered in conjunction with serologic testing methodologies to arrive at a firm diagnosis. In this context of remarkable

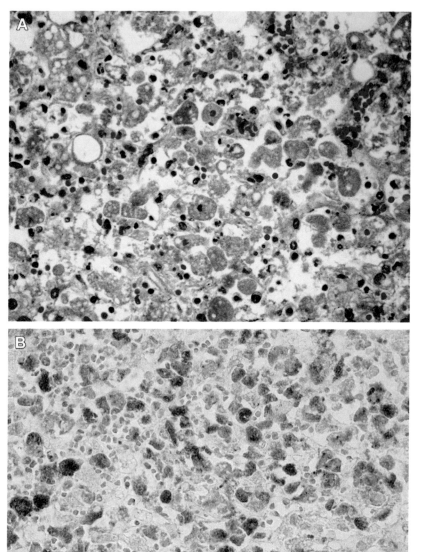

Fig. 12. Yellow fever hepatitis. (*A*) Autopsy section demonstrating marked lobular hepatitis (H&E, original magnification ×100). (*B*) Immunostain for yellow fever antigen confirms the diagnosis (original magnification ×100).

progress, we fully agree with Hofman and colleagues[68] acknowledging pathology as the way to correlate the presence of an infectious agent with the reaction it evokes at the cell and tissue levels.

REFERENCES

1. Theise ND. Liver and gallbladder, [Chapter 18]. In: Kumar V, Abbas AK, Aster JC, editors. Robbins and Cotran pathologic basis of disease. 9th edition. Philadelphia: Elsevier; 2015. p. 821–88.

2. Alves VAF. Acute viral hepatitis, [Chapter 19]. In: Saxena R, editor. Practical hepatic pathology, a diagnostic approach. Philadelphia: Elsevier; 2017. p. 191–210.

3. Zaki S, Alves VA, Hale GL. Non-hepatotropic viral, bacterial and parasitic infections of the liver. In: Burt A, Ferrell L, Hubschner S, editors. MacSween's pathology of the liver. 7th edition. Elsevier; 2017.

4. Gupta E, Ballani N, Kumar M, et al. Role of non-hepatotropic viruses in acute sporadic viral hepatitis and acute-on-chronic liver failure in adults. Indian J Gastroenterol 2015;34:448–52.

5. 2017. Available at: www.cdc.gov/hepatitis/statistics/2015surveillance/index.htm. Accessed January 15, 2018.

6. Aggarwal R, Naik S. Epidemiology of hepatitis E: current status. J Gastroenterol Hepatol 2009;24:1484–93.

7. Bianchi L. Liver biopsy interpretation in hepatitis. Part I. Presentation of critical morphologic features used in diagnosis (glossary). Pathol Res Pract 1983;178:2–19.

8. Drebber U, Odenthal M, Aberle SW, et al. Hepatitis E in liver biopsies from patients with acute hepatitis of clinically unexplained origin. Front Physiol 2013; 4:351.

9. Dias LB Jr, Alves VA, Kanamura C, et al. Fulminant hepatic failure in northern Brazil: morphological, immunohistochemical, and pathogenic aspects of Labrea hepatitis and yellow fever. Trans R Soc Trop Med Hyg 2007;101:831–9.

10. Luedde T, Kaplowitz N, Schwabe RF. Cell death and cell death responses in liver disease: mechanisms and clinical relevance. Gastroenterology 2014;147:765–83.

11. Boyer JL, Klatskin G. Pattern of necrosis in acute viral hepatitis: prognostic value of bridging (subacute hepatic necrosis). N Engl J Med 1970;283: 1063–71.

12. Hanau C, Munoz SJ, Rubin R. Histopathological heterogeneity in fulminant hepatic failure. Hepatology 1995;21:345–51.

13. Scheuer PJ, Maggi G. Hepatic fibrosis and collapse: histological distinction by orcein staining. Histopathology 1980;4:487–90.

14. Hernaez R, Solà E, Moreau R, et al. Acute-on-chronic liver failure: an update. Gut 2017;66:541–53.

15. Fausto N. Liver regeneration and repair: hepatocytes, progenitor cells, and stem cells. Hepatology 2004;39:1477–87.

16. Okuno T, Sano A, Deguchi T, et al. Pathology of acute hepatitis A in humans. Comparison with acute hepatitis B. Am J Clin Pathol 1984;81:162–9.

17. Peron JM, Danjoux M, Kamar N, et al. Liver histology in patients with sporadic acute hepatitis E: a study of 11 patients from South-West France. Virchows Arch 2007;450:405–10.

18. Hewitt PE, Ijaz S, Brailsford SR, et al. Hepatitis E virus in blood components: a prevalence and transmission study in southeast England. Lancet 2014; 384:1766–73.

19. Khuroo MS, Khuroo MS, Khuroo NS. Hepatitis E: discovery, global impact, control and cure. World J Gastroenterol 2016;22:7030–45.

20. Debing Y, Moradpour D, Neyts J, et al. Update on hepatitis E virology: implications for clinical practice. J Hepatol 2016;65:200–12.

21. Kamar N, Selves J, Mansuy JM, et al. Hepatitis E virus and chronic hepatitis in organ-transplant recipients. N Engl J Med 2008;358:811–7.

22. Mufti AR, Reau N. Liver disease in pregnancy. Clin Liver Dis 2012;16:247–69.

23. Gupta P, Jagya N, Pabhu SB, et al. Immunohistochemistry for the diagnosis of hepatitis E virus infection. J Viral Hepat 2012;19:e177–83.

24. Ray MB, Desmet VJ, Bradburne AF, et al. Differential distribution of hepatitis B surface antigen and hepatitis B core antigen in the liver of hepatitis B patients. Gastroenterology 1976;71:462–9.

25. Omata M, Iwama S, Sumida M, et al. Clinico-pathological study of acute non-A, non-B post-transfusion hepatitis: histological features of liver biopsies in acute phase. Liver 1981;1:201–8.

26. Johnson K, Kotiesh A, Boitnott JK, et al. Histology of symptomatic acute hepatitis C infection in immunocompetent adults. Am J Surg Pathol 2007;31: 1754–8.

27. Pessoa MG, Alves VA, Wakamatsu A, et al. Posttransplant recurrent hepatitis C: immunohistochemical detection of hepatitis C virus core antigen and possible pathogenic implications. Liver Int 2008; 28:807–13.

28. Rizzetto M, Canese MG, Arico S, et al. Immunofluorescence detection of new antigen-antibody system (delta/anti-delta) associated to hepatitis B virus in liver and in serum of HBsAg carriers. Gut 1977;18: 997–1003.

29. Farci P, Niro GA. Clinical features of hepatitis D. Semin Liver Dis 2012;32:228–36.

30. Sureau C, Negro F. The hepatitis delta virus: replication and pathogenesis. J Hepatol 2016;64(1 Suppl): S102–16.

31. Fonseca JC, Gayotto LC, Ferreira LC, et al. Labrea hepatitis—hepatitis B and delta antigen expression in liver tissue: report of three autopsy cases. Rev Inst Med Trop Sao Paulo 1985;27: 224–7.

32. Bensabath G, Hadler SC, Soares MC, et al. Hepatitis delta virus infection and Labrea hepatitis: prevalence and role in fulminant hepatitis in the Amazon Basin. JAMA 1987;258:479–83.

33. Mauad T, Hajjar LA, Callegari GD, et al. Lung pathology in fatal novel human influenza A (H1N1) infection. Am J Respir Crit Care Med 2010;181: 72–9.

34. Stumpf MP, Laidlaw Z, Jansen VA. Herpes viruses hedge their bets. Proc Natl Acad Sci U S A 2002; 99:15234–7.

35. Koch DG, Christiansen L, Lazarchick J, et al. Posttransplantation lymphoproliferative disorder—the great mimic in liver transplantation: appraisal of the clinicopathologic spectrum and the role of Epstein-Barr virus. Liver Transpl 2007;13: 904–12.

36. Mellinger JL, Rossaro L, Naugler WE, et al. Epstein-Barr virus (EBV) related acute liver failure: a case series from the US Acute Liver Failure Study Group. Dig Dis Sci 2014;59:1630–7.

37. Ho M. The history of cytomegalovirus and its diseases. Med Microbiol Immunol 2008;197:65–73.

38. Marcelin JR, Beam E, Razonable RR. Cytomegalovirus infection in liver transplant recipients: updates on clinical management. World J Gastroenterol 2014;20:10658–67.

39. Lu DY, Qian J, Easley KA, et al. Automated in situ hybridization and immunohistochemistry for cytomegalovirus detection in paraffin-embedded tissue sections. Appl Immunohistochem Mol Morphol 2009;17:158–64.

40. Agut H. Deciphering the clinical impact of acute human herpesvirus 6 (HHV-6) infections. J Clin Virol 2011;52:164–71.

41. Herrero JI, Quiroga J, Sangro B, et al. Herpes zoster after liver transplantation: incidence, risk factors, and complications. Liver Transpl 2004;10:1140–3.

42. Côté-Daigneault J, Carrier FM, Toledano K, et al. Herpes simplex hepatitis after liver transplantation: case report and literature review. Transpl Infect Dis 2014;16:130–4.

43. Levitsky J, Duddempudi AT, Lakeman FD, et al. Detection and diagnosis of herpes simplex virus infection in adults with acute liver failure. Liver Transpl 2008;14:1498–504.

44. Goodman ZD, Ishak KG, Sesterhenn IA. Herpes simplex hepatitis in apparently immunocompetent adults. Am J Clin Pathol 1986;85:694–9.

45. Jacques SM, Qureshi F. Herpes simplex virus hepatitis in pregnancy: a clinicopathologic study of three cases. Hum Pathol 1992;23:183–7.

46. Norvell JP, Blei AT, Jovanovic BD, et al. Herpes simplex virus hepatitis: an analysis of the published literature and institutional cases. Liver Transpl 2007;13:1428–34.

47. Down C, Mehta A, Salama G, et al. Herpes simplex virus hepatitis in an immunocompetent host resembling hepatic pyogenic abscesses. Case Rep Hepatol 2016;2016:8348172.

48. Ronan BA, Agrwal N, Carey EJ, et al. Fulminant hepatitis due to human adenovirus. Infection 2014;42:105–11.

49. Weidner AS, Panarelli NC, Rennert H, et al. Immunohistochemistry improves the detection of adenovirus in gastrointestinal biopsy specimens from hematopoietic stem cell transplant recipients. Am J Clin Pathol 2016;146(5):627–31.

50. Shimizu Y. Liver in systemic disease. World J Gastroenterol 2008;14:4111–9.

51. Paessler S, Walker DH. Pathogenesis of the viral hemorrhagic fevers. Annu Rev Pathol 2013;8:411–40.

52. Peres LC, Saggioro FP, Dias LB Jr, et al. Infectious diseases in paediatric pathology: experience from a developing country. Pathology 2008;40:161–75.

53. Vieira WT, Gayotto LC, de Lima CP, et al. Histopathology of the human liver in yellow fever with special emphasis on the diagnostic role of the Councilman body. Histopathology 1983;7:195–208.

54. Vasconcelos PF, Luna EJ, Galler R, et al. Serious adverse events associated with yellow fever 17DD vaccine in Brazil: a report of two cases. Lancet 2001;358:91–7.

55. Martin M, Tsai TF, Cropp B, et al. Fever and multisystem organ failure associated with 17D–204 yellow fever vaccination: a report of four cases. Lancet 2001;358:98–104.

56. Samanta J, Sharma V. Dengue and its effects on liver. World J Clin Cases 2015;3:125–31.

57. Teixeira MG, Siqueira JB Jr, Ferreira GL, et al. Epidemiological trends of dengue disease in Brazil (2000-2010): a systematic literature search and analysis. PLoS Negl Trop Dis 2013;7:e2520.

58. 2016. Available at: https://www.cdc.gov/dengue/epidemiology/index.html. Accessed January 15, 2018.

59. Seneviratne SL, Malavige GN, de Silva HJ. Pathogenesis of liver involvement during dengue viral infections. Trans R Soc Tropmed Hyg 2006;100:608–14.

60. Pagliari C, Quaresma JA, Fernandes ER, et al. Immunopathogenesis of dengue hemorrhagic fever: contribution to the study of human liver lesions. J Med Virol 2014;86:1193–7.

61. Enserink M. An obscure mosquito-borne disease goes global. Science 2015;350(6264):1012–3.

62. Weaver SC, Lecuit M. Chikungunya virus and the global spread of a mosquito-borne disease. N Engl J Med 2015;372:1231–9.

63. Martines RB, Ng DL, Greer PW, et al. Tissue and cellular tropism, pathology and pathogenesis of Ebola and Marburg viruses. J Pathol 2015;235(2):153–74.

64. Heeney JL. Ebola: hidden reservoirs. Nature 2015;527(7579):453–5.

65. Zaki SR, Greer PW, Coffield LM, et al. Hantavirus pulmonary syndrome: pathogenesis of an emerging infectious disease. Am J Pathol 1995;146:552–79.

66. Vapalahti O, Mustonen J, Lundkvist A, et al. Hantavirus infections in Europe. Lancet Infect Dis 2003;3:653–61.

67. Katz G, Williams RJ, Burt MS, et al. Hantavirus pulmonary syndrome in the State of Sao Paulo, Brazil, 1993–1998. Vector Borne Zoonotic Dis 2001;1:181–90.

68. Hofman P, Lucas S, Jouvion G, et al. Pathology of infectious diseases: what does the future hold? Virchows Arch 2017;470:483–92.

Nonalcoholic Steatohepatitis
Histopathology Basics Within a Broader Context

Michael H. Schild, DO, Cynthia D. Guy, MD*

KEYWORDS

- Fatty liver disease • Hepatocyte ballooning • Diagnosis

Key points

- At least 5% hepatic steatosis is essential for the diagnosis of nonalcoholic fatty liver disease. Steatosis is often in zone 3 in adults and in zone 1 in children.

- Hepatocyte ballooning is an essential element for the diagnosis of adult nonalcoholic steatohepatitis.

- Mild lobular inflammation and mild portal inflammation are common in nonalcoholic steatohepatitis.

- Nonalcoholic steatohepatitis commonly has pericellular "chicken wire" fibrosis.

- Many of these key features can be absent in cirrhosis (often referred to as "burnt out" steatohepatitis).

ABSTRACT

Nonalcoholic fatty liver disease (NAFLD) is a major health concern and the prevalence continues to increase in many industrialized and developing countries around the world. NAFLD affects adults and children. NAFLD-related cirrhosis is expected to become the top indication for liver transplantation in the near future, and the incidence of NAFLD-related hepatocellular carcinoma is also increasing. Nonalcoholic steatohepatitis is the more severe form of NAFLD. The pathogenesis of NALFD/nonalcoholic steatohepatitis is complex and new concepts continue to evolve. The diagnosis and categorization of nonalcoholic steatohepatitis currently rests on hepatopathologists. Accurate morphologic interpretation is important for therapeutic, prognostic, and investigational purposes.

OVERVIEW

Overweight/obesity and related metabolic conditions are major public health concerns in many parts of the world, including the United States, Europe, the Middle East, Asia, and Latin America.[1] Nonalcoholic fatty liver disease (NAFLD) is the hepatic manifestation of metabolic syndrome, and by definition occurs in the absence of significant alcohol consumption (eg, <20 g/d for women and <30 g/d for men). Metabolic syndrome describes a systemic disorder with at least 3 of 5 of the following: large waist-to-hip ratio (abdominal obesity), high triglyceride level, low high-density lipoprotein cholesterol level, hypertension, and high fasting blood sugar or diabetes mellitus/insulin resistance. NAFLD encompasses a spectrum of hepatic pathology that ranges from isolated steatosis (nonalcoholic fatty liver [NAFL]) to severe

---

Department of Pathology, Duke University, DUHS, Box 3912, Durham, NC 27710, USA
* Corresponding author.
E-mail address: cynthia.guy@duke.edu

Surgical Pathology 11 (2018) 267–285
https://doi.org/10.1016/j.path.2018.02.013

hepatocellular injury with steatosis, inflammation, and ballooning (nonalcoholic steatohepatitis [NASH]). NASH is a more severe and progressive form of NAFLD that is import to diagnose because cirrhosis and hepatocellular carcinoma (HCC) can develop. NASH strongly correlates with hepatic fibrosis. Hepatic steatosis can be diagnosed by imaging studies such as ultrasound examination; however, liver biopsy is the gold standard for the diagnosis of NASH. This review focuses on individual histopathologic lesions used for the diagnosis of NASH and aims to provide a diagnostic roadmap within an epidemiologic and pathobiological context.

EPIDEMIOLOGY

On imaging studies, 25% of adults worldwide are estimated to have NAFLD.[1] Figures are even higher in the Middle East (almost 32%) and South America (30%). Approximately 25% of US adults have NAFLD, equating to 64 million Americans. The estimated incidence of NASH in the general population ranges from 1.5% to 6.5%. NASH is now the leading cause of cirrhosis in the United States and is expected to be the leading indication for liver transplantation by 2020. The negative health and societal impacts of NASH are massive, and the economic burden of NASH and its sequela are projected to be more than $100 billion annually in the United States in direct medical costs.[2]

PATHOGENESIS

NASH is a dynamic disorder that can progress to cirrhosis and HCC, smolder along, or regress to NAFL.[3] The "2-hit" hypothesis of NASH pathogenesis is no longer the pervasive view. In fact, hepatic steatosis is now considered an early and beneficial adaptive response to mitigate lipotoxicity; the incoming and de novo free fatty acids are packaged into relatively inert triacylglycerol.[4]

NASH is a complex disease with a strong genetic component in combination with environmental and nutritional factors (eg, increased consumption of saturated fats, cholesterol, sugars, and processed fructose[5]) and decreased energy expenditure. NAFLD is considered a polygenic and heritable disease[6] with marked interpatient variation regarding disease outcome.[7] The 2 most important genetic modifiers are believed to be *PNPLA3* and *TM6SF2* single nucleotide polymorphisms. Furthermore, an allelic variant of *PNPLA3* has been linked to an increased risk of NAFLD-associated HCC.[8] Ethnicity and gender[9] also influence NASH pathogenesis.

Two major underlying components of NAFLD pathogenesis include obesity and insulin resistance. Other key contributions result from ongoing hepatocellular stress (eg, oxidative stress, endoplasmic reticulum stress, and lipotoxicity), hepatic inflammation, cellular damage, and death (eg, hepatocyte ballooning and apoptosis), with resultant fibrogenesis.[4,10,11]

MICROSCOPIC FEATURES

STEATOSIS

Hepatic lipid droplets are not simply static fat storage depots, but are dynamic organelles composed of a central triacylglycerol core and sterol esters encompassed by a monolayer of phospholipid and proteins.[12] Although the major function of lipid droplets is as an energy reserve, an increasing complexity of lipid droplet biology is now recognized. Although steatosis is regarded a hallmark lesion of NAFLD, growing evidence supports the counterintuitive notion that hepatic triglycerides accumulate as a cytoprotective mechanism against the lipotoxic effects of free fatty acids.[13]

The 2 major forms of hepatic steatosis are macrovesicular and microvesicular. Macrovesicular steatosis is the most common type in NAFLD, and it is used as a component in the 2 most common grading systems (**Table 1**). Macrovesicular steatosis comes in 2 main varieties, large droplet and small droplet. Large droplet steatosis expands to fill the hepatocyte cytoplasm and seems to displace the nucleus to the side (**Fig. 1**). Small droplet steatosis is seen as several small cytoplasmic droplets, and the nucleus is often retained centrally (see **Fig. 1**C). Microvesicular steatosis is often first identified on low-power magnification as an indistinct, pale, eosinophilic area or "patch." Higher power evaluation shows "foamy" cytoplasmic changes (see **Fig. 1**D).

Small patches of microvesicular steatosis in a nonzonal distribution can be seen in a small proportion of NAFLD cases, and has been associated with more severe injury and advanced fibrosis.[14] Extensive microvesicular steatosis has not been described in NAFLD, and if present other etiologies (eg, drug toxicity or Reye syndrome) must be considered.

Macrovesicular steatosis is considered pathologic when it involves more than 5% of hepatocytes. The degree of steatosis is usually assessed in a semiquantitative manner using

Table 1
Comparison of the NASH CRN and FLIP Consortium scoring systems for NAFLD

NASH CRN, NAS	FLIP Consortium NAFLD Scoring System: SAF

Steatosis grade
  The percentage of hepatocytes with macrovesicular steatosis (including large and small droplet forms)
  0: <5%
  1: 5%–33%
  2: 34%–66%
  3: >66%
	Steatosis grade
	  S_0: None
	  S_1: 5%–33%
	  S_2: 34%–66%
	  S_3: >66%

Lobular (acinar) Inflammation
  The average number of foci per 20× objective field
  0: None
  1: <2 foci
  2: 2–4 foci
  3: >4 foci
	Lobular (acinar) Inflammation
	  0: None
	  1: ≤2 foci per 20× objective field
	  2: >2 foci per 20× objective field

Ballooning
  0: None
  1: Few
  2: Many
	Ballooning
	  0: None
	  1: Clusters of hepatocytes with rounded shape and pale and/or reticulated cytoplasm
	  2: Same as score 1 with enlarged hepatocytes (>2× normal size)

NAS (0–8)
  The sum of the scores for steatosis + lobular inflammation + ballooning
	Activity grade (A, 0–4)
	  The sum of the scores for lobular inflammation and ballooning
	  A1: A = 1, mild activity
	  A2: A = 2, moderate activity
	  A3 and A4: A >2, severe activity

Fibrosis stage
  0: No pathologic fibrosis
  1a: Delicate (requires trichrome) centrilobular pericellular fibrosis
  1b: Dense (and visible on hematoxylin and eosin staining) centrilobular pericellular fibrosis
  1c: Periportal pericellular fibrosis
  2: Centrilobular and periportal pericellular fibrosis
  3: Bridging fibrosis
  4: Cirrhosis
	Fibrosis stage (F)
	  F_0: No significant fibrosis
	  F_{1A}: Mild zone 3 perisinusoidal fibrosis
	  F_{1B}: Moderate zone 3 perisinusoidal fibrosis
	  F_{1C}: Portal fibrosis only
	  F_2: Zone 3 and periportal perisinusoidal fibrosis
	  F_3: Bridging fibrosis
	  F_4: Cirrhosis

	SAF score S_{0-3} A_{0-4} F_{0-4}

Abbreviations: CRN, Clinical Research Network; FLIP, Fatty Liver Inhibition of Progression; NAFLD, nonalcoholic fatty liver disease; NAS, Nonalcoholic Fatty Liver Disease Activity Score; NASH, nonalcoholic steatohepatitis; SAF, Steatosis, Activity, and Fibrosis.

low (4× objective) or medium-power (10× objective) magnification. Two of the common scoring systems for NAFLD use the following cutoff values for hepatic steatosis: grade 0, less than 5%; grade 1, 5% to 33%; grade 2, 34%–66%; and grade 3, greater than 66% (**Fig. 2**). It is also important to determine the zonal location, which may provide a clue to the underlying etiology. In adult NAFLD, steatosis often predominates in zone 3 (**Fig. 3**A); however, there are other well-recognized patterns. Panacinar steatosis involves all hepatic zones fairly evenly (**Fig. 3**B). Azonal steatosis is seen as aggregates of steatosis involving zones in an inconsistent manner. Zone 1 steatosis is often seen in pediatric NAFLD (**Fig. 3**C).

Reticulin histochemistry is commonly used in diagnostic liver pathology. Normal hepatic plates are accompanied by delicate reticulin fibers. Reticulin can be crucial for the evaluation

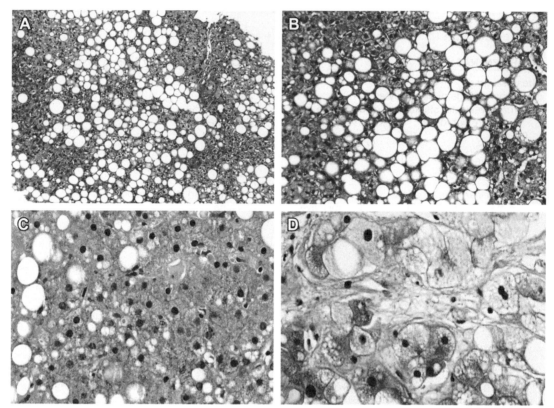

Fig. 1. Macrovesicular and microvesicular steatosis. (*A*) Predominately large droplet macrovesicular steatosis (original magnification ×4; stain: hematoxylin and eosin [H&E]). (*B*) Large lipid droplets fill the cytoplasm. The periphery shows small droplet macrovesicular steatosis (original magnification ×10; stain: H&E). (*C*) Small droplet macrovesicular steatosis (original magnification ×20; stain: H&E). (*D*) Microvesicular steatosis (original magnification ×40; stain: H&E).

of hepatic neoplasms; HCC usually has diminished or absent reticulin. Benign steatotic liver often has diminished reticulin or lacks reticulin (**Fig. 3**D), and this may be a diagnostic pitfall.[15]

LOBULAR INFLAMMATION

A mild amount of lobular (acinar) inflammation is common in NAFLD (**Fig. 4**A), although it is not unusual to see more robust lobular inflammation (**Fig. 4**B). The inflammatory foci are often small, scattered throughout the lobule, and composed of mononuclear cells. Sometimes a small number of neutrophils are admixed. Aggregates of macrophages (microgranulomas) are often seen and these may contain lipid (lipogranulomas). Large well-formed and/or caseating granulomas, however, are not typical in NAFLD and should raise the possibility of an infection or sarcoidosis. Two widely applied scoring systems use a semiquantitative method to grade acinar inflammation (see **Table 1**).

BALLOONING AND MALLORY-DENK BODIES

Hepatocellular ballooning is a principal histologic finding to distinguish NAFL (**Fig. 5**) from NASH. Ballooning is a morphologic manifestation of hepatocellular stress and is classically associated with hepatocyte enlargement, rounded cell contour, cytoplasmic clearing, and reticulation (**Fig. 6**A, B). Normal size or small hepatocytes may show similar changes and can also be considered ballooned.[16,17]

Definitive identification of hepatocyte ballooning on routine hematoxylin and eosin (H&E) staining can sometimes be difficult, as indicated by the less than ideal intraobserver and interobserver agreements.[18,19] Loss of the normal hepatocyte intermediate filament proteins, keratin 8 and 18 (K8/18), by immunohistochemistry (IHC) is an objective marker of ballooning[20] (**Fig. 6**C). Application of K8/18 IHC together with ubiquitin (marking Mallory-Denk bodies) across the spectrum of NAFLD histopathology confirmed the usefulness for the identification of classically enlarged

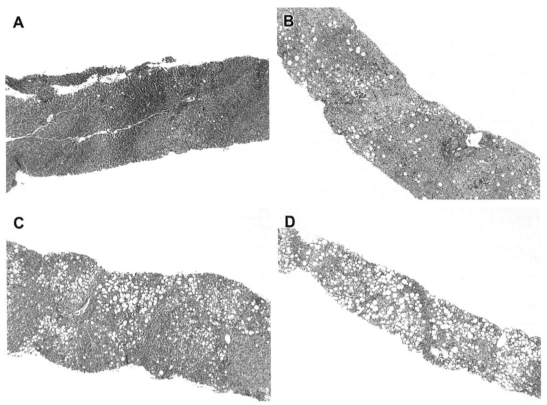

Fig. 2. Steatosis grade. (*A*) Steatosis of less than 5% (original magnification ×2; stain: hematoxylin and eosin [H&E]). (*B*) Grade 1 (5%–33%) steatosis (original magnification ×2; stain: H&E). (*C*) Grade 2 (34%–66%) steatosis (original magnification ×2; stain: H&E). (*D*) Grade 3 (>66%) steatosis (original magnification ×2; stain: H&E).

ballooned hepatocytes.[16] Furthermore, this study demonstrated that small hepatocytes with K8/18 loss and ubiquitin aggregates (Mallory-Denk bodies) are approximately 5 times more numerous than similar but enlarged cells (**Fig.** 6D–F). Both types (large and normal size) are located within fibrous matrix and positively correlate with the H&E ballooning grade and diagnosis of steatohepatitis.[16]

Another IHC method for ballooned hepatocyte identification involves the Hedgehog (Hh) signaling pathway. Hh is a morphogenic signaling network that is activated during many types of acute and chronic liver injury to orchestrate regeneration/repair.[21] Hh ligands (such as Sonic Hh or Indian Hh) promote growth of liver progenitor cells[22] and function as profibrogenic factors.[23,24] Hh signaling is active in NASH.[10,25,26] Injured liver cells produce Hh ligands[27] and release them into the microenvironment.[28] Ballooned hepatocytes (defined by IHC for K8/18) produce Sonic Hh ligand (see **Fig.** 6G, H).[29] Subsequent work using a larger number of human NASH liver biopsy samples confirmed that IHC for Sonic Hh can be used

to identify ballooned hepatocytes, and that Hh pathway activity correlates with histologic severity and degree of fibrosis in NASH.[30] Furthermore, in the PIVENS trial (Pioglitazone versus Vitamin E versus Placebo for the Treatment of Nondiabetic Patients with Nonalcoholic Steatohepatitis), which was sponsored by the National Institute of Diabetes and Digestive and Kidney Diseases, IHC for Sonic Hh+ ballooned hepatocytes correlated with the therapeutic response to vitamin E.[31] Other investigators have shown the usefulness of Sonic Hh IHC for the identification of hepatocyte ballooning and correlated morphometric findings to serologic markers of liver cell injury.[32]

Mallory-Denk bodies are eosinophilic, hyaline cytoplasmic inclusions frequently located near the nucleus.[33] Ballooned hepatocytes frequently, but not always, contain Mallory-Denk bodies.[16,20,33] Mallory-Denk body formation is an orchestrated hepatocellular stress response (eg, oxidative stress and endoplasmic reticulum stress) involving protein misfolding and proteasome overload.[33] It is not currently

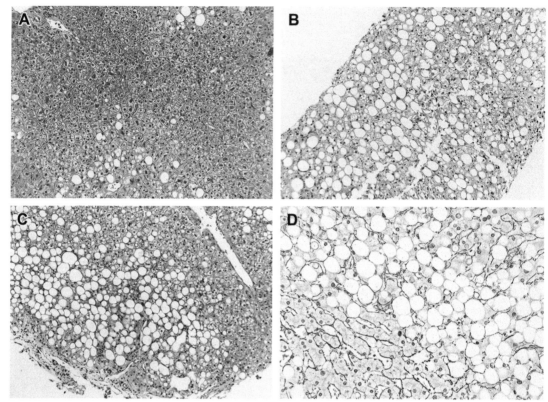

Fig. 3. Steatosis acinar location. (*A*) Centrizonal steatosis (original magnification ×4; stain: hematoxylin and eosin [H&E]). (*B*) Panacinar steatosis (original magnification ×4; stain: H&E). (*C*) Periportal steatosis (original magnification ×4; stain: H&E). (*D*) Reticulin loss around steatotic hepatocytes (original magnification ×10; stain: H&E).

known whether Mallory-Denk bodies are an epiphenomenon of hepatocyte injury, a cytoprotective element, or a contributor to hepatocyte damage.[34] Mallory-Denk body formation is reversible and likely does not reduce hepatocyte viability.[34]

FIBROSIS

Liver fibrosis is a critical histopathologic lesion to evaluate accurately. No other single histologic feature associates with increased liver-related and overall mortality in NAFLD.[35] Liver fibrosis is also the only histologic lesion that independently predicts liver-related morbidity such as ascites, hepatic encephalopathy, and esophageal varices. Hepatic fibrosis results from dysregulated wound healing.[36] One of the primary fibrogenic effectors in the liver is the hepatic stellate cell, which resides in the space of Disse. In healthy livers, the extracellular matrix is dynamic, providing structural and functional stability, and the delicate balance between synthesis and degradation is tightly controlled. However, after chronic fibrogenic injury, extracellular matrix production exceeds degradation and cross-linked

collagenous scar is formed. Cirrhosis can result. Current evidence supports the concept that liver fibrosis is reversible.[37]

A common pattern of fibrosis in NAFLD is perisinusoidal or pericellular "chicken wire" fibrosis (**Fig. 7**). In 1999, a grading and staging system for NAFLD was proposed (Brunt methodology)[38] and this system was modified in in 2005 by the NASH Clinical Research Network.[18] In this system, fibrosis is categorized into stages 0 to 4 (see **Fig. 7, Table 1**). Stage 1A is delicate pericellular/perisinusoidal fibrosis, often seen in zone 3 adjacent to ballooned hepatocytes. Stage 1B is similar to 1A, except that the fibrous stands are thicker and easily recognizable on H&E. Stage 1C is also composed of thin pericellular/perisinusoidal fibrous strands; however, the location is periportal. This form of fibrosis is common in the early stage of pediatric NAFLD. Stage 2 characterizes pericellular scar located both in zone 3 and zone 1. Bridging fibrosis, stage 3, characterizes fibrous matrix which links 2 microscopic anatomic structures. Cirrhosis (stage 4) is the term used when regenerative hepatic nodules are surrounded by fibrous matrix. The acinar

Fig. 4. Lobular inflammation. (*A*) Mild (original magnification ×10; stain: hematoxylin and eosin [H&E]). (*B*) Moderate (original magnification ×10; stain: H&E).

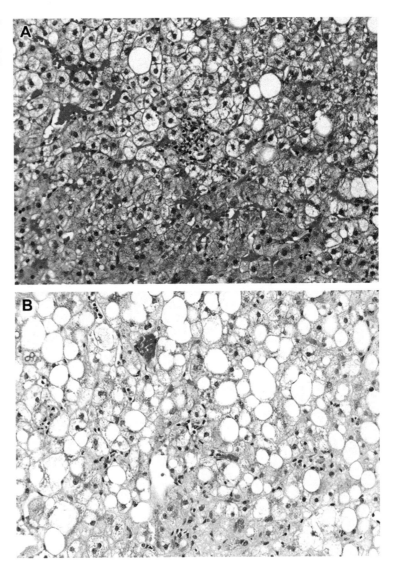

Fig. 5. Nonalcoholic fatty liver. Isolated steatosis without ballooning (original magnification ×10; stain: hematoxylin and eosin).

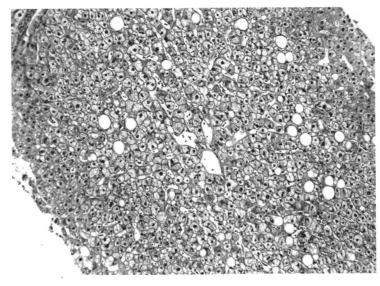

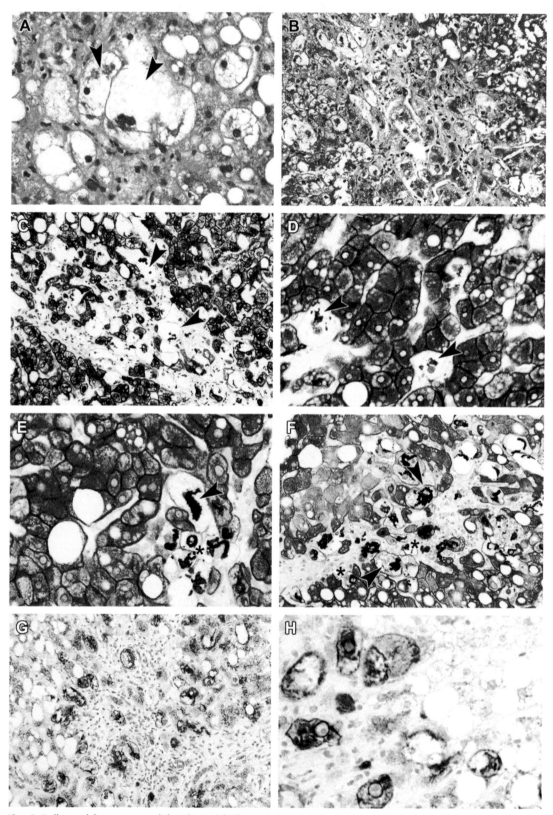

Fig. 6. Ballooned hepatocytes. (*A*) Enlarged ballooned hepatocytes (*arrows;* original magnification ×10; stain: hematoxylin and eosin [H&E]). (*B*) Trichrome with ballooning and pericellular fibrosis (original magnification ×4).

zonal architecture becomes obliterated by cirrhosis; the normal relationships of the portal tracts (and vascular inflow) to the central veins (vascular outflow) are abolished, and portal hypertension can result.

OTHER IMPORTANT HISTOPATHOLOGIC LESIONS SEEN IN NONALCOHOLIC FATTY LIVER DISEASE

Injury and hepatocyte death are present in virtually all liver diseases. Apoptosis is a major category of programmed cell death. Apoptosis is mediated by activated caspases. Apoptotic bodies (also called acidophil bodies) are characterized by oncocytic change, cellular shrinkage, pyknosis and karyorrhexis (**Fig. 8A**). Apoptotic bodies are common in NAFLD, and the number of apoptotic bodies correlates with the degree of lobular inflammation, the ballooning grade, and the diagnostic category of definite NASH.[39] Another morphologic manifestation of cell injury is hepatocyte megamitochondria (**Fig. 8B**).

Much of the morphologic focus in NASH is directed toward the acinar parenchyma in an attempt to characterize the degree of steatosis, inflammation, and hepatocyte injury. Portal inflammation and the ductular reaction have recently come more to the forefront.[40–43] The ductular reaction is a complex process involving hepatic progenitor cells, increased numbers of bile ductules, fibrous matrix, and the inflammation that occurs within the periportal niche; it is a component of liver repair and fibrogenesis. Mild portal inflammation (**Fig. 9A**) is common in NAFLD, but almost 25% of adults and 14% of children show more than mild portal inflammation (**Fig. 9B**).[41] Increased portal inflammation correlates with increased fibrosis stage[41,43] and a ductular reaction.[42,43]

Accurate interpretation of the hepatic microscopic architecture is necessary for appropriate diagnostic categorization. Centrizonal injury and scarring are typical of NASH. Central zone remodeling may result in arteriole formation and a ductular reaction, and both are associated with advanced fibrosis.[44] The centrilobular ductular reaction correlates with fibrosis progression in NASH.[45] Awareness that central zones may contain arterioles and bile ductules may prevent misinterpretation of the histologic pattern of injury.

Hepatocytes normally contain glycogen. Glycogenosis, however, signifies hepatocellular glycogen overload visible by H&E light microscopy as pale, gray, cytoplasmic changes within swollen hepatocytes (**Fig. 10A–C**). The cytoplasm can appear rarefied. Owing to cellular enlargement and cytoplasmic clearing, glycogenosis may be confused with hepatocyte ballooning.[46,47] Glycogen storage disease (see **Fig. 10D**) is an entirely different entity. Glycogenic hepatopathy is another distinct condition that occurs in patients with poorly controlled diabetes mellitus type 1.[48]

PEDIATRIC NONALCOHOLIC FATTY LIVER DISEASE

NAFLD has become the most common cause of chronic liver disease in children of Westernized countries in parallel with the increase in childhood obesity.[49] The histopathologic findings in pediatric NAFLD can differ from adults. Children (typically before puberty) can show zone 1 predominance of macrovesicular steatosis, absence of hepatocyte ballooning, and periportal (rather than centrilobular) pericellular fibrosis (stage 1C pattern; see **Fig. 1C**).[50] Some children with NASH may show the adult pattern of zone 3 steatosis with ballooning, and zone 3 pericellular fibrosis, whereas others may show a combination (overlap) of these patterns.[51]

TWO HISTOPATHOLOGIC SCORING SYSTEMS FOR NONALCOHOLIC FATTY LIVER DISEASE: THE NAFLD ACTIVITY SCORE AND THE STEATOSIS, ACTIVITY, AND FIBROSIS SCORING SYSTEM

Accurate morphologic assessment of NASH is imperative for adequate patient care, research,

---

(*C*) Immunohistochemistry (IHC) for K8/18 (brown chromogen) shows ballooned hepatocytes with Mallory-Denk bodies and loss of keratin (*arrows;* original magnification ×4). (*D*) IHC for K8/18 (brown chromogen) ubiquitin (red chromogen) shows ballooned hepatocytes with Mallory-Denk bodies (*red*) and loss of keratin (*arrows;* original magnification ×10). (*E, F*) IHC for K8/18/ubiquitin shows large ballooned hepatocytes with Mallory-Denk bodies (*arrows*) along with numerous normal size ballooned hepatocytes with Mallory-Denk bodies (*asterisks;* original magnification ×10 and ×4). (*G, H*) IHC for Sonic hedgehog marks ballooned hepatocytes (original magnification ×4 and ×10).

276

and clinical trial evaluations. Histopathologic scoring systems have been developed, and 2 examples are the NAFLD Activity Score (NAS),[18] and the Steatosis, Activity, and Fibrosis scoring system[17] (see **Table 1**).

The NAS was developed for use in clinical trials. It can be applied to liver biopsies from adults and children. The NAS is an unweighted sum of semiquantitative assessments of steatosis,

lobular inflammation, and ballooning. The NAS was never intended to be used to render a diagnosis.[18,52]

In contrast with the NAS, the Steatosis, Activity, and Fibrosis scoring system separates steatosis grade from the activity score (the unweighted sum of the degree of lobular inflammation and ballooning).[17] The Fatty Liver Inhibition of Progression algorithm[17]

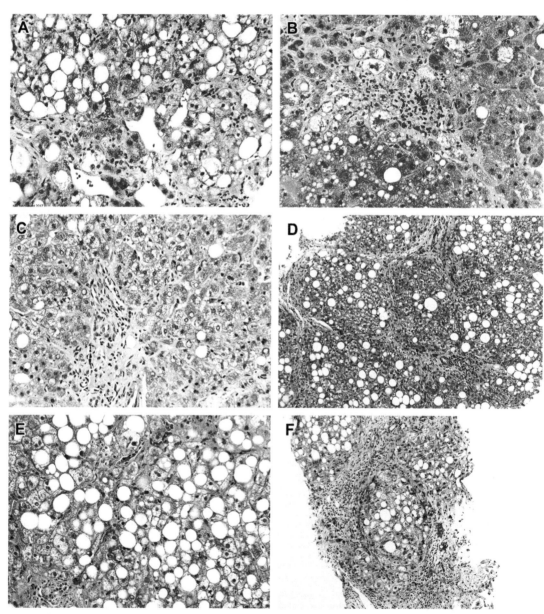

Fig. 7. Fibrosis, Masson trichrome stain. (*A*) Delicate zone 3 pericellular fibrosis (stage 1A; original magnification ×10). (*B*) Thicker zone 3 fibrosis (stage 1B; original magnification ×10). (*C*) Periportal fibrosis (stage 1C; original magnification ×10). (*D*) Central-portal bridging (stage 3; original magnification ×4). (*E*) Portal-portal bridging (stage 3; original magnification ×10). (*F*) Cirrhosis (stage 4; original magnification ×4).

Fig. 8. Common other types of cell death and injury. (*A*) Apoptotic bodies (original magnification ×40; inset original magnification ×60; stain: hematoxylin and eosin [H&E]). (*B*) Megamitochondria (*arrows*; original magnification ×40; stain: H&E).

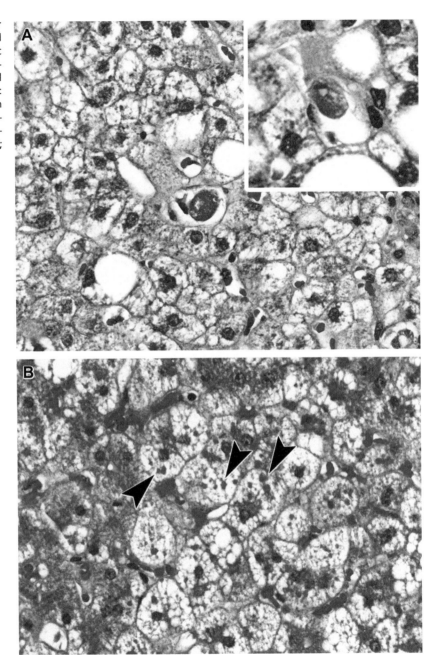

was designed to use the Steatosis, Activity, and Fibrosis score as a backbone for the clinically important distinction between NAFL and NASH. The Fatty Liver Inhibition of Progression algorithm has been shown to improve interobserver agreement in the separation of NAFL from NASH among expert liver pathologists and general pathologists.[53]

DIFFERENTIAL DIAGNOSIS

The diagnosis of steatohepatitis does not directly implicate a single specific etiology. In other words, steatohepatitis does not equate with NASH. Steatohepatitis has a broad differential diagnosis requiring clinical and laboratory correlation. Some of the most common possibilities are discussed herein (and summarized in **Table 2**).

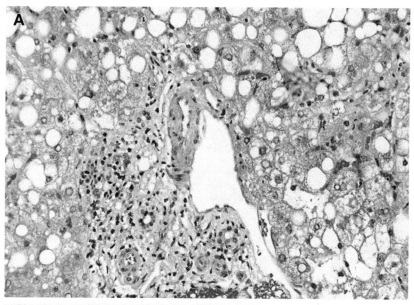

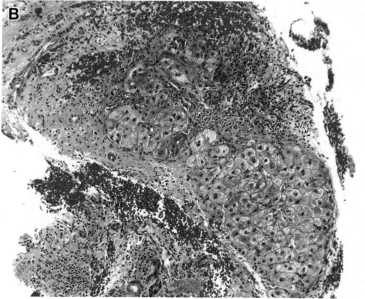

Fig. 9. Portal inflammation. (A) Mild (original magnification ×10; stain: hematoxylin and eosin [H&E]). (B) Moderate (original magnification ×4; stain: H&E).

Pitfalls
FOR THE DIAGNOSIS OF NONALCOHOLIC STEATOHEPATITIS

! Failing to recognize the "pediatric pattern" of NASH. Pediatric NASH often has zone 1 steatosis, lacks ballooning, and has periportal (instead of centrilobular) pericellular chicken wire fibrosis.

! Not recognizing a coexisting/concurrent disease (eg, autoimmune hepatitis [AIH], iron overload disorder, or alpha-1 antitrypsin deficiency).

! Making the diagnosis of steatohepatitis based solely on the presence of ballooning with or without Mallory-Denk bodies. Ballooning hepatocellular injury with Mallory-Denk body production can be seen as a result of many types of cellular injury.

! Failing to recognize mimickers of hepatocyte ballooning such as hepatocellular glycogenosis.

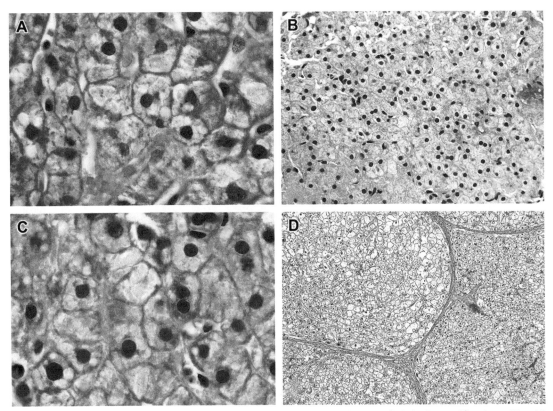

Fig. 10. Glycogenosis. (*A–C*) Hepatocytes with abundant cytoplasmic glycogen (original magnification ×60, ×10, and ×60; stain: hematoxylin and eosin [H&E]). (*D*) Glycogen storage disease type 3B (original magnification ×4; stain: H&E).

Table 2
Differential diagnosis of NASH

NASH vs	Helpful Distinguishing Features or Clinical Information
1. Alcohol-associated liver disease	Ballooning hepatocyte injury tends to be pronounced with "classical" (enlarged) ballooned hepatocytes. Mallory-Denk bodies are often thick and "waxy" or "ropy." Prominent neutrophilic infiltrates can be seen admixed with ballooned hepatocytes or Mallory-Denk bodies (this is referred to as satellitosis). Central veins can be severely injured and scarred or obliterated (this is called central hyaline sclerosis). Canalicular cholestasis can be present.
2. DASH	Distinguishing DASH from NASH requires clinical correlation with a temporally associated drug or medication (eg, amiodarone or irinotecan).
3. CASH	Distinguishing CASH from NASH requires clinical correlation with a temporally associated chemical exposure or toxin (eg, mushrooms, [*Amanita phalloides* "death cap"]). Hepatic steatosis along with necrosis and hemorrhage has been described.
4. Wilson disease	A high clinical suspicion is often required. Helpful laboratory values and clinical findings include a low ceruloplasmin level, elevated 24-h urine copper, Kayser-Fleisher rings (evaluation generally requires an experienced ophthalmologist). A negative liver histochemistry for copper (eg, rhodanine) does not exclude the possibility of Wilson disease.

Abbreviations: CASH, chemical or toxin-associated steatosis and/or steatohepatitis; DASH, drug-induced or drug-associated steatosis and/or steatohepatitis; NASH, nonalcoholic steatohepatitis.

ALCOHOL-ASSOCIATED LIVER DISEASE AND ALCOHOLIC STEATOHEPATITIS

Alcohol-associated liver disease (ALD) shares many histomorphologic features with NAFLD, and both diseases may coexist within a single patient. The extent of alcohol consumption must be carefully documented clinically. Given the large overlap of pathologic changes, it may not be possible to distinguish NAFLD/NASH from ALD/ASH. That being said, ALD can have a variety of lesions not typical of NAFLD.[54] Lesions suggestive of ALD include alcoholic foamy degeneration (essentially pure microvesicular steatosis), fibroobliterative lesions of central veins (central hyaline sclerosis; Fig. 11A), severe zone 3 injury and arteriole formation (Fig. 11B), canalicular cholestasis, and a prominent portal ductular reaction with neutrophils, ballooned hepatocytes with large, thick Mallory-Denk bodies, and surrounding neutrophils (satellitosis).[54]

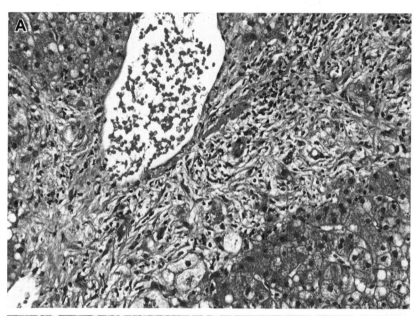

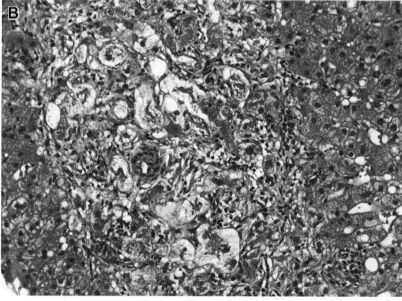

Fig. 11. (A) Alcohol-associated liver disease (ALD) with central hyaline sclerosis (original magnification ×10; stain: hematoxylin and eosin [H&E]). (B) ALD with central arteriole (original magnification ×10; stain: H&E).

WILSON DISEASE

Wilson disease is a monogenic autosomal recessive copper metabolism disorder. The causative gene, *ATP7B*, encodes a copper transporting P-type ATPase. Genetic testing for *ATP7B* mutations is increasingly available. It is now recognized that early-onset (infancy) and late-onset (>70 years of age) presentations can occur.[55] The prevalence of Wilson disease may be greater than previously recognized. Liver biopsy findings in the early stages of Wilson disease include steatosis, hepatocyte ballooning, and Mallory-Denk bodies, and these may be nonzonal as compared with the typical zone 3 location in NASH. In later stages, chronic hepatitis-like features with moderate portal chronic inflammation and periportal fibrosis may be helpful in distinguishing these findings. Prominent lipofuscin and glycogenation of hepatocyte nuclei may also be pronounced. Patients may present with cirrhosis or fulminant hepatic failure. Histochemistry for copper (eg, rhodanine), may be helpful; however, a negative finding does not exclude Wilson disease.

DRUG-ASSOCIATED STEATOHEPATITIS AND CHEMOTHERAPY-ASSOCIATED STEATOHEPATITIS

There are many medications and drugs that can cause hepatic steatosis and steatohepatitis (**Box 1**), and the morphologic features can overlap significantly with NAFLD/NASH. An appropriate clinical history and timeline are necessary to establish chemical or toxin-associated steatosis and/or steatohepatitis/drug-induced or drug-associated steatosis and/or steatohepatitis conclusively. Some histomorphologic clues to suggest medication-induced steatohepatitis are occasionally present.[56] For example, zone 1 ballooned hepatocytes can be seen in amiodarone toxicity. Amiodarone may also cause phospholipidosis—foamy degenerative changes—in hepatocytes and Kupffer cells. Steatosis is often quite mild in amiodarone toxicity in comparison with the prominence of hepatocyte ballooning and Mallory-Denk body formation. Two cardiovascular medications, perhexiline maleate (Pexid, an anti-anginal agent) and diethylaminoethoxyhexestrol (Coralgil, a vasodilator), can cause steatohepatitis and phospholipidosis similar to amiodarone.[56]

NONALCOHOLIC FATTY LIVER DISEASE WITH CONCURRENT DISEASE

Owing to the high prevalence of NAFLD, coexisting diseases may occur; examples include hepatitis C, hepatitis B, human immunodeficiency virus, AIH, ALD, hemochromatosis, alpha-1 antitrypsin deficiency, Wilson disease, and biliary tract diseases. A high degree of awareness of the clinical setting and laboratory values is necessary. Serum autoantibodies, sometimes at high titers, are known to occur in a higher prevalence in NAFLD than in the general population,[57] and these non–organ-specific antibodies can occur in the absence of bona fide autoimmune disease. An accurate diagnosis (NAFLD, AIH, or a combination of NAFLD and AIH) is particularly important because the treatment for AIH may exacerbate NAFLD (eg, glucocorticoids).

PROGNOSIS AND TREATMENT

NAFLD is associated with serious, adverse, interrelated, and bidirectional multiorgan health consequences.[58] The overall morbidity and mortality among patients with NASH is higher than in the general population. The most common causes of death are cardiovascular disease and malignancy, followed by liver-related events. Components of the metabolic syndrome are risk factors for the development of NAFLD/NASH, but it is now becoming increasingly recognized that NAFLD/NASH may precede and contribute to the pathogenesis of the metabolic syndrome.[58] Clinically significant extrahepatic manifestations of NAFLD include obstructive sleep apnea, chronic kidney disease, osteoporosis, colorectal cancer, and iron overload (dysmetabolic iron overload).[58]

Box 1
Medicinal agents causing steatohepatitis

Medications/drugs/therapies that can cause hepatic steatosis and/or steatohepatitis

Irinotecan

Amiodarone

Perhexiline (Pexid)

Diethylaminoethoxyhexestrol (Corilgil)

Total parental nutrition

Methotrexate

Tamoxifen

Steroids

Estrogens

Nifedipine

Total parenteral nutrition

Intestinal bypass surgery

Over the past 30 years, the age-adjusted incidence of HCC in the United States has increased from 1.5 to 4.9 per 100,000 individuals.[59] NAFLD-associated HCC is increasingly being recognized,[60,61] and may occur in a noncirrhotic background.[59]

NAFLD is the fastest growing liver disease in industrialized nations; however, pharmacologic treatment options remain limited. Lifestyle modifications (diet and exercise) persist as the therapeutic backbone, although numerous clinical trials are underway. Bariatric surgery is a therapeutic option advocated by some investigators.

SUMMARY

NAFLD and the metabolic syndrome are prevalent worldwide. They share an interconnected pathogenesis and detrimental outcomes. Accurate histopathologic evaluation of NAFLD/NASH is important and surgical pathologists should be facile with liver biopsy interpretation (**Fig. 12**).

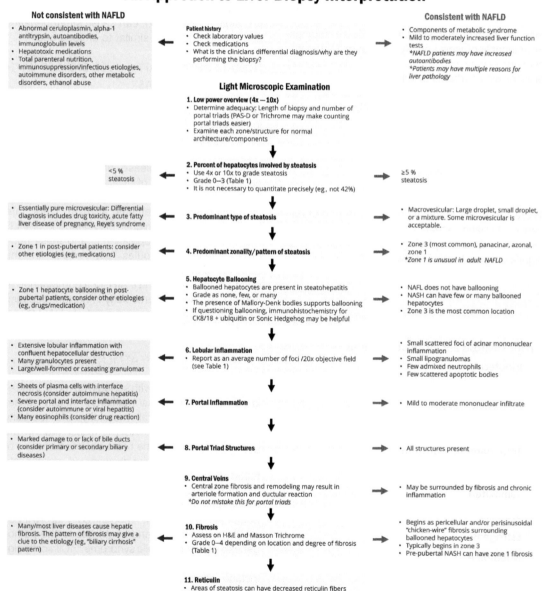

Fig. 12. Diagnostic approach to nonalcoholic fatty liver disease (NAFLD) biopsies. NASH, nonalcoholic steatohepatitis.

REFERENCES

1. Chalasani N, Younossi Z, Lavine JE, et al. The diagnosis and management of nonalcoholic fatty liver disease: practice guidance from the American Association for the Study of Liver Diseases. Hepatology 2018;67(1):328–57.
2. Younossi ZM, Blissett D, Blissett R, et al. The economic and clinical burden of nonalcoholic fatty liver disease in the United States and Europe. Hepatology 2016;64(5):1577–86.
3. Kleiner DE, Brunt EM, Belt PH, et al. Diagnostic patterns and disease activity are related to disease progression and regression in nonalchololic fatty liver disease. Hepatology 2016;64(1 Suppl.): 37A.
4. Hardy T, Oakley F, Anstee QM, et al. Nonalcoholic fatty liver disease: pathogenesis and disease spectrum. Annu Rev Pathol 2016;11:451–96.
5. Abdelmalek MF, Suzuki A, Guy C, et al. Increased fructose consumption is associated with fibrosis severity in patients with nonalcoholic fatty liver disease. Hepatology 2010;51(6):1961–71.
6. Sookoian S, Pirola CJ. Genetic predisposition in nonalcoholic fatty liver disease. Clin Mol Hepatol 2017;23(1):1–12.
7. Anstee QM, Day CP. The genetics of nonalcoholic fatty liver disease: spotlight on PNPLA3 and TM6SF2. Semin Liver Dis 2015;35(3): 270–90.
8. Liu YL, Patman GL, Leathart JB, et al. Carriage of the PNPLA3 rs738409 C >G polymorphism confers an increased risk of non-alcoholic fatty liver disease associated hepatocellular carcinoma. J Hepatol 2014;61(1):75–81.
9. Yang JD, Abdelmalek MF, Pang H, et al. Gender and menopause impact severity of fibrosis among patients with nonalcoholic steatohepatitis. Hepatology 2014;59(4):1406–14.
10. Verdelho Machado M, Diehl AM. Role of hedgehog signaling pathway in NASH. Int J Mol Sci 2016; 17(6), [pii:E857].
11. Bohinc BN, Diehl AM. Mechanisms of disease progression in NASH: new paradigms. Clin Liver Dis 2012;16(3):549–65.
12. Mashek DG, Khan SA, Sathyanarayan A, et al. Hepatic lipid droplet biology: getting to the root of fatty liver. Hepatology 2015;62(3):964–7.
13. Leamy AK, Egnatchik RA, Young JD. Molecular mechanisms and the role of saturated fatty acids in the progression of non-alcoholic fatty liver disease. Prog Lipid Res 2013;52(1):165–74.
14. Tandra S, Yeh MM, Brunt EM, et al. Presence and significance of microvesicular steatosis in nonalcoholic fatty liver disease. J Hepatol 2011;55(3): 654–9.
15. Singhi AD, Jain D, Kakar S, et al. Reticulin loss in benign fatty liver: an important diagnostic pitfall when considering a diagnosis of hepatocellular carcinoma. Am J Surg Pathol 2012;36(5):710–5.
16. Guy CD, Suzuki A, Burchette JL, et al. Costaining for keratins 8/18 plus ubiquitin improves detection of hepatocyte injury in nonalcoholic fatty liver disease. Hum Pathol 2012;43(6):790–800.
17. Bedossa P, Poitou C, Veyrie N, et al. Histopathological algorithm and scoring system for evaluation of liver lesions in morbidly obese patients. Hepatology 2012;56(5):1751–9.
18. Kleiner DE, Brunt EM, Van Natta M, et al. Design and validation of a histological scoring system for nonalcoholic fatty liver disease. Hepatology 2005;41(6):1313–21.
19. Younossi ZM, Gramlich T, Liu YC, et al. Nonalcoholic fatty liver disease: assessment of variability in pathologic interpretations. Mod Pathol 1998; 11(6):560–5.
20. Lackner C, Gogg-Kamerer M, Zatloukal K, et al. Ballooned hepatocytes in steatohepatitis: the value of keratin immunohistochemistry for diagnosis. J Hepatol 2008;48(5):821–8.
21. Omenetti A, Choi S, Michelotti G, et al. Hedgehog signaling in the liver. J Hepatol 2011;54(2):366–73.
22. Ochoa B, Syn WK, Delgado I, et al. Hedgehog signaling is critical for normal liver regeneration after partial hepatectomy in mice. Hepatology 2010; 51(5):1712–23.
23. Jung Y, Brown KD, Witek RP, et al. Accumulation of hedgehog-responsive progenitors parallels alcoholic liver disease severity in mice and humans. Gastroenterology 2008;134(5):1532–43.
24. Omenetti A, Diehl AM. The adventures of sonic hedgehog in development and repair. II. Sonic hedgehog and liver development, inflammation, and cancer. Am J Physiol Gastrointest Liver Physiol 2008;294(3):G595–8.
25. Fleig SV, Choi SS, Yang L, et al. Hepatic accumulation of Hedgehog-reactive progenitors increases with severity of fatty liver damage in mice. Lab Invest 2007;87(12):1227–39.
26. Syn WK, Jung Y, Omenetti A, et al. Hedgehog-mediated epithelial-to-mesenchymal transition and fibrogenic repair in nonalcoholic fatty liver disease. Gastroenterology 2009;137(4):1478–88.e8.
27. Jung Y, Witek RP, Syn WK, et al. Signals from dying hepatocytes trigger growth of liver progenitors. Gut 2010;59(5):655–65.
28. Witek RP, Yang L, Liu R, et al. Liver cell-derived microparticles activate hedgehog signaling and alter gene expression in hepatic endothelial cells. Gastroenterology 2009;136(1):320–30.e2.
29. Rangwala F, Guy CD, Lu J, et al. Increased production of sonic hedgehog by ballooned hepatocytes. J Pathol 2011;224(3):401–10.

30. Guy CD, Suzuki A, Zdanowicz M, et al. Hedgehog pathway activation parallels histologic severity of injury and fibrosis in human nonalcoholic fatty liver disease. Hepatology 2012;55(6):1711–21.

31. Guy CD, Suzuki A, Abdelmalek MF, et al. Treatment response in the PIVENS trial is associated with decreased Hedgehog pathway activity. Hepatology 2015;61(1):98–107.

32. Estep JM, Mehta R, Bratthauer G, et al. Hepatic sonic hedgehog (SHH) expression measured by computer assisted morphometry correlates histologic features of non-alcoholic steatohepatitis (NASH) and circulating markers of apoptosis and cell injury. Hepatology 2016;64(1 Suppl.):1625A.

33. Zatloukal K, French SW, Stumptner C, et al. From Mallory to Mallory-Denk bodies: what, how and why? Exp Cell Res 2007;313(10):2033–49.

34. Ku NO, Strnad P, Zhong BH, et al. Keratins let liver live: mutations predispose to liver disease and crosslinking generates Mallory-Denk bodies. Hepatology 2007;46(5):1639–49.

35. Angulo P, Kleiner DE, Dam-Larsen S, et al. Liver fibrosis, but no other histologic features, is associated with long-term outcomes of patients with nonalcoholic fatty liver disease. Gastroenterology 2015; 149(2):389–97.e10.

36. Lee UE, Friedman SL. Mechanisms of hepatic fibrogenesis. Best Pract Res Clin Gastroenterol 2011; 25(2):195–206.

37. Lee YA, Wallace MC, Friedman SL. Pathobiology of liver fibrosis: a translational success story. Gut 2015;64(5):830–41.

38. Brunt EM, Janney CG, Di Bisceglie AM, et al. Nonalcoholic steatohepatitis: a proposal for grading and staging the histological lesions. Am J Gastroenterol 1999;94(9):2467–74.

39. Yeh MM, Belt P, Brunt EM, et al. Acidophil bodies in nonalcoholic steatohepatitis. Hum Pathol 2016;52: 28–37.

40. Richardson MM, Jonsson JR, Powell EE, et al. Progressive fibrosis in nonalcoholic steatohepatitis: association with altered regeneration and a ductular reaction. Gastroenterology 2007;133(1):80–90.

41. Brunt EM, Kleiner DE, Wilson LA, et al. Portal chronic inflammation in nonalcoholic fatty liver disease (NAFLD): a histologic marker of advanced NAFLD-Clinicopathologic correlations from the nonalcoholic steatohepatitis Clinical Research Network. Hepatology 2009;49(3):809–20.

42. Skoien R, Richardson MM, Jonsson JR, et al. Heterogeneity of fibrosis patterns in non-alcoholic fatty liver disease supports the presence of multiple fibrogenic pathways. Liver Int 2013;33(4):624–32.

43. Gadd VL, Skoien R, Powell EE, et al. The portal inflammatory infiltrate and ductular reaction in human nonalcoholic fatty liver disease. Hepatology 2014; 59(4):1393–405.

44. Gill RM, Belt P, Wilson L, et al. Centrizonal arteries and microvessels in nonalcoholic steatohepatitis. Am J Surg Pathol 2011;35(9):1400–4.

45. Zhao L, Westerhoff M, Pai RK, et al. Centrilobular ductular reaction correlates with fibrosis stage and fibrosis progression in non-alcoholic steatohepatitis. Mod Pathol 2018;31(1):150–9.

46. Kleiner DE, Behling C, Guy CD, et al. Glycogenosis is associated with measures of insulin resistance in adults with nonalcoholic fatty liver disease. Mod Pathol 2012;25:416A.

47. Guy CD, Brunt EM, Behling C, et al. Hepatic glycogenosis in children with NAFLD: a different disease than glycogenic hepatopathy. Mod Pathol 2012;25: 414A.

48. Torbenson M, Chen YY, Brunt E, et al. Glycogenic hepatopathy: an underrecognized hepatic complication of diabetes mellitus. Am J Surg Pathol 2006; 30(4):508–13.

49. Berardis S, Sokal E. Pediatric non-alcoholic fatty liver disease: an increasing public health issue. Eur J Pediatr 2014;173(2):131–9.

50. Schwimmer JB, Behling C, Newbury R, et al. Histopathology of pediatric nonalcoholic fatty liver disease. Hepatology 2005;42(3):641–9.

51. Carter-Kent C, Yerian LM, Brunt EM, et al. Nonalcoholic steatohepatitis in children: a multicenter clinicopathological study. Hepatology 2009;50(4): 1113–20.

52. Brunt EM, Kleiner DE, Wilson LA, et al, NASH Clinical Research Network (CRN). Nonalcoholic fatty liver disease (NAFLD) activity score and the histopathologic diagnosis in NAFLD: distinct clinicopathologic meanings. Hepatology 2011; 53(3):810–20.

53. Bedossa P, FLIP Pathology Consortium. Utility and appropriateness of the Fatty Liver Inhibition of Progression (FLIP) algorithm and Steatosis, Activity, and Fibrosis (SAF) score in the evaluation of biopsies of nonalcoholic fatty liver disease. Hepatology 2014;60(2):565–75.

54. Yeh MM, Brunt EM. Pathological features of fatty liver disease. Gastroenterology 2014;147(4):754–64.

55. Bandmann O, Weiss KH, Kaler SG. Wilson's disease and other neurological copper disorders. Lancet Neurol 2015;14(1):103–13.

56. Ramachandran R, Kakar S. Histological patterns in drug-induced liver disease. J Clin Pathol 2009; 62(6):481–92.

57. Vuppalanchi R, Gould RJ, Wilson LA, et al. Clinical significance of serum autoantibodies in patients with NAFLD: results from the nonalcoholic steatohepatitis Clinical Research Network. Hepatol Int 2012; 6(1):379–85.

58. VanWagner LB, Rinella ME. Extrahepatic manifestations of nonalcoholic fatty liver disease. Curr Hepatol Rep 2016;15(2):75–85.

59. Pocha C, Kolly P, Dufour JF. Nonalcoholic fatty liver disease-related hepatocellular carcinoma: a problem of growing magnitude. Semin Liver Dis 2015; 35(3):304–17.

60. Starley BQ, Calcagno CJ, Harrison SA. Nonalcoholic fatty liver disease and hepatocellular carcinoma: a weighty connection. Hepatology 2010;51(5): 1820–32.

61. Ma C, Zhang Q, Greten TF. Nonalcoholic fatty liver disease promotes hepatocellular carcinoma through direct and indirect effects on hepatocytes. FEBS J 2018;285(4):752–62.

Chronic Hepatitis C and Direct Acting Antivirals

Maria Westerhoff, MD[a],*, Joseph Ahn, MD, MS, MBA[b]

KEYWORDS

• Hepatitis C • Directly acting antivirals • Transient elastography • Liver biopsy • Diagnostic criteria
• Histology

Key points

- HCV is the most common blood borne viral infection in the United States.

- HCV patients with comorbidities, such as alcohol use, NASH, and hepatitis B coinfection are more likely to undergo liver biopsy. Hence, pathologists should keep in mind that concomitant effects of these factors may be seen on histology.

- Histologic features of chronic HCV hepatitis include dense lymphoid aggregates in the portal tracts with mild interface activity. Severe necroinflammatory activity is unusual in chronic HCV and should prompt consideration of another or additional disease entity.

- Cure rates with direct acting antivirals are now more than 90% in most cases. The risk for HCC, however, still persists and underscores the need for continued HCC surveillance.

- Persistent inflammation may be found even after achieving sustained virologic response due to treatment. Regression of fibrosis can also occur.

ABSTRACT

The hepatitis C virus (HCV) is the most common blood-borne infection in the United States and is the most common cause of end-stage liver disease requiring liver transplant. Over the last 10 years, direct acting antiviral therapies have revolutionized HCV treatment, increasing the cure rates from less than 50% to more than 90% in those who reach access to care. This article is an overview for pathologists and clinicians covering the histologic findings of HCV as well as direct acting antiviral therapy.

HEPATITIS C VIRUS OVERVIEW

The hepatitis C virus (HCV) is the most common blood-borne infection in the United States, affecting up to 3.5 to 4 million Americans.[1] It is also the most common cause of end-stage liver disease requiring liver transplant.[2] HCV poses an underrecognized public health challenge and remains undiagnosed in most of those infected (up to 70%).[3,4] Furthermore, since 2007, HCV has surpassed the human immunodeficiency virus (HIV) as a cause of death in the United States, and contributed to a growing health care access and outcome disparity because it disproportionately affects those who are homeless, living below the poverty level, incarcerated, or with a history of injection drug use or alcohol abuse. The irony is that over the last 10 years, a revolution in HCV treatment with directly acting antiviral (DAA) therapies has occurred, increasing the cure rates from less than 50% to more than 90% in those who are able to traverse gaps in current practice from infection to diagnosis to access to care. This article provides an overview of HCV for pathologists and clinicians with a specific focus on DAAs and histologic findings of HCV.

---

[a] University of Michigan, 1301 Catherine Street, 5231 Medical Science Building 1, Ann Arbor, MI 48104, USA;
[b] Oregon Health & Science University, 3181 SW Sam Jackson Park Road, Mail Code L-461, Portland, OR 97239, USA
* Corresponding author.
E-mail address: mariawesterhoff@gmail.com

Surgical Pathology 11 (2018) 287–296
https://doi.org/10.1016/j.path.2018.02.002

RISK FACTORS FOR HEPATITIS C VIRUS

Risk factors for HCV are well known, including injection drug use, high-risk sexual exposures, blood transfusions, tattoo placement, hemodialysis, occupation as a health care worker, and vertical transmission. Risk factors for progression of hepatic fibrosis include host factors, such as older age at infection, male gender, duration of infection, iron overload (hemochromatosis), and most importantly and within patient control, alcohol and tobacco use. Other factors include immunosuppression; hepatic steatosis associated with alcoholic and nonalcoholic fatty liver disease; diabetes mellitus (DM); coinfection with hepatitis B virus (HBV); and viral factors, such as genotype 3 and alanine aminotransferase (ALT) elevation as shown in **Box 1**.[5] Given the growing prevalence of nonalcoholic steatohepatitis (NASH) in the United States, providers must be aware of the concomitant risk it poses on those already infected with HCV in increasing the risk of hepatic

---

Box 1
Factors influencing liver fibrosis

Host

- Duration of infection

- Age at infection greater than 40 years old

- Gender (male)

Toxins

- ETOH consumption

- Tobacco/cannabis use

- Iron overload

Immunosuppression

- HIV coinfection

- Organ transplant

Liver-related factors

- HBV coinfection

- ALT elevation

- Fibrosis

- Genotype 3

Metabolic factors

- Steatosis

- Insulin resistance

Viral load is NOT predictive

From Feld JJ, Liang TJ. Hepatitis C: identifying patients with progressive liver injury. Hepatology 2006 43(S1): S195; with permission.

---

fibrosis, cirrhosis, and hepatocellular carcinoma (HCC). Furthermore, it is important for pathologists to recognize that it is these patients with comorbidities, such as alcohol use, NASH, DM, and HBV, or HIV coinfection who are more likely to undergo a biopsy of the liver, so that assessment for and awareness of concomitant effects of these factors are taken into account on histologic interpretation.

The incubation period of HCV is on average 6 to 8 weeks, and only a small minority (~20%) of patients present symptomatically with nonspecific complaints of malaise or fatigue, with only rare development of jaundice. Chronic infection occurs in approximately 60% to 85% of those acutely infected, but once established, the natural history of HCV is progressive. Over a period of 20 to 40 years, patients with chronic HCV progress to cirrhosis in at least 20%. Once cirrhosis is established, the risk of HCC remains elevated at more than 1% to 4% a year, and the risk of hepatic decompensation at 3% to 6% per year. Patients with HCC or hepatic decompensation face a high risk of death without liver transplantation.[6–8] Despite the recent groundbreaking strides in DAA development, the United States still faces the prospect of an important incidence of decompensated cirrhosis and HCC as a result of the aging of the "Baby Boomers" (born between 1945–1965), who have a more than three-fold higher prevalence of HCV than the rest of the US population, and thus are at a higher risk for such HCV complications.[9]

Like those with acute infection, most patients with chronic HCV hepatitis have no symptoms, with gradual and incremental development of fatigue as the main complaint, until cirrhosis and end-stage liver disease develop, at which point ascites, hepatic encephalopathy, and jaundice can occur. Extrahepatic manifestations of HCV include mixed cryoglobulinemia, porphyria cutanea tarda, polyarteritis nodose, and association with DM and lymphoma (**Fig. 1**).

Abnormal liver function tests are the most common mode of alerting providers to the presence of HCV infection, and thus, the Centers for Disease Control and Prevention has recommended testing for HCV in those at risk, including those with injection drug use history, abnormal liver enzymes, and those born between 1945 and 1965 (**Box 2**).[10] A positive anti-HCV antibody indicates exposure to HCV but does not distinguish between active or resolved infection, and is also not protective toward reinfection. Because false-positive serologic testing can occur, it is imperative for a confirmatory HCV RNA test to be performed.[11] An HCV genotype is then obtained to guide treatment

Fig. 1. Extrahepatic manifestations of HCV. RA, rheumatoid arthritis.

- While primary site clinical infection with HCV = liver, can develop related disease at other sites. These include:
  a. Mixed cryoglobulinemia
  b. Porphyria cutanea tarda
  c. Polyarteritis Nodosa

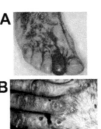

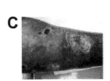

- Lichen planus, Thyroid disease, Sjogren's, RA, Vasculitis
- Association with DM, B cell non-Hodgkin Lymphoma

selection and in cases where patients have previously been treated with DAAs, viral resistance panels are available to identify mutations that may increase resistance to DAAs.

DIRECTLY ACTING ANTIVIRAL THERAPY

Unlike previous interferon-based treatment regimens that acted by generally stimulating the patient's immune response against HCV, DAAs "directly" act to inhibit the protein components of the HCV virus (**Fig. 2**). Currently DAAs are available in four main categories based on their target: (1) NS3/4A protease inhibitors, (2) nucleotide NS5B polymerase inhibitors, (3) nonnucleoside NS5B polymerase inhibitors, and (4) NS5A replication complex inhibitors (**Table 1**).[12]

Box 2
Centers for Disease Control and Prevention testing recommendations for chronic HCV infection

Persons for whom HCV testing is recommended
Adults born during 1945 to 1965

HCV testing recommended for those who

- Currently inject drugs
- Ever injected drugs, including those who injected once or a few times many years ago
- Persons with selected medical conditions, including persons
  ○ Who received clotting factor concentrates produced before 1987
  ○ Who were ever on long-term hemodialysis
  ○ With persistently abnormal ALT levels
  ○ Who have HIV infection
- Were prior recipients of transfusions or organ transplants, including persons who
  ○ Were notified they received blood from a donor who later tested positive for HCV infection
  ○ Received a transfusion of blood, blood components, or organ transplant before July 1992

HCV testing based on a recognized exposure is recommended for

- Health care, emergency medical, and public safety workers after needle sticks, sharps, or mucosal exposures to HCV-positive blood
- Children born to HCV-positive women

Note: For persons who might have been exposed to HCV within the past 6 months, testing for HCV RNA or follow-up testing for HCV antibody is recommended.

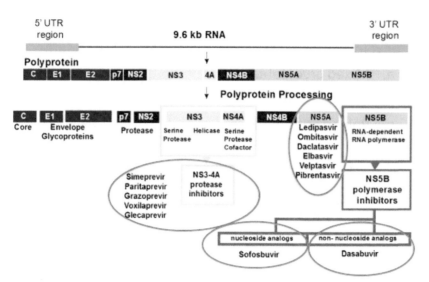

Fig. 2. Direct-acting anti-virals targets. (*From* McGovern B, Abu Dayyeh B, Chung RT. Avoiding therapeutic pitfalls: the rational use of specifically targeted agents against hepatitis C infection. Hepatology 2008;48:1702; with permission.)

The reader is directed to www.hcvguidelines.org for the latest update on specific prescribing recommendations, because that is outside the purview of this article. The efficacy of the latest generation of DAAs approved in 2017 approach nearly 100% for treatment-naive patients, and more than 90% for those who have been previously treated with earlier-generation DAAs. The main limitation of DAA therapy has been their cost, precluding universal or even widespread use, such that a minority of patients achieve cure, or sustained virologic response (SVR) (Fig. 3). Emerging issues in HCV therapy with DAAs that had not previously been recognized with interferon-based therapies include the risks of HBV reactivation and the persistence of active HCV histologic changes in liver transplant recipients who achieve SVR.

HBV reactivation has been reported in patients with HBV/HCV coinfection, not on suppressive HBV therapy, with severity ranging from mild to fulminant liver injury. In addition, patients without active HBV, but previous exposure, denoted by a positive anti-HB core antibody, have been reported to suffer HBV reactivation.[13] As such, clinicians caring for patients with HCV have been recommended to test for HBV with HBV surface antigen, anti-HB surface antibody, and anti-HB core antibody before initiating HCV DAA therapy. For patients with a positive HB surface antigen or positive anti-HB core antibody, monitoring HBV DNA levels during therapy and with any rise in liver function tests is recommended. In addition, patients with active HBV are advised to be treated with oral HBV therapies before or at the time of DAA therapy initiation (www.hcvguidelines.org). Pathologists evaluating liver biopsies obtained from patients with HCV on DAAs with elevated liver

Table 1
DAA options

Food and Drug Administration Approval	NS3/4A Protease Inhibitor	Nucleotide NS5B Polymerase Inhibitor	Nonnucleoside NS5B Polymerase Inhibitor	NS5A Replication Complex Inhibitor	Other
2013		Sofosbuvir			± Ribavirin
2014		Sofosbuvir		Ledipasvir	± Ribavirin
2014	Simeprevir	Sofosbuvir			
2014	Paritaprevir		Dasabuvir	Ombitasvir	± Ribavirin
2015		Sofosbuvir		Daclatasvir	± Ribavirin
2016	Grazoprevir			Elbasvir	± Ribavirin
2016		Sofosbuvir		Velpatasvir	± Ribavirin
2017	Voxilaprevir	Sofosbuvir		Velpatasvir	
2017	Glecaprevir			Pibrentasvir	
2018	Grazoprevir	Uprifosbuvir		Ruzasvir	

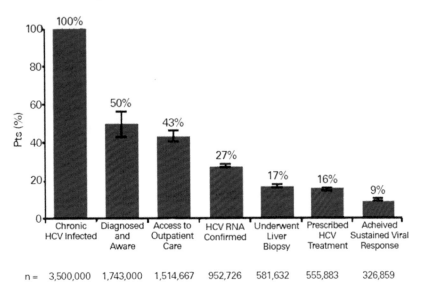

Fig. 3. Gaps in current practice in regards to hepatitis C. Only ~43% of patients with HCV have access to outpatient care and 9% achieve SVR. (*From* Yehia BR, Schranz AJ, Umscheid CA, et al. The treatment cascade for chronic hepatitis C virus infection in the United States: a systematic review and meta-analysis. PLoS One 2014; 9:e101554; with permission.)

enzymes should consider the possibility of HBV reactivation.

Pathologists need to be aware of persistent histologic changes typically associated with active HCV despite the lack of detection of serum HCV RNA in patients who have achieved SVR. Sixty-five allograft liver biopsy specimens from patients who received a liver transplant for chronic HCV were evaluated in one study.[14] Even after treatment and documented SVR, 69% of the liver biopsy specimens had features of active HCV infection. Further polymerase chain reaction testing of the liver tissue itself revealed that in 31 of 32 specimens analyzed there were undetectable HCV RNA levels after SVR. Pathologists should be aware of the patient's SVR status as they conduct histologic examinations and be cognizant to the extremely small, but reported cases of HCV recurrence despite serologic confirmation of undetectable HCV RNA. Clinicians should continue to monitor patients after achieving SVR, and obtain HCV RNA testing in those patients with recurrent elevated liver function tests.

HISTOLOGIC EXAMINATION FOR HEPATITIS C VIRUS

Historically, patients diagnosed with chronic HCV underwent a liver biopsy to evaluate for inflammatory activity and stage of fibrosis, because these

were used to guide therapeutic decisions and initiation of surveillance for HCC and esophageal varices. Despite the great utility of histologic examination of the liver sampling error remains an important limitation. In addition, the risks of complications, such as hemorrhage, pain, and misdirected sampling of the gallbladder, kidney, lung, or bowels, promoted interest in noninvasive alternatives to liver biopsy. From a practical standpoint, the perception of the liver biopsy as being a high-risk procedure, coupled with its low reimbursement, has stimulated the move of the procedure from the realm of gastroenterologists and hepatologists to the radiology suite. Furthermore, the perception of interpretation variability by pathologists contributed to the pursuit of serologic and radiologic alternatives.[15]

Alternatives to liver biopsy include use of routine laboratory studies, such as serum ALT, aspartate aminotransferase, and platelet count to calculate the APRI Score (ALT/aspartate aminotransferase divided by the platelet count) and the Fibrosis 4 Score and proprietary fibrosis blood tests.[16] However, serologic tests for fibrosis are limited in their ability to detect minimal or mild fibrosis. Nevertheless, their noninvasive nature and repeatability have lent to their increased use in clinical practice.

A more recent development has been transient elastography (TE), which is an ultrasound-based measurement of shear wave velocity through the liver correlated to liver stiffness, and thus fibrosis

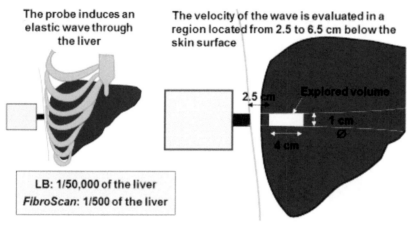

The probe induces an elastic wave through the liver

The velocity of the wave is evaluated in a region located from 2.5 to 6.5 cm below the skin surface

2.5 cm

Explored volume

1 cm Ø

4 cm

LB: 1/50,000 of the liver
FibroScan: 1/500 of the liver

Fig. 4. Transient elastography.

(Fig. 4). Higher stiffness of the liver has been correlated with worsening fibrosis on histologic examination.[17] Practical considerations limiting the use of TE include factors that inhibit correct placement of the TE probe, such as obesity, ascites, tight intercostal spaces, and a nonfasting state. Its main limitation, however, is that it does not directly assess the degree of ongoing HCV associated neuroinflammatory activity or allow detection of a superimposed pathologic state as possible by liver biopsy. False-positive results can be caused by factors that worsen liver stiffness, including acute hepatitis, hepatic congestion from congestive heart failure or outflow obstruction, or alcoholic steatohepatitis. An important advantage of TE is that it samples a larger volume of the liver at 1/500 compared with 1/50,000 for liver biopsy. In addition, it is safer and less expensive than a liver biopsy, which facilitates serial examinations. It is important to recognize that each chronic disease state (eg, HBV, alcoholic liver disease, HCV) differs in cutoffs for fibrosis levels,[18] and in those with superimposed hepatic insults (eg, HCV and alcoholic steatohepatitis, HCV and NASH, or HCV and HBV infection) accurate evaluation by TE may not be possible. Because these are the patients who often require periodic assessment liver biopsy remains an important diagnostic tool. Magnetic resonance elastography is available, but is currently not widely used for assessment of HCV-associated fibrosis given the high cost and limited availability.

Liver biopsy in patients with HCV remains the primary modality to evaluate for concomitant diseases, such as NASH and autoimmune hepatitis, and to assess the degree of ongoing neuroinflammatory activity. It has particular use in the post–liver transplant setting where there are multiple competing diagnostic considerations that might impact interpretation of other diagnostic tests. In addition, liver biopsy is widely available, whereas TE and magnetic resonance elastography still have limited availability. Thus, histologic examination of liver specimens from patients with HCV remains pertinent and the skills of pathologists for expert interpretation remain in demand. **Table 2** shows a generalized comparison between the three diagnostic modalities.

HISTOLOGIC FINDINGS IN ACUTE HEPATITIS C VIRUS HEPATITIS

Patients with acute HCV hepatitis are not routinely biopsied because they are often asymptomatic and do not present for clinical attention (**Table 3**). Pathologists may encounter such a biopsy in situations where acute HCV is not suspected and unrecognized because HCV antibody testing is negative (too early for antibody development) and the HCV polymerase chain reaction has not been obtained. The histologic features of acute hepatitis C are similar to that seen in other acute viral hepatitis, with lobular changes predominating over that of portal inflammation seen prominently in chronic hepatitis. The lobular necroinflammatory changes include clusters of swollen, pale hepatocytes; inflammatory cell foci usually of lymphocytes and macrophages in areas of hepatocyte dropout; and scattered acidophil bodies. Acidophil bodies are apoptotic hepatocytes that display deeply eosinophilic cytoplasm and, if present, hyperchromatic and shrunken nuclei. Finally, cholestatic changes have been described in the setting of acute HCV infection, with bile ductular reaction, minimal macrovesicular steatosis, and cholestasis.[19]

HISTOLOGIC FINDINGS IN CHRONIC HEPATITIS C VIRUS HEPATITIS

In contrast to acute HCV hepatitis, chronic HCV hepatitis has predominantly portal inflammation with dense lymphoid aggregates.[20,21] Mild

Table 2
Comparison of liver biopsy and noninvasive markers of fibrosis

Factor	Liver Biopsy	Serum Markers	Elastography
Cost	~$2000	Laboratory cost	Machine investment $130,000; staff time
Risks	Present	Minimal, phlebotomy	None
Contraindications	Multiple: bleeding diathesis, obesity, ascites, extrahepatic biliary obstruction	Conditions with high rate of false positivity	Patient needs to be able to lay still, ascites, volume overload, obesity
Accuracy	80%	60%–80%	60%–95%
System requirements	Operator, pathology laboratory, pathologist	Clinical laboratory, phlebotomy, materials	Machine, staff, time
Specimen adequacy	16-gauge needle; length of liver fragment at least 15 mm with >12 portal tracts	Blood sample	Staff time
False positives	Interobserver variability	Sepsis, nonhepatic inflammation, hemolysis, thrombocytopenia	Obesity, narrow ribs, ascites, heart failure, volume overload
False negatives	Interobserver variability	Varies per test	Various
Time for results	24–72 h minimum	1–2 h minimum laboratory, 1–2 wk for results	15–45 min

interface hepatitis, characterized by lymphocytes spilling over from portal tracts into the lobules past the limiting plate, is common. Bile duct damage can also be seen.[20] Severe necroinflammatory activity is not usual in hepatitis C and should prompt consideration for the presence of another concomitant condition, such as autoimmune hepatitis. Lobular features include scattered foci of lymphocytes and acidophil bodies. Mild macrovesicular steatosis may be present, especially in HCV genotype 3 infection.[22,23] Nonnecrotizing lobular granulomas are only rarely seen in the context of hepatitis C.[24,25]

Fibrosis involving portal tracts and extending into the lobules is best assessed on connective tissue stains, such as the Masson trichrome. Fibrous septa eventually connect portal tract to portal tract and portal tract to central vein. Cirrhosis is predominantly macronodular. There is potential for regression of liver fibrosis in patients who have achieved SVR (**Figs. 5–7**). Histologic evidence for this in previously cirrhotic patients includes the

Table 3
Pathologic features of hepatitis C

	Acute	Chronic
Portal inflammation	+/−	++
Lobular changes	+++	+
Cholestasis	+/−	−
Acidophil bodies	+	+
Notes	• Looks like acute hepatitis of other causes (not specific to HCV) • Lobular disarray, inflammatory foci, hepatocyte dropout • No portal fibrosis	• Dense portal mononuclear inflammatory infiltrates with mild interface activity • Scattered lobular inflammation and acidophil bodies • Can have portal fibrosis

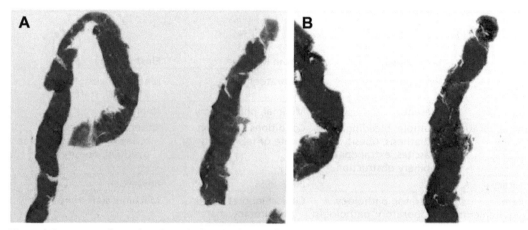

Fig. 5. (*A*) Hematoxylin and eosin stain (original magnification ×20) for a liver biopsy in a patient with chronic HCV before treatment. This biopsy shows prominent portal-based lymphoid aggregates typical of chronic hepatitis. (*B*) Masson trichrome stain (original magnification ×20) of the same case shows established cirrhosis.

presence of thin incomplete fibrous septa with vague parenchymal nodularity, abnormal approximation of portal tracts to central veins, abnormal portal tracts missing veins, and hepatic veins with prolapsed hepatocytes.[26] In one study of 97 patients who achieved SVR, liver fibrosis regressed in 45%, remained stable in 48%, and progressed in 6%, after an average 5.8 years following treatment.[27] Of note, 12% of the studied cohort had HCC, with a higher rate in those with progressive fibrosis compared with those with regressed or stable fibrosis. The cumulative incidence of HCC in this SVR cohort was 4.1%, 14.0%, and 20.3% at 5, 10, and 15 years, respectively.

Another study of 96 patients with treated HCV cirrhosis and more than 10 years follow-up reported regression of fibrosis in 19% of the study population (METAVIR stage 0, 1, or 2, reduced from a baseline of METAVIR stage 4).[28] Again, SVR did not prevent the development of HCC in 9% of their study group, but was more likely to occur in those with cirrhosis. One patient continued to have persistent viremia, but had regression of fibrosis and long-term absence of liver disease complications, suggesting that

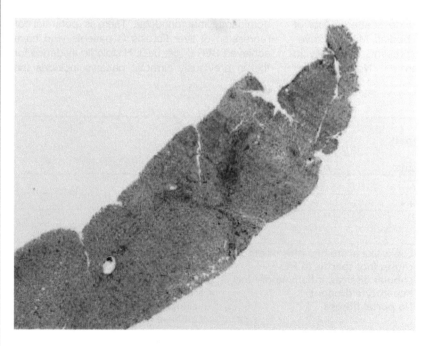

Fig. 6. Hematoxylin and eosin stain (original magnification ×XXX) of a biopsy from the same patient as that seen in **Fig. 5**, 1 year post-treatment and with sustained viral response. The biopsy continues to show prominent lymphoid aggregates, which to a pathologist unaware of treatment status, may be erroneously diagnosed as ongoing chronic hepatitis.

Fig. 7. Masson trichrome stain (original magnification ×XXX) in the same patient as that seen in **Figs. 5** and **6**, 2 years post-treatment and SVR. In contrast to the cirrhotic findings in **Fig. 5**, this biopsy shows regression of fibrosis, with thin, perforated fibrous septa.

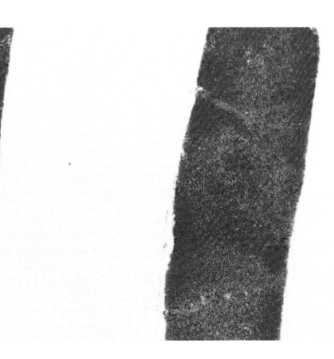

control of hepatic necroinflammatory activity is more important to fibrosis regression than complete viral clearance. Fibrosis regression was found to be a common result in a prospective study of cirrhotic HCV patients successfully treated with PEGylated interferon and ribavirin.[29] In this study, patients underwent pretreatment and post-treatment liver biopsies that were examined using digital morphometric and immunohistochemical methods. Sixty-one percent of their 38 patients achieved a decrease of at least one METAVIR staging score point in the post-treatment liver biopsy. However, comparable data for DAAs with large sample sizes and long-term follow-up are not yet available.

In regards to DAAs and HCC, there were several initially reported studies with small numbers of patients that suggested that treatment might actually increase the risk of HCC.[30–32] However, follow-up larger studies including one with more than 22,000 DAA-treated patients showed that the incidence of HCC in patients who achieved SVR was considerably lower than those who did not achieve SVR, with a 76% reduction in risk for cancer by DAA treatment.[33] Therefore, emphasis should be placed on treating patients with HCV before progression to cirrhosis, because risk of HCC in DAA-induced SVR patients was found to be 4.7-fold higher in patients with cirrhosis than those without cirrhosis. Furthermore, despite SVR with DAAs, the absolute risk of HCC persists; there is an annual incidence of 0.90%. This underscores the importance of ongoing HCC surveillance for patients with cirrhosis.

SUMMARY

HCV infection is the most common reason for liver transplantation in the United States. Only a few decades after its discovery, curing HCV has become a reality with DAAs, which have an impressive efficacy for eliciting viral clearance. Pathologists may face two challenges: properly diagnosing chronic HCV hepatitis in light of the disparity between viral clearance and histologic activity, and determining fibrosis regression. Nevertheless, the risk for HCC is not completely eradicated even with the use of DAA. It is hoped that the burden for donor liver transplants, however, will be reduced with the efficacy of DAA in curbing end-stage liver disease.

REFERENCES

1. Denniston MM, Jiles RB, Drobeniuc J, et al. Chronic hepatitis C virus infection in the United States, National Health and Nutrition Examination Survey 2003 to 2010. Ann Intern Med 2014;160(5):293–300.
2. OPTN/SRTR 2015 annual data report: introduction. Am J Transplant 2017;17(Suppl 1):11–20.
3. Yehia BR, Schranz AJ, Umscheid CA, et al. The treatment cascade for chronic hepatitis C virus infection in the United States: a systematic review and meta-analysis. PLoS One 2014;9:e101554.
4. Ly KN, Xing J, Klevens RM, et al. The increasing burden of mortality from viral hepatitis in the United

States between 1999 and 2007. Ann Intern Med 2012;156(4):271–8.

5. Feld JJ, Liang TJ. Hepatitis C: identifying patients with progressive liver injury. Hepatology 2006; 43(S1):S194–206.

6. National Institutes of Health Consensus Development Conference Statement: management of hepatitis C 2002 (June 10-12, 2002). Gastroenterology 2002;123(6):2082–99.

7. Serfaty L, Aumaitre H, Chazouilleres O, et al. Determinants of outcome of compensated hepatitis C virus-related cirrhosis. Hepatology 1998;27: 1435–40.

8. Fattovich G, Giustina G, Degos F, et al. Morbidity and mortality in compensated cirrhosis type C: a retrospective follow-up study of 384 patients. Gastroenterology 1997;112:463–72.

9. Jacobson IM, Davis GL, El-Serag H, et al. et al. Prevalence and challenges of liver diseases in patients with chronic hepatitis C virus infection. Clin Gastroenterol Hepatol 2010;8:924–33.

10. Available at: https://www.cdc.gov/hepatitis/hcv/ guidelinesc.htm. Accessed September 26, 2017.

11. AASLD/IDSA HCV Guidance Panel. Hepatitis C guidance: AASLD-IDSA recommendations for testing, managing, and treating adults infected with hepatitis C virus. Hepatology 2015;62(3):932–54.

12. McGovern B, Abu Dayyeh B, Chung RT. Avoiding therapeutic pitfalls: the rational use of specifically targeted agents against hepatitis C infection. Hepatology 2008;48:1700–12.

13. Collins JM, Raphael KL, Terry C, et al. Hepatitis B virus reactivation during successful treatment of hepatitis C virus with sofosbuvir and simeprevir. Clin Infect Dis 2015;61:1304–6.

14. Whitcomb E, Choi WT, Jerome KR, et al. Biopsy specimens from allograft liver contain histologic features of hepatitis C virus infection after virus eradication. Clin Gasteroenterol Hepatol 2017; 15:1279–85.

15. Czaja AJ, Carpenter HA. Optimizing diagnosis from the medical liver biopsy. Clin Gasteroenterol Hepatol 2007;5:898–907.

16. Chou R, Wasson N. Blood tests to diagnose fibrosis or cirrhosis in patients with chronic hepatitis C virus infection: a systematic review. Ann Intern Med 2013; 158:807–20.

17. Tapper EB, Castera L, Afdhal NH. FibroScan (vibration-controlled transient elastography): where does it stand in the United States practice. Clin Gasteroenterol Hepatol 2015;13:27–36.

18. Afdhal NH, Bonder A. Biopsy no more; changing the screening and diagnostic algorithm for hepatitis C. Clin Gasteroenterol Hepatol 2013;11: 309–10.

19. Johnson K, Kotiesh A, Boitnott JK, et al. Histology of symptomatic acute hepatitis C infection in immunocompetent adults. Am J Surg Pathol 2007; 31(11):1754–8.

20. Bach N, Thung SN, Schaffner F. The histological features of chronic hepatitis C and autoimmune chronic hepatitis: a comparative analysis. Hepatology 1992; 15(4):572–7.

21. Lefkowitch JH, Schiff ER, Davis GL, et al. Pathological diagnosis of chronic hepatitis C: a multicenter comparative study with chronic hepatitis B. The Hepatitis Interventional Therapy Group. Gastroenterology 1993;104(2):595–603.

22. Gordon A, McLean CA, Pedersen JS, et al. Hepatic steatosis in chronic hepatitis B and C: predictors, distribution and effect on fibrosis. J Hep 2005;43(1):38–44.

23. Mihm S, Fayyazi A, Hartmann H, et al. Analysis of histopathological manifestations of chronic hepatitis C virus infection with respect to virus genotype. Hepatology 1997;25(3):735–9.

24. Emile JF, Sebagh M, Fe ray C, et al. The presence of epithelioid granulomas in hepatitis C virus-related cirrhosis. Hum Pathol 1993;24(10):1095–7.

25. Ozaras R, Tahan V, Mert A, et al. The prevalence of hepatic granulomas in chronic hepatitis C. J Clin Gastroenterol 2004;38(5):449–52.

26. Wanless IR, Nakashima E, Sherman M. Regression of human cirrhosis. Morphologic features and the genesis of incomplete septal cirrhosis. Arch Pathol Lab Med 2000;124(11):1599–607.

27. Tachi Y, Hirai T, Miyata A, et al. Progressive fibrosis significantly correlates with hepatocellular carcinoma in patients with a sustained virological response. Hepatol Res 2015;45:238–46.

28. Mallet V, Gilgenkrantz H, Serpaggi J, et al. Brief communication: the relationship of regression of cirrhosis to outcome in chronic hepatitis C. Ann Intern Med 2008;149(6):399–403.

29. D'Ambrosio R, Aghemo A, Rumi MG, et al. A morphometric and immunohistochemical study to assess the benefit of a sustained virological response in hepatitis C virus patients with cirrhosis. Hepatology 2012;56(2):532–43.

30. Reig M, Marino Z, Perello C, et al. Unexpected high rate of early tumor recurrence in patients with HCV-related HCC undergoing interferon-free therapy. J Hepatol 2016;65:719–26.

31. Conti F, Buonfiglioli F, Scuteri A, et al. Early occurrence and recurrence of hepatocellular carcinoma in HCV related cirrhosis treated with direct-acting antivirals. J Hepatol 2016;65:727–33.

32. Ravi S, Axley P, Jones D, et al. Unusually high rates of hepatocellular carcinoma after treatment with direct-acting antiviral therapy for hepatitis C related cirrhosis. Gastroenterology 2017;152:911–2.

33. Kanwal F, Kramer J, Asch SM, et al. Risk of hepatocellular cancer in HCV patients treated with direct acting antiviral agents. Gastroenterology 2017;153: 996–1005.

Recent Advances in the Histopathology of Drug-Induced Liver Injury

David E. Kleiner, MD, PhD

KEYWORDS

- Hepatotoxicity • Acute hepatitis • Autoimmune hepatitis • Hepatic necrosis • Cholestasis

Key points

- Liver biopsy provides clinically useful information on differential diagnosis and character of injury in drug-induced liver injury (DILI).
- The pattern of injury on biopsy relates to the etiologic differential diagnosis, including both drug and nondrug causes.
- Recent reports of DILI show several themes, including injury from herbals and dietary supplements and from traditional pharmaceuticals.
- A variety of immunomodulatory agents have been associated with DILI in recent years, most associated with an autoimmune hepatitis-like injury.

ABSTRACT

Drug-induced liver injury (DILI) is constantly changing as new drugs are approved and as new herbals and dietary supplements (HDS) reach the market. The pathologist plays a key role in the evaluation of DILI by classifying and interpreting the histologic findings considering patients' medical history and drug exposure. The liver biopsy findings may suggest alternative explanations of the injury and additional testing that should be performed to exclude non-DILI causes. Recent reports of iatrogenic liver injury are reviewed with attention to immunomodulatory and antineoplastic agents as well as reports of injury associated with HDS use.

Abbreviations

AIH	Autoimmune hepatitis
CTLA-4	Cytotoxic T-lymphocyte antigen-4
CVID	Common variable immunodeficiency
DIAIH	Drug-induced autoimmune hepatitis
DILI	Drug-induced liver injury
DILIN	Drug-Induced Liver Injury Network
HDS	Herbal and dietary supplements
LDO	Large duct obstruction
PBC	Primary biliary cholangitis
PFIC	Progressive familial intrahepatic cholestasis
TNF	Tumor necrosis factor
VBDS	Vanishing bile duct syndrome

OVERVIEW

Drug-induced liver injury (DILI) is one of the more challenging areas in liver pathology. The complexity

Conflict of Interest Declaration: The author reports no conflicts of interest.

Financial Support: This review was supported by the Intramural Research Program of the NIH, National Cancer Institute.

Laboratory of Pathology, National Cancer Institute, 10 Center Drive, Building 10, Room 2S235, MSC1500, Bethesda, MD 20892, USA

E-mail address: kleinerd@mail.nih.gov

Surgical Pathology 11 (2018) 297–311
https://doi.org/10.1016/j.path.2018.02.009
1875-9181/18/Published by Elsevier Inc.

of the challenge derives from multiple sources. There are more than 350 separate drugs that have been associated with some risk of liver injury in the publicly available reference Web site LiverTox (livertox.nlm.nih.gov).[1] Each drug may have one or more characteristic clinical presentations and patterns of injury. In well more than half of these drugs, the type of injury (clinical and/or histologic) has only been the subject of case reports or small series, so the worldwide published experience is very limited. Overall, the incidence of DILI is low, with population-based incidence rates that vary from 8.1 per 100,000 over a 3-year period in France[2] to 19.1 per 100,000 over a 2-year period in Iceland.[3] The incidence of DILI due to any individual drug is difficult to estimate but is certainly much lower. Liver biopsies are not performed on all cases of DILI. In the US Drug Induced Liver Injury Network (DILIN), biopsies were performed in only about 50% of cases and were available for central review in only about 33%.[4] In a similar clinical network established across Spain to register cases of DILI, biopsy results were only available in about 25% of cases.[5] Thus, the potential biopsy material available for review to any one pathologist will be limited, even at busy academic medical centers. The challenge is compounded by comorbidities that affect the liver and by polypharmacy. Pathologists, as the expert interpreters of tissue findings, must strive to discern the diagnostic possibilities and to offer alternative, non-DILI possibilities for the injury. This review covers both the basic evaluation of the liver biopsy in cases of suspected DILI as well as some of the recent published information on DILI histology.

EVALUATION OF THE LIVER BIOPSY

Because a liver biopsy is not a required part of the workup for a case of suspected DILI, the clinician submitting the biopsy will likely have questions about the cause of the liver injury. They may be looking for the pathologist to confirm their clinical suspicion of DILI when most of the other possibilities have been excluded or DILI may be only one of several possible etiologic considerations. In some cases, the drug may be providing a clear therapeutic benefit and the clinician may be looking for guidance as to whether the drug may be safely continued, as in the case of methotrexate. Finally, DILI might not be suspected at all but might be suggested by the pathologist.

Fig. 1 diagrams an approach to the liver biopsy in cases of suspected DILI.[6] It is best to start with an unbiased evaluation of the liver pathology to determine a pattern of injury. The liver, like other organs, shows stereotyped responses to injury that can be

organized into particular patterns related to differential diagnosis. Hans Popper and colleagues[7] were the first to categorize DILI in this fashion, dividing cases into 6 histologic patterns of injury: zonal necrosis, hepatitis with or without cholestasis, acute hepatitislike with or without massive necrosis, simple cholestasis, reactive hepatitis, and steatosis. The US DILIN used a larger classification of 18 categories in its blinded review of cases of suspected DILI. Table 1 organizes the patterns of injury into those that have been most commonly observed in studies of acute DILI and those that are less common. In this DILIN study, necro-inflammatory and cholestatic patterns accounted for 86% of the cases,[8] whereas all but one of the cases in Popper and colleagues' study[7] and 95% of the cases in Andrade and colleagues' study[5] could be placed into one of these 7 patterns. The steatotic patterns are relatively rare. Macrovesicular steatosis and steatohepatitis present with modest elevations of aminotransferases and normal bilirubin and so fail to meet the protocol entry requirements,[9] whereas drug-induced microvesicular steatosis is restricted to a limited list of agents that primarily injure mitochondria.[10] The vascular injury patterns are also uncommon in the large cohort studies, which may also relate to case selection bias and a limited number of implicated agents.[11] The patterns of glycogenosis,[12,13] ground-glass cell change,[14] and inclusions[15,16] may sometimes be associated with sufficient laboratory abnormalities to result in a biopsy but are uncommon in the cohort studies.

Once the biopsy has been evaluated for the pattern of injury, and the severity of the lesions has been assessed, the pathologist should establish the non-DILI histologic differential diagnosis (see Table 1). This process can be analyzed with respect to the clinical history and laboratory and imaging findings. The emphasis should be placed on identifying a non-DILI explanation for the injury, as DILI should always be a diagnosis of exclusion. Depending on the clinical evaluation before liver biopsy, additional testing may be suggested by the histologic injury pattern. Checklists of information recommended for publication of DILI cases can be used to identify potentially useful tests.[17] If DILI cannot be excluded, the possibility that DILI caused the injury can be entertained. The patients' list of medications can be evaluated for suspects based on several factors, including the temporal exposure to the medication and the likelihood of the medication to cause the pattern of injury observed. Drugs tend to be associated with some injury patterns more than others. For example, minocycline is usually associated with noncholestatic hepatitis patterns, occasionally with cholestatic hepatitis and not associated with zonal necrosis or acute cholestasis.[8,18]

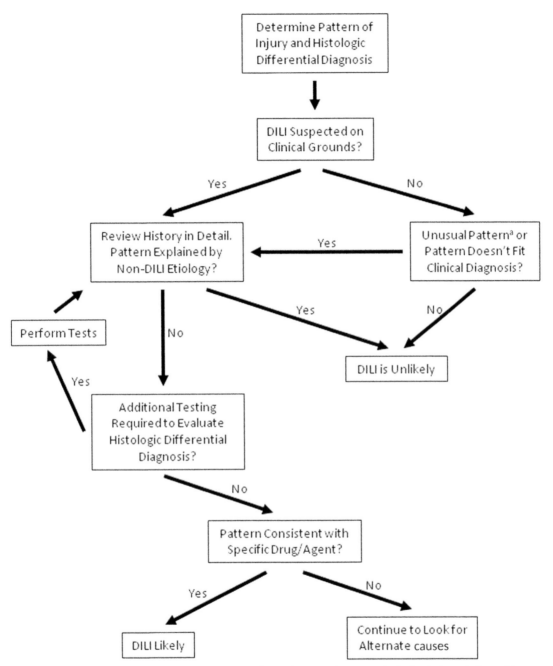

Fig. 1. Algorithm for biopsy evaluation in suspected DILI. [a] Unusual patterns include cholestatic hepatitis, combination patterns (eg, cholestasis with steatohepatitis), and patterns with eosinophils, granulomas and necrosis. (*From* Kleiner DE. Liver histology in the diagnosis and prognosis of drug-induced liver injury. Clin Liver Dis 2014;4(1):12–16.)

RECENT REPORTS OF HISTOLOGIC INJURY PATTERNS IN DRUG-INDUCED LIVER INJURY

The primary literature remains a major reference point for pathologists for information on patterns of liver injury that may be associated with particular agents. However, most of the literature is fragmented, with the primary data scattered across the breadth of the medical literature in the form of case reports and small series. Only a portion of the literature describes the results of liver biopsies, and fewer still show photomicrographs of the

Table 1
Common and uncommon patterns of injury in drug-induced liver injury

Pattern	Characteristic Features	Caveats	Non-DILI Causes Common	Non-DILI Causes Uncommon
Common Patterns				
Zonal coagulative necrosis	Zone 3 or 1 coagulative necrosis, usually without significant inflammation	Steatosis may be seen in the non-necrotic parenchyma; should examine veins for changes of venoocclusive disease	Hypoxic-ischemic injury	
Submassive to massive necrosis	Extensive panacinar necrosis, variable inflammation	Often a consequence of severe acute hepatitis	Fulminant viral or autoimmune hepatitis	Herpetic or adenoviral hepatitis
Acute (lobular) hepatitis	Lobular-dominant inflammation with/without confluent or bridging necrosis; no cholestasis	Mild presentations overlap with nonspecific reactive hepatitis	Acute viral or autoimmune hepatitis	Graft-vs-host disease
Chronic (portal) hepatitis	Portal-dominant inflammation, interface hepatitis (also includes mononucleosis pattern), with or without portal-based fibrosis; no cholestasis	Mild presentations overlap with nonspecific reactive hepatitis	Chronic viral or autoimmune hepatitis	Early PBC, EBV hepatitis, CVID, hepatitis A
Cholestatic hepatitis	Acute or chronic hepatitis pattern plus zone 3 cholestasis	Often an inverse relationship between the severity of inflammation and severity of cholestasis	Acute viral hepatitis (acute form), acute LDO	Graft-vs-host disease, PFIC
Acute cholestasis (intrahepatic, canalicular)	Hepatocellular and/or canalicular cholestasis in zone 3; may show duct injury, but little inflammation	May be completely normal hepatocytes or may be ballooned in areas of cholestasis	Sepsis, acute LDO, postsurgical cholestasis,	Benign recurrent intrahepatic cholestasis
Chronic cholestasis	Periportal cholate stasis, periportal fibrosis, copper accumulation, duct sclerosis or injury, duct loss	Zone 3 cholestasis may also be seen	PBC, sclerosing cholangitis, chronic LDO	Ischemic cholangitis, idiopathic ductopenia, PFIC

Uncommon Patterns

Pattern	Description	Comment		
Granulomatous hepatitis	Inflammation dominated by granulomas (usually non-necrotizing), portal or lobular	Granulomas are usually nonfibrogenic and may be mixed with lymphocytes or eosinophils	Sarcoidosis, PBC, fungal or mycobacterial infection	Atypical bacterial or rickettsial infection
Steatosis, microvesicular	Predominantly microvesicular steatosis, inflammation variable	May see small groups of hepatocytes with microvesicular steatosis in the context of other injury patterns		Cholesterol ester storage disease and variants, alcoholic foamy degeneration, fatty liver of pregnancy
Steatosis, macrovesicular	Predominantly macrovesicular steatosis without significant portal or lobular inflammation, no cholestasis	Vacuoles may be variably sized but cells should not have a foamy appearance	Obesity, diabetes, alcohol	Lipodystrophy
Steatohepatitis	Zone 3 ballooning injury, sinusoidal fibrosis, Mallory bodies, variable inflammation and steatosis, no cholestasis	Ballooning should not be the cell swelling sometime seen with cholestasis	Obesity, diabetes, alcohol	Lipodystrophy
Sinusoidal obstruction syndrome/venoocclusive disease	Occlusion or loss of central veins, thrombosis, with or without central hemorrhage and necrosis	Masson trichrome stains useful to identify occluded central veins		Environmental toxins
Hepato-portal sclerosis	Disappearance of portal veins	Often a subtle finding unless there are clear occlusive changes in the portal veins		Environmental toxins
Nodular regenerative hyperplasia	Diffuse nodular transformation, with or without mild inflammation and sinusoidal fibrosis	Should always be in the differential when minimal changes are apparent on the routine stain	Collagen vascular diseases, CVID, lymphoproliferative diseases	
Sinusoidal dilation/peliosis	Sinusoidal alterations with/without mild lobular inflammation, sinusoidal fibrosis	Sinusoidal dilation may be associated with atrophic hepatocyte plates	Central venous hypertension	

(continued on next page)

Table 1
(continued)

Pattern	Characteristic Features	Caveats	Non-DILI Causes	
			Common	Uncommon
Glycogenosis	Diffuse hepatocyte swelling with very pale bluish-gray cytoplasm		Type 1 diabetes	
Ground-glass change	Diffuse homogenization of cell cytoplasm due to induction of smooth endoplasmic reticulum			
Hepatocellular inclusions (poly-glucosan like bodies)	Discrete cytoplasmic inclusions that stain variably with periodic-acid Schiff			

Abbreviations: CVID, common variable immunodeficiency; EBV, Epstein-Barr virus; LDO, large duct obstruction; PBC, primary biliary cholangitis; PFIC, progressive familial intrahepatic cholestasis.

findings. **Table 2** summarizes such reports published since 2015 in the English literature along with the patterns of injury extracted from the articles using the written descriptions and photomicrographs according to the classification presented in **Table 1**.

HERBALS AND DIETARY SUPPLEMENTS

Although a large number of different agents are reported, several themes emerge. First, while most of the reports concern prescription-based pharmaceuticals, the second largest category are herbals and dietary supplements (HDSs). HDSs encompass a broad category of agents that includes vitamin and mineral supplements, fish oils, plant extracts, ethnic traditional medicines and proprietary commercial products. In the United States, HDSs are consumed by half or more of the US population[19]; the US Food and Drug Administration may only require limited safety testing of new products before marketing.[20] Like more conventional medications, there have been numerous case reports and small series implicating HDSs with liver injury. In a study drawn from the US DILIN cohort, Navarro and colleagues[21] identified 136 cases (15%) out of 839 patients who had liver injury due to HDSs. They divided this group into those with injury due to HDS marketed for bodybuilding (45 cases), HDSs marketed for other purposes (85 cases), and patients who were taking both types of HDSs at the time of the injury (6 cases). In comparing the bodybuilding HDS cases with the nonbodybuilding HDSs cases and DILI due to conventional medications, there was no difference in the rate of hospitalization; but the cases of injury due to nonbodybuilding HDSs were much more likely to develop evidence of acute liver failure or undergo liver transplantation than either of the other two groups. The types of nonbodybuilding HDSs implicated in cases that led to death or transplantation spanned the full variety of these agents, from weight-loss and energy-boosting supplements to Asian herbal remedies to multivitamins. Several recent studies have focused on acute hepatitis and liver failure associated with proprietary mixtures of HDSs, such as Herbalife[22,23] and OxyELITE Pro.[24,25] It is often difficult or impossible to identify the component of the mixture that might be the causal agent or if 2 or more of the components are interacting to cause injury. Acute hepatitis and cholestatic hepatitis are the patterns of injury most frequently associated with these compounds (**Fig. 2**A).

On the other hand, although bodybuilding HDSs were associated with a high rate of hospitalizations

Table 2
Case reports and small series reporting iatrogenic hepatic injury findings, 2015 to 2017

Author, Year	Implicated Agent	Histologic Patterns[a]
Pharmaceutical Agents		
Slim et al,[57] 2015	Acetaminophen	Cholestatic hepatitis
Eder et al,[58] 2015	Agomelatine	Chronic hepatitis
Taylor et al,[59] 2016	Anakinra	Acute hepatitis
Kumar[60] 2015	Artemisinin	Cholestatic hepatitis
Carrascosa et al,[61] 2015	Atorvastatin	Chronic hepatitis
Yun et al,[62] 2016	Bicalutamide	Cholestatic hepatitis
Chintamaneni et al,[63] 2016	Bupivacaine	Cholestatic hepatitis (2)
Kumagai et al,[64] 2016	Camostat mesilate and/or benzbromarone	Chronic hepatitis (AIH-like)
Pisapia et al,[65] 2015	Clopidogrel	Acute hepatitis with cholestasis
Bessone et al,[66] 2016	Cyproterone acetate	Submassive to massive necrosis (3), acute hepatitis with cholestasis (2), AIH-like chronic hepatitis (1), cirrhosis (1)
Miyashima et al,[67] 2016	Daclatasvir/asunaprevir	Acute on chronic hepatitis with eosinophilia
Bohm et al,[68] 2016	Febuxostat	Acute cholestasis
Harati et al,[69] 2016	Hydralazine	Acute hepatitis with zone 3 necrosis
Bjornsson et al,[38] 2015	Infliximab	Acute hepatitis (3), mild reactive hepatitis (1), acute cholestasis (1)
Parra et al,[39] 2015	Infliximab	Acute hepatitis with necrosis
Shelton et al,[41] 2015	Infliximab	AIH-like hepatitis (6)
Rodrigues et al,[40] 2015	Infliximab (7), adalimumab (1)	AIH-like chronic hepatitis (8)
Villamil et al,[70] 2015	Interferon beta 1a	AIH-like acute hepatitis
Kim et al,[71] 2016	Iodine-131	Acute hepatitis
Johncilla et al,[44] 2015	Ipilimumab	Acute hepatitis (9), acute cholangitis (1)
Jung et al,[72] 2016	Levocetirizine	Chronic hepatitis
Salvado et al,[73] 2015	Masitinib	AIH-like acute hepatitis
Stelzer et al,[74] 2015	Mesalazine	Granulomatous hepatitis
Davidov et al,[32] 2016	Methylprednisolone	Acute hepatitis with zone 3 necrosis
Grilli et al,[33] 2015	Methylprednisolone	Chronic hepatitis with incomplete cirrhosis
Oliveira et al,[34] 2015	Methylprednisolone	Hepatitis with zone 3 necrosis
Sakamura et al,[75] 2017	Multi-agent chemotherapy	Venoocclusive disease
Antezana et al,[46] 2015	Natalizumab	Acute hepatitis with zone 3 necrosis
Bernardes et al,[76] 2015	Nimesulide	Acute hepatitis with extensive necrosis
Kumar[77] 2015	Oral contraceptives	Sinusoidal dilation
Conrad et al,[78] 2016	Sertraline	Ductal paucity
Dyson et al,[79] 2016	Sofosbuvir	Cholestatic acute hepatitis (superimposed on underlying cirrhosis) (2)
Aygun et al,[51] 2016	Temozolomide	Cholestatic hepatitis

(continued on next page)

Table 2
(continued)

Author, Year	Implicated Agent	Histologic Patterns[a]
Balakrishnan et al,[52] 2016	Temozolomide	Cholestatic hepatitis with ductopenia
Grieco et al,[53] 2015	Temozolomide	Acute cholestasis
Herbals and Dietary Supplements		
Brazeau et al,[27] 2015	Anabolic steroid supplement	Sinusoidal dilation
Yokomori eta l,[80] 2016	Freshwater clam extract supplement	Acute cholestasis
Corey et al,[81] 2016	Garcinia cambogia	Acute hepatitis with massive necrosis
Jin et al,[82] 2015	Herbal medication (not specified)	Nodular regenerative hyperplasia
Rios et al,[22] 2016	Herbalife products	Hepatoportal sclerosis (2)
Alhaddad et al,[83] 2016	Khat	Cholestatic hepatitis (1), chronic hepatitis (1), possible confounding prior liver disease
Mahamoud et al,[84] 2016	Khat	Chronic hepatitis, bridging fibrosis
Gedela et al,[85] 2016	Kombucha tea	Chronic hepatitis
Hayashi et al,[86] 2016	Multiple dietary supplements	Acute hepatitis with zone 3 necrosis
Heidemann et al,[24] 2016	OxyELITE Pro	Massive necrosis (2), severe hepatitis with necrosis (1), cholestatic hepatitis (1)
Occupational and Recreational Agents		
Atayan et al,[87] 2015	Ecstasy	Zonal necrosis
Ito et al,[88] 2016	Organic solvents	Acute hepatitis

[a] Numbers in parentheses indicate case numbers when multiple cases are reported.

(71%), none of these patients died or required liver transplantation. Bodybuilding agents sometimes contain anabolic steroids, which have been associated with several patterns of injury, most commonly with acute cholestasis or cholestatic hepatitis[26] along with sinusoidal dilation[27] and peliosis hepatis[28] (**Fig. 2B**). They have also been associated with hepatocellular tumors, particularly hepatocellular adenomas.[29] The mechanism of cholestasis in these cases is poorly understood; but it is strongly associated with 17-alpha alkylation of the steroid backbone,[30] perhaps in individuals with bile salt transporter mutations.[31]

IMMUNOMODULATING AGENTS AND DRUG-INDUCED AUTOIMMUNE HEPATITIS

Among the pharmaceutical agents listed in **Table 2**, there are several agents that stand out. There are several drugs used to control the immune system, including methylprednisolone, the anti–tumor necrosis factor (TNF) agents infliximab and adalimumab, the anti–cytotoxic T-lymphocyte antigen-4 (CTLA-4) agent ipilimumab, and the anti-alpha 4 integrin antibody natalizumab. Methylprednisolone was the subject of 3 case reports,[32–34] 2 of which showed the same injury pattern: (acute) hepatitis with zonal necrosis. Corticosteroids have been associated with steatosis and may exacerbate underlying chronic hepatitis, but methylprednisolone in particular has been associated with an autoimmunelike hepatitis after several weeks of therapy.[35,36] The mechanism of this paradoxic injury is unknown.

The anti-TNF agents infliximab, adalimumab, and etanercept are all potent antiinflammatory drugs that are used to treat inflammatory bowel disease and various rheumatic conditions. Infliximab and adalimumab are monoclonal antibodies that bind to and block TNF alpha. Etanercept is a soluble form of the TNF alpha receptor that binds to TNF alpha circulating in the serum. All 3 of these agents have been associated with severe acute liver injury[37] and can cause reactivation of hepatitis B. Two newer members of the class, certolizumab and golimumab, have not yet been reported to cause serious liver injury, but may have the same potential as the other monoclonal

Fig. 2. Examples of HDS injury. (*A*) Acute hepatitis associated with a green tea–containing supplement. There is diffuse parenchymal injury with inflammation, hepatocyte swelling, and rosette formation (hematoxylin-eosin [H&E], original magnification ×100). (*B*) Acute cholestasis associated with anabolic steroids. Numerous bile plugs are present in canaliculi (H&E, original magnification ×600). (*Courtesy of* the US Drug-Induced Liver Injury Network Durham, NC.)

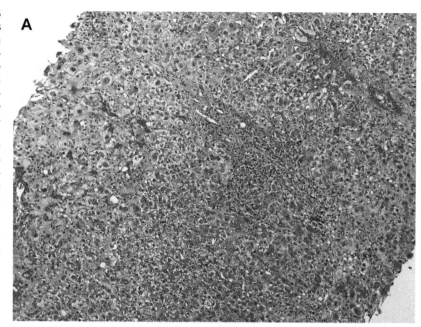

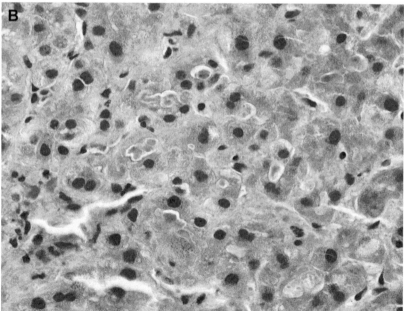

antibodies. Infliximab is the best studied, with most cases reported in the literature. Ghabril and colleagues[37] summarized the experience in the US DILIN with their report of 6 cases of anti-TNF DILI. In their summary of published cases, 26 were due to infliximab, whereas etanercept and adalimumab each accounted for 4 cases. The most common histologic pattern of infliximab DILI is acute or chronic hepatitis with features of autoimmune hepatitis (AIH) (**Fig. 3**). These patients frequently have elevated titers of antinuclear antibodies and sometime other serologic findings as well. Other patterns that have been observed in some cases include hepatocellular necrosis without an associated infiltrate and acute cholestasis.[37] Of the 20 cases of anti-TNF agents published in the last 2.5 years, 18 showed hepatitis, which was usually described as autoimmunelike, whereas there was only one case of acute cholestasis and one mild reactive hepatitis.[38–41]

Ipilimumab and tremelimumab are monoclonal antibody agents directed against CTLA-4. CTLA-4 is an immune checkpoint protein that inhibits the activation of cytotoxic T lymphocytes and results in

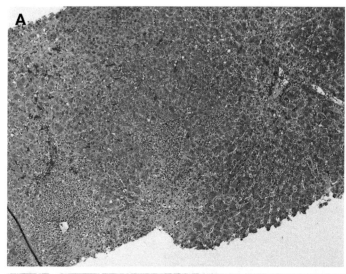

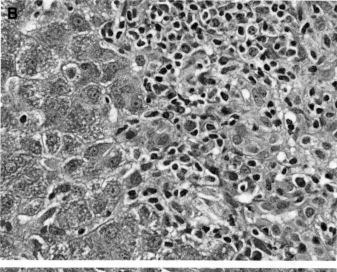

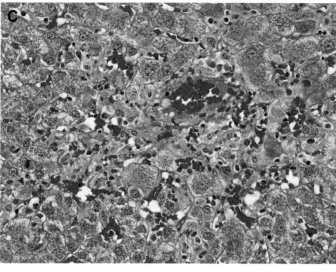

Fig. 3. Autoimmune hepatitis-like injury from infliximab. (*A*) Dense portal inflammation with zone 3 inflammation is evident from low power (hematoxylin-eosin [H&E], original magnification ×100). (*B*) Interface hepatitis with plasma cells (H&E, original magnification ×600). (*C*) Peri-venular inflammation with hepatocyte dropout (H&E, original magnification ×400). (*Courtesy of* the US Drug-Induced Liver Injury Network, Durham, NC.)

persistent activation of these immune cells. Ipilimumab in particular has been associated with a variety of autoimmunelike reactions with a minority of cases involving the liver.[42,43] The series reported by Johncilla and colleagues[44] described a panlobular hepatitis with central vein endothelialitis (Fig. 4). About half of the cases had a prominent plasma cell infiltrate. Of note, several patients also had received nivolumab, another type of immune-checkpoint inhibitor; combination therapy has been associated with an increased number of immune-related adverse events.[45] None of the patients in this series had serologic markers of AIH, in contrast to idiopathic AIH and the anti-TNF agents.

Natalizumab interferes with immune responses by blocking migration of lymphocytes to areas of inflammation. It is used in the treatment of multiple sclerosis and inflammatory bowel disease, and its use has been associated with an increased risk of central nervous system infection by polyomaviruses. Postmarketing surveillance has resulted in several reports of liver injury to regulatory agencies, but only a few case reports have been published.[46] In the case reported by Antezana and colleagues,[46] there was a lymphoplasmacytic infiltrate in the portal areas with interface hepatitis as well as hepatocyte dropout in zone 3. Serology was positive only for low titers of anti–smooth muscle antibody and anti–F-actin. The hepatitis resolved without corticosteroid treatment as documented by a follow-up liver biopsy. They summarized 11 cases from the literature, 7 of which had liver biopsies. All had autoimmunelike infiltrates, and 4 of the 7 also had positive serologies.

The cases of DILI described earlier raise the difficult issue of distinguishing idiopathic AIH from drug-induced AIH (DIAIH). Both conditions are diagnoses of exclusion and often require a liver biopsy for confirmation. The incidence of AIH is low, about 1.9 per 100,000,[47] in the range of the overall incidence of DILI. There are several drugs that have been associated with either clinical or histologic presentation mimicking AIH. These drugs include nitrofurantoin, minocycline, hydralazine, methyldopa, and the statins. In a large retrospective study, Bjornsson and colleagues[48] examined 261 patients with AIH and identified 24 (9%) cases of AIH that seemed to be medication related. In most of these cases, the implicated drug was nitrofurantoin or minocycline. There were few differences between the histology of the DIAIH cases and the rest of the AIH cases except that none of the DIAIH cases were cirrhotic. A study from the US DILIN cohort examined cases of nitrofurantoin, minocycline, hydralazine, and methyldopa because these are the drugs most commonly associated with DIAIH.[18] Although most of the minocycline and nitrofurantoin

cases presented with a serologic finding of AIH, only half of the hydralazine and methyldopa cases had positive serologies. Not all the cases had typical AIH pathology either; 29% of the cases showed cholestatic hepatitis. Hisamochi and colleagues[49] investigated a cohort of 16 DILI cases with AIH-like findings on biopsy and divided them into 2 groups based on whether they relapsed after an initial treatment period, a finding that was suggested by Bjornsson and colleagues'[48] study as a differentiation factor between idiopathic AIH and DIAIH. They identified no clinical or histologic differences between these two groups, but the sample size was small. Nevertheless, liver biopsy remains a useful tool, particularly in cases in which either the clinical presentation or the histologic findings do not fit with idiopathic AIH. Cholestasis in a suspected DIAIH case has been suggested as a finding in favor of a drug cause.[50]

TEMOZOLOMIDE AND VANISHING BILE DUCT SYNDROME

Three of the recent case reports concern temozolomide, an antineoplastic alkylating agent mainly used in the treatment of gliomas.[51–53] Temozolomide mainly causes cholestatic patterns of injury, spanning from acute cholestasis to cholestatic hepatitis to chronic cholestasis with ductopenia. Bile duct injury with a high incidence of significant bile duct loss characterizes most of the cases. In a study of 4 cases by Grant and colleagues,[54] 3 demonstrated at least mild ductopenia and the fourth showed bile duct injury. Because the drug is used to treat a highly lethal malignancy, it is difficult to understand the long-term hepatic implications of the duct loss; but at the very least, patients are deprived of a potentially effective medication if they recover from the hepatic injury. In general, vanishing bile duct syndrome (VBDS) is a diagnosis associated with a poor prognosis. In a recent series of 26 patients with VBDS due to DILI, 7 patients either underwent liver transplant or died in follow-up, despite treatment with corticosteroids and ursodiol.[55] Even if the liver survives, recovery is likely to be delayed. Patients with liver enzyme abnormalities persisting more than a year after onset are more likely to show chronic cholestatic changes with or without ductopenia than any other pattern of injury.[56]

THE PATHOLOGIST'S ROLE IN THE EVALUATION OF SUSPECTED DRUG-INDUCED LIVER INJURY

The first job of the pathologist is always the careful evaluation of histologic changes. When a liver

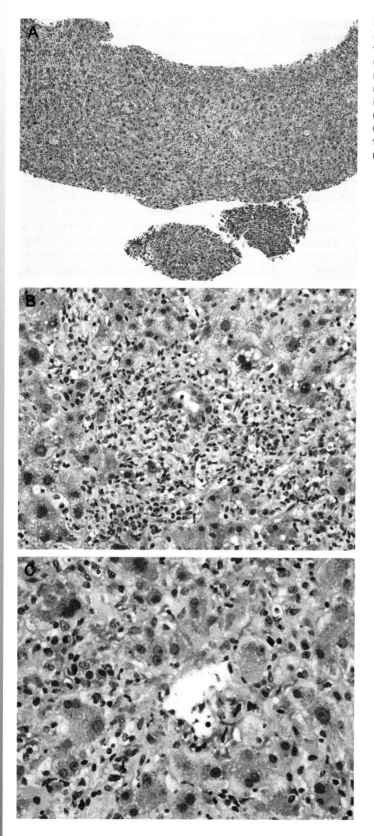

Fig. 4. Injury associated with ipilimumab. (*A*) Diffuse parenchyma and portal inflammation without necrosis (hematoxylin-eosin [H&E], original magnification ×100). (*B*) Portal inflammation with bile duct injury and increased numbers of eosinophils (H&E, original magnification ×400). (*C*) Peri-venular inflammation with focal endothelialitis (H&E, original magnification ×600).

biopsy is performed in a case of suspected DILI, determination of drug involvement becomes a collaborative effort between the pathologist and the patients' physician. With expert interpretation of histologic findings, the liver biopsy can identify alternate causes and raise or lower the likelihood of a particular drug injury based on reported patterns. As **Table 2** suggests, the histologic landscape of findings is constantly changing as new drugs are approved and cases are published. The histologic findings may influence clinical decision-making. Additional testing may be indicated. Both the histologic pattern of injury and the severity of injury (inflammation, necrosis, fibrosis, cholestasis, vascular) should be clearly communicated in the written report, and the pathologist may consider supplementing the interpretation as new clinical information is generated in the follow-up. Although DILI may be one of the more challenging areas of hepatic pathology, the potential clinical benefit of a carefully interpreted biopsy is incalculable and is well worth the extra time investment that the case may require.

REFERENCES

1. Bjornsson ES, Hoofnagle JH. Categorization of drugs implicated in causing liver injury: critical assessment based on published case reports. Hepatology 2016;63(2):590–603.
2. Sgro C, Clinard F, Ouazir K, et al. Incidence of drug-induced hepatic injuries: a French population-based study. Hepatology 2002;36(2):451–5.
3. Bjornsson ES, Bergmann OM, Bjornsson HK, et al. Incidence, presentation, and outcomes in patients with drug-induced liver injury in the general population of Iceland. Gastroenterology 2013;144(7): 1419–25, 1425.e1–3. [quiz: e19–20].
4. Chalasani N, Fontana RJ, Bonkovsky HL, et al. Causes, clinical features, and outcomes from a prospective study of drug-induced liver injury in the United States. Gastroenterology 2008;135(6): 1924–34, 1934.e1–4.
5. Andrade RJ, Lucena MI, Fernandez MC, et al. Drug-induced liver injury: an analysis of 461 incidences submitted to the Spanish registry over a 10-year period. Gastroenterology 2005;129(2):512–21.
6. Kleiner DE. Liver histology in the diagnosis and prognosis of drug-induced liver injury. Clin Liver Dis 2014;4(1):12–6.
7. Popper H, Rubin E, Cardiol D, et al. Drug-induced liver disease: a penalty for progress. Arch Intern Med 1965;115:128–36.
8. Kleiner DE, Chalasani NP, Lee WM, et al. Hepatic histological findings in suspected drug-induced liver injury: systematic evaluation and clinical associations. Hepatology 2014;59(2):661–70.
9. Chalasani N, Bonkovsky HL, Fontana R, et al. Features and outcomes of 899 patients with drug-induced liver injury: The DILIN prospective study. Gastroenterology 2015;148(7):1340–52.e7.
10. Begriche K, Massart J, Robin MA, et al. Drug-induced toxicity on mitochondria and lipid metabolism: mechanistic diversity and deleterious consequences for the liver. J Hepatol 2011;54(4):773–94.
11. Gitlin N. Drug-induced hepatic vascular abnormalities. Clin Liver Dis 1998;2:591–606.
12. Iancu TC, Shiloh H, Dembo L. Hepatomegaly following short-term high-dose steroid therapy. J Pediatr Gastroenterol Nutr 1986;5(1):41–6.
13. Torbenson M, Chen YY, Brunt E, et al. Glycogenic hepatopathy: an underrecognized hepatic complication of diabetes mellitus. Am J Surg Pathol 2006; 30(4):508–13.
14. Aiges HW, Daum F, Olson M, et al. The effects of phenobarbital and diphenylhydantoin on liver function and morphology. J Pediatr 1980;97(1):22–6.
15. Wisell J, Boitnott J, Haas M, et al. Glycogen pseudo-ground glass change in hepatocytes. Am J Surg Pathol 2006;30(9):1085–90.
16. Lefkowitch JH, Lobritto SJ, Brown RS Jr, et al. Ground-glass, polyglucosan-like hepatocellular inclusions: a "new" diagnostic entity. Gastroenterology 2006;131(3):713–8.
17. Fontana RJ, Seeff LB, Andrade RJ, et al. Standardization of nomenclature and causality assessment in drug-induced liver injury: summary of a clinical research workshop. Hepatology 2010;52(2):730–42.
18. de Boer YS, Kosinski AS, Urban TJ, et al. Features of autoimmune hepatitis in patients with drug-induced liver injury. Clin Gastroenterol Hepatol 2017;15(1): 103–12.e2.
19. Bailey RL, Gahche JJ, Lentino CV, et al. Dietary supplement use in the United States, 2003-2006. J Nutr 2011;141(2):261–6.
20. Dietary supplements Silver Spring, MD: U.S. Food and Drug Administration. 2017. Available at: https:// www.fda.gov/Food/DietarySupplements/default.htm. Accessed September 5, 2017.
21. Navarro VJ, Barnhart H, Bonkovsky HL, et al. Liver injury from herbals and dietary supplements in the U.S. Drug-Induced Liver Injury Network. Hepatology 2014;60(4):1399–408.
22. Rios FF, Rodrigues de Freitas LA, Codes L, et al. Hepatoportal sclerosis related to the use of herbals and nutritional supplements. Causality or coincidence? Ann Hepatol 2016;15(6):932–8.
23. Stickel F, Droz S, Patsenker E, et al. Severe hepatotoxicity following ingestion of Herbalife nutritional supplements contaminated with Bacillus subtilis. J Hepatol 2009;50(1):111–7.
24. Heidemann LA, Navarro VJ, Ahmad J, et al. Severe acute hepatocellular injury attributed to OxyELITE Pro: a case series. Dig Dis Sci 2016;61(9):2741–8.

25. Foley S, Butlin E, Shields W, et al. Experience with OxyELITE pro and acute liver injury in active duty service members. Dig Dis Sci 2014;59(12):3117–21.

26. Elsharkawy AM, McPherson S, Masson S, et al. Cholestasis secondary to anabolic steroid use in young men. BMJ 2012;344:e468.

27. Brazeau MJ, Castaneda JL, Huitron SS, et al. Case report of supplement-induced hepatitis in an active duty service member. Mil Med 2015;180(7):e844–6.

28. Kou T, Watanabe M, Yazumi S. Hepatic failure during anabolic steroid therapy. Gastroenterology 2012;143(6):e11–2.

29. Ishak KG. Hepatic lesions caused by anabolic and contraceptive steroids. Semin Liver Dis 1981;1(2):116–28.

30. Bond P, Llewellyn W, Van Mol P. Anabolic androgenic steroid-induced hepatotoxicity. Med Hypotheses 2016;93:150–3.

31. El Sherrif Y, Potts JR, Howard MR, et al. Hepatotoxicity from anabolic androgenic steroids marketed as dietary supplements: contribution from ATP8B1/ABCB11 mutations? Liver Int 2013;33(8):1266–70.

32. Davidov Y, Har-Noy O, Pappo O, et al. Methylprednisolone-induced liver injury: case report and literature review. J Dig Dis 2016;17(1):55–62.

33. Grilli E, Galati V, Petrosillo N, et al. Incomplete septal cirrhosis after high-dose methylprednisolone therapy and regression of liver injury. Liver Int 2015;35(2):674–6.

34. Oliveira AT, Lopes S, Cipriano MA, et al. Induced liver injury after high-dose methylprednisolone in a patient with multiple sclerosis. BMJ Case Rep 2015;2015, [pii:bcr2015210722].

35. Caster O, Conforti A, Viola E, et al. Methylprednisolone-induced hepatotoxicity: experiences from global adverse drug reaction surveillance. Eur J Clin Pharmacol 2014;70(4):501–3.

36. Marino M, Morabito E, Altea MA, et al. Autoimmune hepatitis during intravenous glucocorticoid pulse therapy for Graves' ophthalmopathy treated successfully with glucocorticoids themselves. J Endocrinol Invest 2005;28(3):280–4.

37. Ghabril M, Bonkovsky HL, Kum C, et al. Liver injury from tumor necrosis factor-alpha antagonists: analysis of thirty-four cases. Clin Gastroenterol Hepatol 2013;11(5):558–64.e3.

38. Bjornsson ES, Gunnarsson BI, Grondal G, et al. Risk of drug-induced liver injury from tumor necrosis factor antagonists. Clin Gastroenterol Hepatol 2015;13(3):602–8.

39. Parra RS, Feitosa MR, Machado VF, et al. Infliximab-associated fulminant hepatic failure in ulcerative colitis: a case report. J Med Case Rep 2015;9:249.

40. Rodrigues S, Lopes S, Magro F, et al. Autoimmune hepatitis and anti-tumor necrosis factor alpha therapy: a single center report of 8 cases. World J Gastroenterol 2015;21(24):7584–8.

41. Shelton E, Chaudrey K, Sauk J, et al. New onset idiosyncratic liver enzyme elevations with biological therapy in inflammatory bowel disease. Aliment Pharmacol Ther 2015;41(10):972–9.

42. Beck KE, Blansfield JA, Tran KQ, et al. Enterocolitis in patients with cancer after antibody blockade of cytotoxic T-lymphocyte-associated antigen 4. J Clin Oncol 2006;24(15):2283–9.

43. Kleiner DE, Berman D. Pathologic changes in ipilimumab-related hepatitis in patients with metastatic melanoma. Dig Dis Sci 2012;57(8):2233–40.

44. Johncilla M, Misdraji J, Pratt DS, et al. Ipilimumab-associated hepatitis: clinicopathologic characterization in a series of 11 cases. Am J Surg Pathol 2015;39(8):1075–84.

45. Postow MA, Chesney J, Pavlick AC, et al. Nivolumab and ipilimumab versus ipilimumab in untreated melanoma. N Engl J Med 2015;372(21):2006–17.

46. Antezana A, Sigal S, Herbert J, et al. Natalizumab-induced hepatic injury: a case report and review of literature. Mult Scler Relat Disord 2015;4(6):495–8.

47. Boberg KM, Aadland E, Jahnsen J, et al. Incidence and prevalence of primary biliary cirrhosis, primary sclerosing cholangitis, and autoimmune hepatitis in a Norwegian population. Scand J Gastroenterol 1998;33(1):99–103.

48. Bjornsson E, Talwalkar J, Treeprasertsuk S, et al. Drug-induced autoimmune hepatitis: clinical characteristics and prognosis. Hepatology 2010;51(6):2040–8.

49. Hisamochi A, Kage M, Ide T, et al. An analysis of drug-induced liver injury, which showed histological findings similar to autoimmune hepatitis. J Gastroenterol 2016;51(6):597–607.

50. Suzuki A, Brunt EM, Kleiner DE, et al. The use of liver biopsy evaluation in discrimination of idiopathic autoimmune hepatitis versus drug-induced liver injury. Hepatology 2011;54(3):931–9.

51. Aygun C, Altinok AY, Cakir A, et al. Acute temozolomide induced liver injury: mixed type hepatocellular and cholestatic toxicity. Acta Gastroenterol Belg 2016;79(4):487–9.

52. Balakrishnan A, Ledford R, Jaglal M. Temozolomide-induced biliary ductopenia: a case report. J Med Case Rep 2016;10:33.

53. Grieco A, Tafuri MA, Biolato M, et al. Severe cholestatic hepatitis due to temozolomide: an adverse drug effect to keep in mind. Case report and review of literature. Medicine (Baltimore) 2015;94(12):e476.

54. Grant LM, Kleiner DE, Conjeevaram HS, et al. Clinical and histological features of idiosyncratic acute liver injury caused by temozolomide. Dig Dis Sci 2013;58(5):1415–21.

55. Bonkovsky HL, Kleiner DE, Gu J, et al. Clinical presentations and outcomes of bile duct loss caused by drugs and herbal and dietary supplements. Hepatology 2017;65(4):1267–77.

56. Fontana RJ, Hayashi PH, Barnhart H, et al. Persistent liver biochemistry abnormalities are more common in older patients and those with cholestatic drug induced liver injury. Am J Gastroenterol 2015;110(10):1450–9.

57. Slim R, Fathallah N, Aounallah A, et al. Paracetamol-induced Stevens Johnson syndrome and cholestatic hepatitis. Curr Drug Saf 2015;10(2):187–9.

58. Eder P, Permoda-Osip A, Majewski P, et al. Agomelatine-induced liver injury in a patient with choledocholithiasis. Acta Neuropsychiatr 2015;27(1):56–9.

59. Taylor SA, Vittorio JM, Martinez M, et al. Anakinra-induced acute liver failure in an adolescent patient with Still's disease. Pharmacotherapy 2016;36(1):e1–4.

60. Kumar S. Cholestatic liver injury secondary to artemisinin. Hepatology 2015;62(3):973–4.

61. Carrascosa MF, Salcines-Caviedes JR, Lucena MI, et al. Acute liver failure following atorvastatin dose escalation: is there a threshold dose for idiosyncratic hepatotoxicity? J Hepatol 2015;62(3):751–2.

62. Yun GY, Kim SH, Kim SW, et al. Atypical onset of bicalutamide-induced liver injury. World J Gastroenterol 2016;22(15):4062–5.

63. Chintamaneni P, Stevenson HL, Malik SM. Bupivacaine drug-induced liver injury: a case series and brief review of the literature. J Clin Anesth 2016;32:137–41.

64. Kumagai J, Kanda T, Yasui S, et al. Autoimmune hepatitis following drug-induced liver injury in an elderly patient. Clin J Gastroenterol 2016;9(3):156–9.

65. Pisapia R, Abdeddaim A, Mariano A, et al. Acute hepatitis associated with clopidogrel: a case report and review of the literature. Am J Ther 2015;22(1):e8–13.

66. Bessone F, Lucena MI, Roma MG, et al. Cyproterone acetate induces a wide spectrum of acute liver damage including corticosteroid-responsive hepatitis: report of 22 cases. Liver Int 2016;36(2):302–10.

67. Miyashima Y, Honma Y, Miyagawa K, et al. Daclatasvir and asunaprevir combination therapy-induced hepatitis and cholecystitis with coagulation disorder due to hypersensitivity reactions. Intern Med 2016; 55(24):3595–601.

68. Bohm M, Vuppalanchi R, Chalasani N. Febuxostat-induced acute liver injury. Hepatology 2016;63(3): 1047–9.

69. Harati H, Rahmani M, Taghizadeh S. Acute cholestatic liver injury from hydralazine intake. Am J Ther 2016;23(5):e1211–4.

70. Villamil A, Mullen E, Casciato P, et al. Interferon beta 1a-induced severe autoimmune hepatitis in patients with multiple sclerosis: report of two cases and review of the literature. Ann Hepatol 2015;14(2):273–80.

71. Kim CW, Park JS, Oh SH, et al. Drug-induced liver injury caused by iodine-131. Clin Mol Hepatol 2016;22(2):272–5.

72. Jung MC, Kim JK, Cho JY, et al. A case of levocetirizine-induced liver injury. Clin Mol Hepatol 2016;22(4):495–8.

73. Salvado M, Vargas V, Vidal M, et al. Autoimmune-like hepatitis during masitinib therapy in an amyotrophic lateral sclerosis patient. World J Gastroenterol 2015; 21(36):10475–9.

74. Stelzer T, Kohler S, Marques Maggio E, et al. An unusual cause of febrile hepatitis. BMJ Case Rep 2015;2015, [pii:bcr2014205857].

75. Sakumura M, Tajiri K, Miwa S, et al. Hepatic sinusoidal obstruction syndrome induced by non-transplant chemotherapy for non-Hodgkin lymphoma. Intern Med 2017;56(4):395–400.

76. Bernardes SS, Souza-Nogueira A, Moreira EG, et al. Nimesulide-induced fatal acute liver failure in an elderly woman with metastatic biliary adenocarcinoma. A case report. Sao Paulo Med J 2015; 133(4):371–6.

77. Kumar S. Oral contraceptive-induced hepatic sinusoidal dilatation. Dig Liver Dis 2015;47(6): e10.

78. Conrad MA, Cui J, Lin HC. Sertraline-associated cholestasis and ductopenia consistent with vanishing bile duct syndrome. J Pediatr 2016;169: 313–5.e1.

79. Dyson JK, Hutchinson J, Harrison L, et al. Liver toxicity associated with sofosbuvir, an NS5A inhibitor and ribavirin use. J Hepatol 2016;64(1):234–8.

80. Yokomori H, Yamazaki H, Oda M. Freshwater clam extract supplement-induced acute cholestasis. Hepatology 2016;63(2):665–6.

81. Corey R, Werner KT, Singer A, et al. Acute liver failure associated with Garcinia cambogia use. Ann Hepatol 2015;15(1):123–6.

82. Jin SM, Song SH, Cho YH, et al. A case of nodular regenerative hyperplasia of the liver combined with toxic hepatitis. Korean J Gastroenterol 2015;65(1): 52–6.

83. Alhaddad OM, Elsabaawy MM, Rewisha EA, et al. Khat-induced liver injuries: a report of two cases. Arab J Gastroenterol 2016;17(1):45–8.

84. Mahamoud HD, Muse SM, Roberts LR, et al. Khat chewing and cirrhosis in Somaliland: case series. Afr J Prim Health Care Fam Med 2016;8(1):e1–4.

85. Gedela M, Potu KC, Gali VL, et al. A case of hepatotoxicity related to kombucha tea consumption. S D Med 2016;69(1):26–8.

86. Hayashi M, Abe K, Imaizumi H, et al. Drug-induced liver injury with autoimmune features complicated with hemophagocytic syndrome. Clin J Gastroenterol 2016;9(3):150–5.

87. Atayan Y, Cagin YF, Erdogan MA, et al. Ecstasy induced acute hepatic failure. Case reports. Acta Gastroenterol Belg 2015;78(1):53–5.

88. Ito D, Tanaka T, Akamatsu N, et al. Recurrent acute liver failure because of acute hepatitis induced by organic solvents: a case report. Medicine (Baltimore) 2016;95(1):e2445.

Pathologic Features of Hereditary Cholestatic Diseases

Andrew D. Clouston, MBBS, PhD, FRCPA*

KEYWORDS

- Liver pathology • Neonatal cholestasis • Bile canalicular transporter disorders • Alagille syndrome

---

Key points

- An obstructive appearance with ductular reaction can occur in cystic fibrosis, ATP-binding cassette B4 (ABCB4) deficiency, and, uncommonly, in alpha-1-antitrypsin (A1AT) deficiency and Alagille syndrome (early in the disease course).

- In neonates, A1AT deficiency often does not have typical globules in the hepatocytes and instead shows cholestasis and, in some cases, duct loss.

- As well as progressive biliary cirrhosis in children, bile canalicular transporter deficiency can have a milder disease phenotype that includes recurrent cholestasis, intrahepatic cholestasis of pregnancy, chronic cholestatic liver function tests with a mild ductular reaction on biopsy, low phospholipid-associated cholelithiasis with early gallstones, or unexplained late biliary cirrhosis in adults. In severe disease, the level of the γ–glutamyl transferase and the histologic pattern helps to distinguish the likely transporter deficiency.

ABSTRACT

The inherited diseases causing conjugated hyperbilirubinemia are diverse, with variability in clinical severity, histologic appearance, and time of onset. The liver biopsy appearances can also vary depending on whether the initial presentation is in the neonatal period or later. Although many of the disorders have specific histologic features in fully developed and classic cases, biopsies taken early in the disease course may be nonspecific, showing either cholestatic hepatitis or an obstructive pattern of injury requiring close correlation with the laboratory and clinical findings to reach the correct diagnosis. Additionally, increased understanding of the range of hepatic changes occurring in mild deficiencies of bile canalicular transporter proteins suggest that these disorders, particularly ABCB4 deficiency, may be more common than previously recognized; improved awareness should prompt further investigation.

OVERVIEW

Inherited cholestatic diseases are a group of disorders that commonly present early in life and are characterized clinically by conjugated hyperbilirubinemia. Although most have one or more pathognomonic histopathologic features in classic cases, the initial biopsy may not demonstrate these; therefore, the diseases need to be actively considered in a differential diagnosis and the biopsies correlated with the clinical, laboratory, and genetic data. Particularly in the neonate and infant, there are a limited number of reaction patterns. An obstructive appearance with ductular reaction, portal inflammation, edema, and cholestasis can occur not only in biliary but also in metabolic disorders, such as alpha-1-antitrypsin

---

Disclosure Statement: The author has no financial or competing conflicts of interest to disclose.
Faculty of Medicine, University of Queensland, Herston Road, Brisbane, Queensland 4006, Australia
* Envoi Specialist Pathologists, 5/38 Bishop Street Kelvin Grove, Queensland 4059, Australia.
E-mail address: andrewclouston@envoi.com.au

1875-9181/18/Crown Copyright © 2018 Published by Elsevier Inc. All rights reserved.

surgpath.theclinics.com

Abbreviations	
A1AT	Alpha-1-antitrypsin
ABCB4	ATP-binding cassette B4
ABCB11	ATP-binding cassette B11
BRIC	Benign recurrent intrahepatic cholestasis
BSEP	Bile pump export pump
CF	Cystic fibrosis
CFTR	Cystic fibrosis transmembrane conductance regulator
DR	Ductular reaction
FXR	Farnesoid X receptor
HCC	Hepatocellular carcinoma
LPAC	Low phospholipid-associated cholelithiasis
MDR3	Multidrug resistance P-glycoprotein 3
PC	Phosphatidylcholine
PFIC	Progressive familial intrahepatic cholestasis
Pi	Protease inhibitor
γ-GT	γ-Glutamyl transferase

(A1AT) deficiency. Other diseases present as neonatal hepatitis with hepatocyte swelling, giant cell transformation and inflammation, and parenchymal cholestasis.

The histologic patterns may vary between neonates, children, and adults because of several factors. Early clinical manifestations often lead to biopsy before the disease pattern has fully manifested itself, such as A1AT deficiency causing cholestatic changes before characteristic globules develop after 3 months. The maturity of the liver also plays a role particularly in the very young; neonatal factors, such as narrow bile ducts, an incompletely developed biliary tree, slow bile flow, immaturity of bile acid profile, and variable maturity of hepatocytes and cholangiocytes, can exacerbate cholestasis at this time.[1] Duct loss and portal fibrosis can be early changes and may develop quickly in the very young.[1,2] Finally, factors such as the severity of the genetic anomaly and age-associated variation in response to injury modify the biopsy appearances.[1]

It has become clear in recent years that bile acids play an important role in many cholestatic liver disorders and their transporters may be affected by several inherited conditions.[3] The hydrophobic bile acids are osmotically active and have a key role in bile drainage in the canaliculi and proximal bile ductules. They are also toxic, so dysregulation of their secretion or failure to be incorporated into protective

micelles in the bile can lead to direct hepatocellular or biliary injury. Mild manifestations of abnormal canalicular biliary transporters can be clinically silent or very slowly progressive, precipitated by external factors, such as hormones, drugs, or inflammation. It is probable that many of these patients remain undiagnosed, but increased awareness and access to genetic testing could see an increase in recognition. A bicarbonate barrier or umbrella at the luminal surface of the cholangiocytes, maintained particularly by the cystic fibrosis (CF) transmembrane conductance regulator (CFTR) chloride channel, is also important for cholangiocyte protection.[4]

CYSTIC FIBROSIS

CF is a common multi-organ hereditary disease affecting mainly lung and pancreatic function and occurring in about 1 in 3000 births.[5] It is caused by mutation in the gene encoding CTFR, an ATP-dependent chloride channel promoting chloride/bicarbonate exchange. Although almost 2000 mutations are described, about two-thirds are due to a phenylalanine deletion (F508del).[6,7]

The mutations in CF result in clinical manifestations of variable severity.[6] Defective function of the CTFR channel causes altered biliary transport of bile acids and also affects the bicarbonate umbrella at the cholangiocyte surface.[4] This results in duct plugging by inspissated secretions and also toxicity to cholangiocytes and hepatocytes, leading to inflammation, ductular proliferation and activation of myofibroblasts to produce fibrosis.[8,9]

Improved therapy and, thus, life span has seen an increase in the number of cases of adult CF liver disease, particularly when revised diagnostic criteria are used[10,11]; it is now seen in about a third of patients,[6,11] although causes only 2.5% of deaths. In those developing significant liver disease it occurs relatively early, with initial manifestations generally developing before 18 years of age and most presenting before the age of 10.[5,12] Neonatal hepatitis can also occur.[13] Advanced cases are characterized by portal hypertension more often than synthetic failure[8]; it was suggested recently that portal venous obliterative lesions possibly caused by gut inflammation[14] could be playing a role, discussed further later. A primary sclerosing cholangitis-like appearance may be seen on imaging (magnetic resonance cholangiopancreatography [MRCP]) with intrahepatic and extrahepatic strictures and beading.[15]

PATHOLOGY

Liver biopsy has a role in CF management but is used variably and is more commonly performed in pediatric cases.[8,11] Steatosis is the most common change, occurring not as a result of the *CTFR* mutation but rather because of nutritional and endocrine aberrations.[6] Luminal inspissated eosinophilic mucin in the small bile ducts are commonly but not invariably seen, and these are the pathognomonic feature. Causing obstruction, these can lead to biopsy appearances of a marked obstructive pattern early in life. More commonly, there is the development of a ductular reaction, portal inflammation, periductal neutrophilia, and variable portal fibrosis with bridging fibrous septa (**Fig. 1**).

The diagnosis of fibrosing liver disease without biopsy can be difficult.[9] The presence of fibrous septa on biopsy seems to be an important feature and in a series of pediatric cases predicted the later development of portal hypertension.[8] As is typical of biliary disorders, this fibrosis can be variable, unpredictable, and patchy. Dual passes of the biopsy needle increase the detection of portal fibrosis; if performed, a third of cases will show differing fibrosis stages in the 2 biopsies, sometimes varying by up to 2 stages.[8] It is recommended that fibrosis staging be performed only if 5 or more portal areas are present in the biopsy.[8] The literature on CF refers to focal biliary fibrosis (sometimes called *focal biliary cirrhosis*), which may progress in some cases to multi-lobular biliary cirrhosis.

As mentioned earlier, portal hypertension is an important late clinical outcome. In one study it developed in 71% of children who had bridging fibrous septa on index biopsy.[8] Importantly, it can be associated with a noncirrhotic liver; recent evidence suggests that this does not reflect sampling error but rather that vascular liver disease may be occurring silently in some patients more frequently than previously recognized. In a relatively large study of long-surviving adults with CF liver disease, only one liver biopsy was performed and it showed nodular regenerative hyperplasia.[11] A recent European case series of 8 patients with CF and severe portal hypertension found that none were cirrhotic. Transjugular liver biopsies or explants showed obliterative portal veno-pathy with loss of vein branches from many portal tracts, para-portal shunt vessels (ectopic portal veins), centrilobular sinusoidal dilation, and nodular regenerative hyperplasia.[14] Some showed portal calcification in areas of lost portal veins, which could sometimes be detected radiologically. There was also centrilobular hepatocytic expression of keratin-7 immunohistochemically in some patients, possibly reflecting a reaction to ischemia. The vascular changes coexisted with chronic biliary obstructive changes, including cholate stasis in some cases.[14]

ALPHA-1-ANTITRYPSIN DEFICIENCY

A1AT is a serine protease inhibitor (Pi) produced mainly but not exclusively in hepatocytes. It is encoded by *SERPINA1*, which has more than 200 genetic variants.[16] The normal gene product, PiM, has important clinical variants with the two

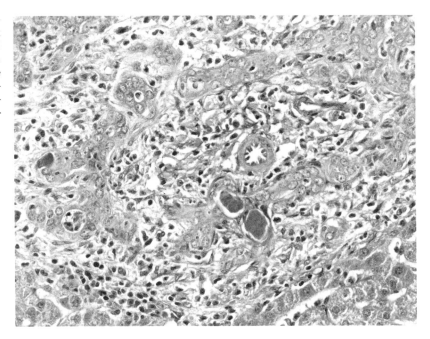

Fig. 1. CF. Eosinophilic inclusions in the bile duct lumens are accompanied by a ductular reaction and portal fibrosis in the explant from an 8-year-old child (hematoxylin-eosin, original magnification ×200).

most important being the PiZ and PiS allelic variants. Because of codominant expression, the amount of circulating Pi reflects expression by both alleles, with deficiency inherited as an autosomal recessive condition. Liver disease occurs through the accumulation of the abnormal Pi protein in hepatocytes, occurring in 1 in 3500 births[17] and affecting mainly Caucasians.

The pathogenesis of the liver and lung diseases in A1AT deficiency differs. The reduced Pi in serum results in tissue destruction by unopposed neutrophil elastases in the lung, particularly in smokers. Conversely, in the liver, the injury is caused by protein misfolding and, crucially, polymerization in the endoplasmic reticulum of the hepatocytes, causing direct toxic injury.[17] The PiZ isoform is most prone to polymerization, as are the rare variants M_{duarte} and M_{malton}. PiS, the second most common mutant, does not polymerize at a clinically significant rate when inherited homozygously (PiSS) so does not form globules; but when coinherited with the Z allele (PiSZ), heteropolymers are formed and liver disease may occur.[16]

The clinical presentation of A1AT deficiency is bimodal, occurring in either the neonatal or adult periods and is highly variable, ranging from neonatal cholestasis to acute liver failure (rarely) or later as chronic hepatitis and cirrhosis emerging in adulthood.[17,18]

About 10% of individuals develop neonatal cholestasis, and reasons for this presentation are unclear but may relate to immaturity of the biliary secretory function. In many cases it is self-limited, and by late adolescence most affected patients have regained normal liver chemistry tests.[17] However, up to a quarter of them develop progressive liver disease during childhood.[19,20] An indolent chronic hepatitis progressing to cirrhosis develops in up to 30% of those surviving long-term into late adulthood,[18] with a distinct male predominance. Hepatocellular carcinoma (HCC) has been described in up to 40% of cirrhotic patients.[18]

PATHOLOGY

Cytoplasmic eosinophilic globules of polymerized A1AT within periportal hepatocytes are the typical diagnostic feature and are seen by periodic acid Schiff staining after diastase digestion (Fig. 2). The globules are generally not apparent before 12 weeks of age, although the increased A1AT may be detectable by immunoperoxidase staining before this.[2,20] The globules may be irregularly distributed and are variable in size. The presence of typical globules occurs not only in homozygous patients but can also rarely accumulate in large numbers in heterozygous patients, so correlation with the phenotype is required.

Because globules are not usually seen before 12 weeks of age, neonates expressing the disease show biopsy appearances mimicking neonatal hepatitis or extrahepatic biliary atresia.[20] Cholestasis, ductular reaction, and fibrosis can all be seen, giving a picture similar to large duct obstruction. Periportal steatosis may be a diagnostic clue.[20] Inflammation is generally mild and can be accompanied by extramedullary hematopoiesis. In up to 10% there is a paucity of bile ducts[20] and accumulation of copper-associated protein (Fig. 2C). The prognosis is poorer if jaundice is prolonged for more than 6 weeks and if the biopsy shows a marked ductular reaction, severe fibrosis with extensive bridging fibrosis, or cirrhosis.[19]

In older children or adults, the histology is generally nonspecific apart from the presence of globules. Mild portal inflammation, variable fibrosis, or cirrhosis can be seen. Cirrhotic patients are at an increased risk for primary liver cancer.[21]

DISORDERS OF BILE CANALICULAR TRANSPORTERS (FAMILIAL INTRAHEPATIC CHOLESTASIS AND RELATED DISORDERS)

PATHOGENESIS

Bile salt translocation across the canalicular membrane is a critical function of the hepatocyte. Bile salts are needed for emulsification and digestion of fat in the intestinal lumen and are also important for producing bile flow in the canaliculi. Several transporter proteins play a role in bile formation.[22] Bile acids (making up 50% of the bile) are transported by ATP-binding cassette B11 (ABCB11) (also called bile salt export pump [BSEP]). Because bile acids are toxic to canalicular membranes once transported, a second component, phosphatidylcholine (PC) comprising 25% of the bile, is secreted to form micelles with the bile acids and secreted cholesterol. This secretion is achieved by flopping PC from the inner cell membrane leaflet to the outer leaflet on the canalicular luminal surface where it is released into the bile.[22] The floppase performing this is ABCB4 (also called multidrug resistance P-glycoprotein 3 [MDR3]). This phospholipid transfer causes an unacceptable degree of membrane instability, so a third protein ATP8B1 (also called FIC1) transports phosphatidylserine in the other direction from the outer to inner leaflet, stabilizing the canalicular membrane.[22] All 3 transporters are needed for normal bile formation and flow.

Fig. 2. A1AT deficiency. (*A*) In a 5-year-old girl, cytoplasmic eosinophilic globules are visible in hepatocytes and there is cholestasis (hematoxylin-eosin [H&E], original magnification ×400). (*B*) Globules of polymerized A1AT are highlighted by Periodic acid–Schiff–diastase (PASD) staining (PASD, original magnification ×400). (*C*) Explant showing extensive bile duct loss (H&E, original magnification ×200).

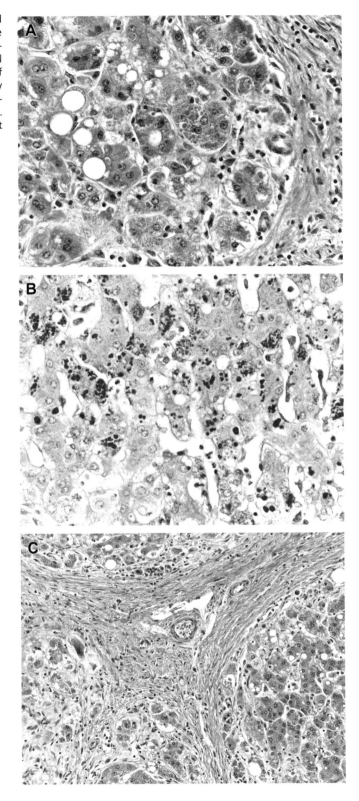

Expression of the bile acid/canalicular transporter proteins is regulated by orphan nuclear receptors, particularly farnesoid X receptor (FXR).[23] These nuclear receptors can be downregulated or blocked by estrogen and progesterone metabolites.[24,25] When the transporters are already defective, any further reduced expression induced by these hormones (pregnancy, oral contraceptive pill) or inflammatory cytokines can then precipitate frank cholestatic disease. As therapeutic targets, FXR and other nuclear receptors can be upregulated by agonists, such as ursodeoxycholic acid, thereby upregulating the canalicular transporter proteins.

Loss of ABCB4-transported PC leads to defective micelle formation and bile acid–induced injury to the canalicular and bile duct luminal surface. Additionally, cholesterol (4% of the bile) is not incorporated into micelles and becomes lithogenic, leading to precipitation with calculus formation and possibly direct cholesterol crystal injury to biliary cells.

Inherited disorders of the bile canalicular transporters are probably under-recognized, and their clinical expressions continue to be clarified. The classic form, also termed *progressive familial intrahepatic cholestasis* (PFIC), includes a heterogeneous group of autosomal recessive diseases, which are now characterized by identifying the specific deficient transporter due to mutations in the genes encoding ATP8B1, ABCB11, or ABCB4 (**Table 1**). Homozygous or compound heterozygous mutations with marked loss of activity result in early and severe cholestatic disease that can progress to fibrosis and cirrhosis.[26] Rare cases of low γ-glutamyl transferase (γ-GT)–associated PFICs (so-called PFIC 4–6) have been ascribed to mutations in other genes, such as *TJP2* (encoding tight junction protein 2), *NR1H4* (encoding FXR), and *MYO5B* (encoding myosin 5b).[3]

Heterozygosity and mutations causing a milder phenotype are probably more common than currently recognized; the functional outcome of different mutations is quite variable, presenting as a range of cholestatic disorders, including benign recurrent intrahepatic cholestasis (BRIC), cholestasis precipitated by external factors, such as pregnancy or drugs, or ill-defined and mild cholestatic liver tests.[2,27–29] It is very useful to carefully interrogate the family history if this disease is being considered, because extended family members can have related disorders.

CLINICAL MANIFESTATIONS

Progressive Familial Intrahepatic Cholestasis

ATP8B1 and ABCB11 deficiencies are characterized by low or normal γ-GT levels despite the cholestasis. ATP8B1 deficiency, previously called PFIC1, Byler disease, or Greenland familial cholestasis, presents in the first few months of life but progresses slowly over years, developing fibrosis and then cirrhosis.[29] ABCB11 deficiency (PFIC2) is also seen in the neonatal period, with marked pruritus, jaundice, and rapid progression to cirrhosis, often by 2 years of age. Serum transaminases are higher because of retained toxic bile acids causing prominent hepatocellular injury. There is an increased incidence of HCC and cholangiocarcinoma, seen in up to 15%, particularly in those with ABCB11 deficiency.[29,30] Apparent recurrence of disease in individuals who have undergone a transplant is described after the emergence of anti-ABCB11 (anti-BSEP) antibodies, recognizing the previously unseen protein.[31] ABCB4 deficiency in its severe form usually presents later, with an elevated γ-GT, which is a useful distinguishing feature from the other two disorders. Some present in the first year,[3]

Table 1
Progressive familial intrahepatic cholestasis

Disorder	ATP8B1 Deficiency	ABCB11 Deficiency	ABCB4 Deficiency
Other names	PFIC1 Byler disease FIC1 deficiency	PFIC2 BSEP deficiency	PFIC3 MDR3 deficiency
Gene product	ATP8B1 FIC1	ABCB11 BSEP	ABCB4 MDR3
γ-GT level	Low or normal	Low or normal	Elevated
Histologic pattern	Bland cholestasis	Neonatal hepatitis	Obstructive DR
Electron microscopy	Coarse granular bile (Byler bile)	Nonspecific	Nonspecific
Fibrosis progression	Slow	Rapid	Moderate

Abbreviations: DR, ductular reaction; γ-GT, γ-glutamyl transferase.

but the mean age of presentation is around 3 years old.[29]

Manifestations of Milder Disease

BRIC is a rare disorder caused by *ATP8B1* or *ABCB11* mutations that have milder clinical expression, characterized by episodes of jaundice lasting weeks to months, which may be precipitated by external factors, such as infection, fever, drugs, or hormones.[3] These episodes resolve spontaneously.

Milder forms of ABCB4 deficiency can be seen in adults, often in carriers of a heterozygous *ABCB4* mutation. As only a single gene copy is required for disease expression, the inheritance is dominant, so that horizontal and vertical pedigrees often have evidence of cholestatic diseases of various types. Studies have suggested that mutations in *ABCB4* can manifest as[32] intrahepatic cholestasis of pregnancy,[33] drug-induced cholestasis, unexplained episodic jaundice, unexplained chronic cholestatic liver tests, adult cryptogenic cirrhosis with biliary features, adult ductopenia, and low phospholipid-associated cholelithiasis (LPAC) syndrome.

LPAC syndrome is characterized by biliary symptoms before 40 years of age, recurrent symptoms after cholecystectomy, recurrent hepatolithiasis/microlithiasis, and a normal MRCP.[34] The recurrent pain and intrahepatic microlithiasis are due to the precipitation of free cholesterol crystals due to the lack of PC and failure to form micelles with bile acids.

Intrahepatic cholestasis of pregnancy has been linked to ABCB4 deficiency in about 15% of (usually more severe) cases, and this is the best-characterized genetic link. Other candidate genes with less convincing evidence of involvement include *ABCB11*, *ATP8B1*, *ABCC2* (encoding MRP2), and *NR1H4* (encoding FXR).[35]

PATHOLOGY: SEVERE DISEASE IN INFANTS AND CHILDREN

ATP8B1 Deficiency

Affected infants develop bland canalicular cholestasis with little inflammation.[2,20,36] Fibrosis develops slowly and can progress to cirrhosis over a period of years, usually developing in the first or second decade.[2,29,36] If this disease is suspected, a part of the biopsy should be fixed in glutaraldehyde for electron microscopy to demonstrate the loss of canalicular microvilli and distention by characteristic, coarsely granular bile (Byler bile).[36] Ideally the biopsy should be taken when the child is not on exogenous bile acid therapy.[36]

ABCB11 Deficiency

This disease is initially characterized by a nonspecific neonatal hepatitis pattern. In addition to cholestasis, there is hepatocyte swelling, giant cell change, lobular inflammation, and, often, extramedullary hematopoiesis (**Fig. 3**).[2,36–38] Centrilobular fibrosis is also commonly found.[37] Portal inflammation, a ductular reaction, and fibrosis can be present, particularly as the disease progresses; cirrhosis develops within a year or two. The histologic picture is not specific, but immunohistochemistry has a role, showing absent or reduced ABCB11 expression in the canaliculi of most cases (**Fig. 3B**).[37,38]

ABCB4 Deficiency

The histologic picture of severe ABCB4 deficiency has an obstructive biliary pattern (**Fig. 4**) with a prominent ductular reaction.[39] Periductal inflammation, fibrosis, and copper accumulation occur as the disease progresses, although the tempo and severity vary between individuals.[3] Immunohistochemical loss of ABCB4 expression is well established in the diagnosis, but the protein may remain detectable even when not or only poorly functional, so that only about 50% of those affected show diagnostic absent or faint canalicular staining.[29]

PATHOLOGY: MILDER DISEASE IN ADULTS

The recognition of the role of bile canalicular transporter defects in a range of cholestatic diseases continues to unfold and is probably best characterized for ABCB4 deficiency. If homozygous mutation causes severe disease in 1 in 100,000 births,[40] the frequency of heterozygosity is expected to be around 1 in 300. The milder disease that occurs in some heterozygotes usually requires an additional insult, such as hormonal changes or drugs for disease expression, and has diverse patterns. In some cases individual patients have been documented to show several disease patterns at different times of disease evolution.

ABCB4 mutations have been linked to about 15% of cases of intrahepatic cholestasis of pregnancy. As well as canalicular cholestasis seen in drug- and pregnancy-associated cholestasis, other relatively subtle histologic manifestations are being described in mildly affected patients. Understanding this is useful to make sense of unusual biopsies where a classic picture is not seen. For example, some cases of drug-induced jaundice show bile duct injury and loss instead of canalicular cholestasis (**Fig. 5**). A recent study of liver findings in 13 adults with proven heterozygous

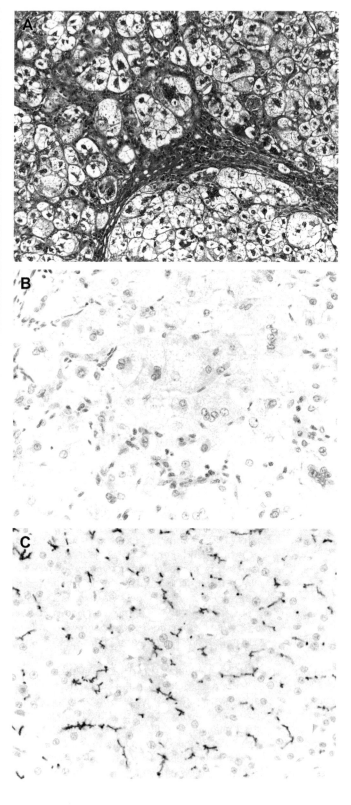

Fig. 3. ABCB11 (BSEP) deficiency. (*A*) There is hepatocyte swelling, giant cell transformation, and extensive fibrosis (hematoxylin-eosin, original magnification ×200). (*B*) Loss of ABCB11 staining in canaliculi. (*C*) Normal control (*B, C* ABCB11 immunoperoxidase, original magnification ×400). (*Courtesy of* Dr Andrew Clouston and Dr Nicole Graf, Westmead Children's Hospital, Sydney. The photos were taken by Dr Andrew Clouston.)

Fig. 4. ABCB4 (MDR3) deficiency. (A) Biliary cirrhosis pattern in the explant of an 8-year-old girl. Her father subsequently developed similar cirrhosis due to more indolent disease (hematoxylin-eosin, original magnification ×40). (B) Loss of normal canalicular expression of ABCB4. (C) Normal ABCB4 (MDR3) staining pattern (B, C ABCB4 immunoperoxidase, original magnification ×400).

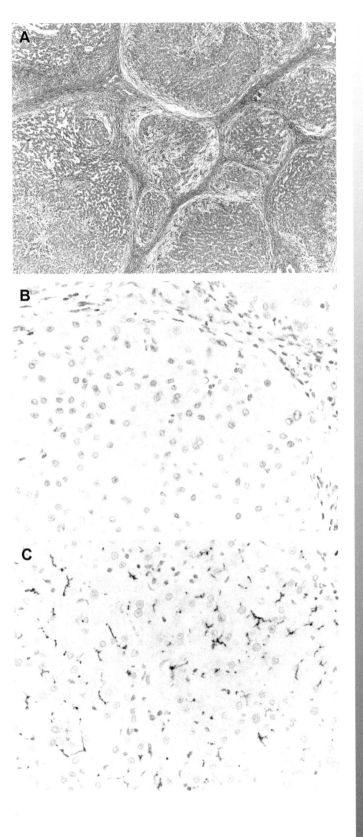

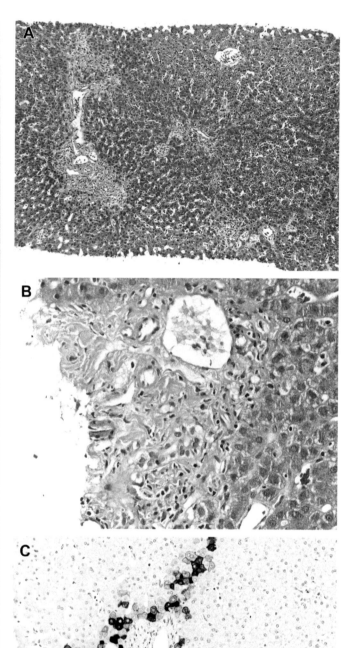

Fig. 5. Mild ABCB4 deficiency. (*A*) This 19-year-old woman developed jaundice after commencing oral contraceptive pill. Her biopsy shows biliary injury, a mild ductular reaction, and focal bile duct loss (hematoxylin-eosin [H&E], original magnification ×40). (*B*) There is vacuolation and mild inflammation of the biliary epithelium. There was not the expected canalicular cholestasis. Gene testing found heterozygous mutation of the *ABCB4* gene (H&E, original magnification ×200). (*C*) Keratin-7 immunostaining shows duct loss and periportal hepatocyte staining (keratin-7 immunoperoxidase, original magnification ×100).

mutations[41] found that most biopsies from patients with ABCB4 mutations had a ductular reaction, mild portal inflammation, and fibrosis. In 3 patients aggregates of cholesterol crystals (or spaces where the crystals had dissolved) were identified, and the presence of frank hepatolithiasis was associated with biliary dysplasia and subsequent cholangiocarcinoma in one case. Two of 13 biopsies showed obliterative duct scars,[41] commonly regarded as a feature that is suggestive of primary sclerosing cholangitis. Progression to cirrhosis was rare. In another study of patients with unexplained cholestatic liver tests, ABCB4 mutations were found in 34% of cases; liver biopsy usually showed portal fibrosis and a ductular reaction.[42] In the author's hands and others,[41,43] ABCB4/MDR3 immunoperoxidase staining of the canalicular membrane is generally normal in these mild cases of cholestatic disease, contrasting with the frequent diminution of canalicular staining that characterizes full-blown severe disease (PFIC3).

In summary, there is a range of mild cholestatic or biliary changes, such as ductular reaction, mild portal fibrosis, and a biliary gestalt, that occur on a background of chronic cholestatic liver chemistry tests, where the usual tests for primary biliary cholangitis, primary sclerosing cholangitis, and large duct obstruction are negative. Some of these represent mild ABCB4 deficiency disease. A careful family history is required; if this is suggestive, then genetic testing is worth considering.

BILE ACID SYNTHETIC DISORDERS

The primary disorders of bile acid synthesis are rare inherited defects of enzymes leading to the inadequate formation of normal bile acids, causing poor bile flow, toxic injury to hepatocytes, and malabsorption of fat-soluble vitamins. There are 9 known defects[44] profiled in more detail elsewhere.[20,45]

The hallmark clinical features are low serum γ-GT, normal or low serum bile acids, and, often, absence of pruritus (except in 3βHSD deficiency), despite the presence of marked jaundice.[20,45] The combined defects are distinctly rare and account for only 1% to 2% of neonatal cholestasis. In most of the disorders there is a good response to oral bile acid therapy. Zellweger syndrome, also known as cerebrohepatorenal syndrome, is characterized by disrupted peroxisomal biosynthesis secondary to mutations in one of the PEX genes, affecting the last step of bile acid synthesis.[45] Affected individuals have craniofacial and bony abnormalities, chronic liver disease, and a progressive course leading to death by 2 years of age.

The pathologic changes can vary with age and the affected gene. Neonates develop giant cell hepatitis that can be persistent, canalicular cholestasis, portal inflammation, and variable fibrosis, with progression of the fibrosis in older children.[20] In Zellweger syndrome, the cholestatic and hepatocellular changes are accompanied by increased iron storage and progressive fibrosis.[45]

ALAGILLE SYNDROME

Alagille syndrome (arteriohepatic dysplasia) is a multisystem disorder that, in liver, is characterized by a paucity of intrahepatic bile ducts due to a failure of normal duct morphogenesis during liver growth. The paucity is defined as a bile duct/portal tract ratio of less than 0.5.[46,47] It is an autosomal dominant disorder resulting from mutations in JAG1 (94% of cases) or the gene for its receptor NOTCH2 (2%).[48]

The syndrome affects multiple organs and, as well as bile duct paucity, there can be heart malformations, characteristic facies, butterfly vertebrae, and eye abnormalities (posterior embryotoxon). The penetrance is variable,[48] and 70% of cases represent spontaneous mutations.[20] This disorder accounts for about 5% to 10% of neonatal cholestasis,[47] with a variable prognosis that is more favorable in children whose cholestasis resolves, although 25% will progress.[20]

PATHOGENESIS

Notch-2 signaling in cholangiocytes, triggered by binding to the Jagged-1 ligand expressed on portal mesenchymal cells, is a key pathway for arborization of the intrahepatic biliary tree.[48] Early cholangiogenesis during fetal life develops from the ductal plate, which forms from bipotential hepatoblasts.[49] Impaired Notch signaling did not prevent ductal plate formation in a rodent model (though did impair it somewhat)[50] but had much more impact later, so it seems to be more important in the second phase of bile duct branching and elongation, particularly after the disappearance of the ductal plates in the neonatal period.[49] Because of this phenomenon, bile ducts can be present in the central portion of the liver in some cases, with marked paucity more peripherally.[46,49,51]

PATHOLOGY

In an adequate biopsy with at least 6 portal tracts, bile duct paucity can be diagnosed when the bile duct/portal tract ratio is less than 0.5 because ducts are present in greater than 90% of portal tracts in the normal pediatric liver (**Fig. 6**).[20,47,52] Before 4 months of age, when about two-thirds

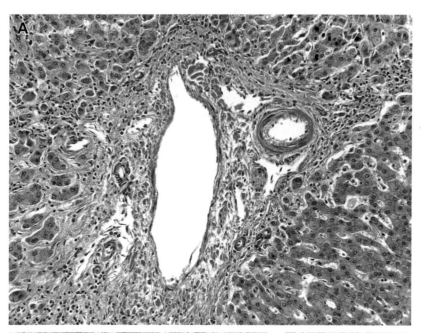

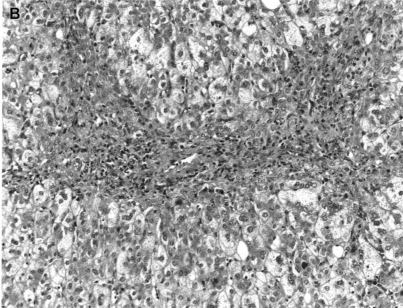

Fig. 6. Alagille syndrome. (*A*) There is absence of bile ducts in portal areas. Despite the marked cholestasis, no ductular reaction is seen and inflammation is only mild (hematoxylin-eosin [H&E], original magnification ×200). (*B*) Early proliferative phase of Alagille syndrome in a 4-month-old boy. There is a prominent ductular reaction at the periphery of the portal tract, but no anatomic duct is seen near the hepatic artery branch at the center of the figure (H&E, original magnification ×200).

of patients present, bile duct paucity is found in many cases.[47] One series of Alagille syndrome biopsies found an average duct/portal ratio of 0.126.[52]

However, up to a quarter of early biopsies show either a biliary obstructive picture resembling biliary atresia or a neonatal hepatitis pattern[20,46,47,53] without obviously reduced duct numbers. The presence of a prominent periportal ductular reaction even when the anatomic ducts are absent can be a significant problem, masking the duct paucity and closely mimicking biliary atresia (**Fig. 6B**).

Additional biopsy changes can include cholestasis, extramedullary hematopoiesis, giant cell change, and early copper accumulation. Keratin-7 immunostaining may be of use to show the reduced duct count if not obscured by a ductular reaction, and this will also stain the periportal hepatocytes. There may be mild lymphocytic inflammation of the remaining bile ducts,[46,49] but this does not seem to be the cause of duct paucity. Older children with Alagille syndrome can also be identified using CD10 immunostaining. Expression of CD10 along the hepatocyte canalicular membrane is physiologically absent before the 2 years of age but is seen throughout the lobules after this.[54] In Alagille syndrome, the expression fails to occur at the expected age and lack of canalicular CD10 persists in older children with the syndrome.[54]

Although there can be a confounding ductular reaction in some cases, generally the portal tracts without bile ducts appear relatively bland without a ductular reaction, and fibrosis is variable or often absent (Fig. 6A).[20,49] Arteries with muscular thickening have been described.[49] Central nodular masses form in about 30% of children before 10 years of age, probably representing a hyperplastic response in regions where there are more preserved bile ducts that have formed earlier in fetal development (see earlier discussion).[49,51] HCC, considered a rare complication in Alagille syndrome,[55] has been described in some children[56,57] as well as adults.

ACKNOWLEDGMENTS

The author thanks Dr Catherine Campbell for reviewing the article and Dr Nicole Graf for providing case material.

REFERENCES

1. Wells RG. Hepatic fibrosis in children and adults. Clin Liver Dis 2017;9:99–101.
2. Morotti RA, Jain D. Pediatric cholestatic disorders: approach to pathologic diagnosis. Surg Pathol Clin 2013;6:205–25.
3. Reichert MC, Hall RA, Krawczyk M, et al. Genetic determinants of cholangiopathies: molecular and systems genetics. Biochim Biophys Acta 2018, [Epub ahead of print].
4. Beuers U, Hohenester S, de Buy Wenniger LJ, et al. The biliary HCO3- umbrella: a unifying hypothesis on pathogenetic and therapeutic aspects of fibrosing cholangiopathies. Hepatology 2010;52:1489–96.
5. Debray D, Kelly D, Houwen R, et al. Best practice guidance for the diagnosis and management of cystic fibrosis-associated liver disease. J Cyst Fibros 2011;10(Suppl 2):S29–36.
6. Herrmann U, Dockter G, Lammert F. Cystic fibrosis-associated liver disease. Best Pract Res Clin Gastroenterol 2010;24:585–92.
7. Wilschanski M, Durie PR. Patterns of GI disease in adulthood associated with mutations in the CFTR gene. Gut 2007;56:1153–63.
8. Lewindon PJ, Shepherd RW, Walsh MJ, et al. Importance of hepatic fibrosis in cystic fibrosis and the predictive value of liver biopsy. Hepatology 2011; 53:193–201.
9. Pereira TN, Walsh MJ, Lewindon PJ, et al. Paediatric cholestatic liver disease: diagnosis, assessment

10. Gillespie CD, O'Reilly MK, Allen GN, et al. Imaging the abdominal manifestations of cystic fibrosis. Int J Hepatol 2017;2017:5128760.
11. Koh C, Sakiani S, Surana P, et al. Adult-onset cystic fibrosis liver disease: diagnosis and characterization of an underappreciated entity. Hepatology 2017;66: 591–601.
12. Flass T, Narkewicz MR. Cirrhosis and other liver disease in cystic fibrosis. J Cyst Fibros 2013;12: 116–24.
13. Parisi GF, Di Dio G, Franzonello C, et al. Liver disease in cystic fibrosis: an update. Hepat Mon 2013;13:e11215.
14. Witters P, Libbrecht L, Roskams T, et al. Liver disease in cystic fibrosis presents as non-cirrhotic portal hypertension. J Cyst Fibros 2017;16:e11–3.
15. Durieu I, Pellet O, Simonot L, et al. Sclerosing cholangitis in adults with cystic fibrosis: a magnetic resonance cholangiographic prospective study. J Hepatol 1999;30:1052–6.
16. Bals R. Alpha-1-antitrypsin deficiency. Best Pract Res Clin Gastroenterol 2010;24:629–33.
17. Fairbanks KD, Tavill AS. Liver disease in alpha 1-antitrypsin deficiency: a review. Am J Gastroenterol 2008;103:2136–41.
18. Eriksson S. Alpha 1-antitrypsin deficiency and liver cirrhosis in adults. An analysis of 35 Swedish autopsied cases. Acta Med Scand 1987;221:461–7.
19. Francavilla R, Castellaneta SP, Hadzic N, et al. Prognosis of alpha-1-antitrypsin deficiency-related liver disease in the era of paediatric liver transplantation. J Hepatol 2000;32:986–92.
20. Quaglia A, Roberts EA, Torbenson M. Developmental and inherited liver disease. In: Burt AD, Ferrell LD, Hubscher SG, editors. MacSween's pathology of the liver. 7th edition. Edinburgh (United Kingdom): Churchill Livingstone Elsevier; 2017. p. 111–274.
21. Rudnick DA, Perlmutter DH. Alpha-1-antitrypsin deficiency: a new paradigm for hepatocellular carcinoma in genetic liver disease. Hepatology 2005;42: 514–21.
22. Linton KJ. Lipid flopping in the liver. Biochem Soc Trans 2015;43:1003–10.
23. Ghonem NS, Assis DN, Boyer JL. Fibrates and cholestasis. Hepatology 2015;62:635–43.
24. Abu-Hayyeh S, Papacleovoulou G, Lovgren-Sandblom A, et al. Intrahepatic cholestasis of pregnancy levels of sulfated progesterone metabolites inhibit farnesoid X receptor resulting in a cholestatic phenotype. Hepatology 2013;57:716–26.
25. Milona A, Owen BM, Cobbold JF, et al. Raised hepatic bile acid concentrations during pregnancy in mice are associated with reduced

farnesoid X receptor function. Hepatology 2010; 52:1341–9.

26. Jacquemin E, De Vree JM, Cresteil D, et al. The wide spectrum of multidrug resistance 3 deficiency: from neonatal cholestasis to cirrhosis of adulthood. Gastroenterology 2001;120:1448–58.

27. Gordo-Gilart R, Hierro L, Andueza S, et al. Heterozygous ABCB4 mutations in children with cholestatic liver disease. Liver Int 2016;36:258–67.

28. Srivastava A. Progressive familial intrahepatic cholestasis. J Clin Exp Hepatol 2014;4:25–36.

29. van der Woerd WL, van Mil SW, Stapelbroek JM, et al. Familial cholestasis: progressive familial intrahepatic cholestasis, benign recurrent intrahepatic cholestasis and intrahepatic cholestasis of pregnancy. Best Pract Res Clin Gastroenterol 2010;24: 541–53.

30. Knisely AS, Strautnieks SS, Meier Y, et al. Hepatocellular carcinoma in ten children under five years of age with bile salt export pump deficiency. Hepatology 2006;44:478–86.

31. Keitel V, Burdelski M, Vojnisek Z, et al. De novo bile salt transporter antibodies as a possible cause of recurrent graft failure after liver transplantation: a novel mechanism of cholestasis. Hepatology 2009; 50:510–7.

32. Davit-Spraul A, Gonzales E, Baussan C, et al. The spectrum of liver diseases related to ABCB4 gene mutations: pathophysiology and clinical aspects. Semin Liver Dis 2010;30:134–46.

33. Wasmuth HE, Glantz A, Keppeler H, et al. Intrahepatic cholestasis of pregnancy: the severe form is associated with common variants of the hepatobiliary phospholipid transporter ABCB4 gene. Gut 2007;56:265–70.

34. Poupon R, Rosmorduc O, Boelle PY, et al. Genotype-phenotype relationships in the low-phospholipid-associated cholelithiasis syndrome: a study of 156 consecutive patients. Hepatology 2013;58: 1105–10.

35. Geenes V, Williamson C. Intrahepatic cholestasis of pregnancy. World J Gastroenterol 2009;15: 2049–66.

36. Bull LN, Carlton VE, Stricker NL, et al. Genetic and morphological findings in progressive familial intrahepatic cholestasis (Byler disease [PFIC-1] and Byler syndrome): evidence for heterogeneity. Hepatology 1997;26:155–64.

37. Evason K, Bove KE, Finegold MJ, et al. Morphologic findings in progressive familial intrahepatic cholestasis 2 (PFIC2): correlation with genetic and immunohistochemical studies. Am J Surg Pathol 2011;35: 687–96.

38. Davit-Spraul A, Fabre M, Branchereau S, et al. ATP8B1 and ABCB11 analysis in 62 children with normal gamma-glutamyl transferase progressive familial intrahepatic cholestasis (PFIC): phenotypic differences between PFIC1 and PFIC2 and natural history. Hepatology 2010;51:1645–55.

39. Davit-Spraul A, Gonzales E, Baussan C, et al. Progressive familial intrahepatic cholestasis. Orphanet J Rare Dis 2009;4:1.

40. Gonzales E, Spraul A, Jacquemin E. Clinical utility gene card for: progressive familial intrahepatic cholestasis type 3. Eur J Hum Genet 2014;22:

41. Wendum D, Barbu V, Rosmorduc O, et al. Aspects of liver pathology in adult patients with MDR3/ABCB4 gene mutations. Virchows Arch 2012;460:291–8.

42. Ziol M, Barbu V, Rosmorduc O, et al. ABCB4 heterozygous gene mutations associated with fibrosing cholestatic liver disease in adults. Gastroenterology 2008;135:131–41.

43. Sannier A, Ganne N, Tepper M, et al. MDR3 immunostaining on frozen liver biopsy samples is not a sensitive diagnostic tool for the detection of heterozygous MDR3/ABCB4 gene mutations. Virchows Arch 2012;460:535–7, [author reply: 539].

44. Sokol RJ. Reloading against rare liver diseases. J Pediatr Gastroenterol Nutr 2010;50:9–10.

45. Sundaram SS, Bove KE, Lovell MA, et al. Mechanisms of disease: inborn errors of bile acid synthesis. Nat Clin Pract Gastroenterol Hepatol 2008;5: 456–68.

46. Dahms BB, Petrelli M, Wyllie R, et al. Arteriohepatic dysplasia in infancy and childhood: a longitudinal study of six patients. Hepatology 1982;2:350–8.

47. Subramaniam P, Knisely A, Portmann B, et al. Diagnosis of Alagille syndrome-25 years of experience at King's College Hospital. J Pediatr Gastroenterol Nutr 2011;52:84–9.

48. Masek J, Andersson ER. The developmental biology of genetic Notch disorders. Development 2017;144: 1743–63.

49. Libbrecht L, Spinner NB, Moore EC, et al. Peripheral bile duct paucity and cholestasis in the liver of a patient with Alagille syndrome: further evidence supporting a lack of postnatal bile duct branching and elongation. Am J Surg Pathol 2005;29:820–6.

50. Sparks EE, Huppert KA, Brown MA, et al. Notch signaling regulates formation of the three-dimensional architecture of intrahepatic bile ducts in mice. Hepatology 2010;51:1391–400.

51. Rougemont AL, Alvarez F, McLin VA, et al. Bile ducts in regenerative liver nodules of Alagille patients are not the result of genetic mosaicism. J Pediatr Gastroenterol Nutr 2015;61:91–3.

52. Herman HK, Abramowsky CR, Caltharp S, et al. Identification of bile duct paucity in Alagille syndrome: using CK7 and EMA immunohistochemistry as a reliable panel for accurate diagnosis. Pediatr Dev Pathol 2016;19:47–50.

53. Kahn EI, Daum F, Markowitz J, et al. Arteriohepatic dysplasia. II. Hepatobiliary morphology. Hepatology 1983;3:77–84.

54. Byrne JA, Meara NJ, Rayner AC, et al. Lack of hepatocellular CD10 along bile canaliculi is physiologic in early childhood and persistent in Alagille syndrome. Lab Invest 2007;87:1138–48.

55. Lykavieris P, Hadchouel M, Chardot C, et al. Outcome of liver disease in children with Alagille syndrome: a study of 163 patients. Gut 2001;49: 431–5.

56. Bhadri VA, Stormon MO, Arbuckle S, et al. Hepatocellular carcinoma in children with Alagille syndrome. J Pediatr Gastroenterol Nutr 2005;41: 676–8.

57. Rabinovitz M, Imperial JC, Schade RR, et al. Hepatocellular carcinoma in Alagille's syndrome: a family study. J Pediatr Gastroenterol Nutr 1989; 8:26–30.

Primary Biliary Cholangitis and Autoimmune Hepatitis

Raul S. Gonzalez, MD[a],*, Kay Washington, MD, PhD[b]

KEYWORDS

- Primary biliary cholangitis • Primary biliary cirrhosis • Autoimmune hepatitis • Biliary disease
- Chronic hepatitis • Overlap syndrome • Autoantibodies • Differential diagnosis

---

Key points

- Primary biliary cholangitis is an autoimmune disorder that usually presents with increased alkaline phosphatase and serum IgM, along with antimitochondrial antibodies.

- Liver biopsy in primary biliary cholangitis shows nonsuppurative cholangitis, along with mild to moderate portal inflammation. Granulomatous destruction of bile ducts may be present.

- Patients with autoimmune hepatitis have increased AST, ALT, and IgG. Serologic findings include antinuclear and anti–smooth muscle antibodies.

- Moderate chronic inflammation in portal tracts and lobules is seen in autoimmune hepatitis. Occasional features include hepatocyte rosette-like regeneration and emperipolesis. Patients may have fibrosis or cirrhosis at presentation.

- Primary biliary cholangitis and autoimmune hepatitis can occur in the same patient (overlap), and they can also mimic one another both clinically/serologically and histologically, necessitating careful judgment.

ABSTRACT

Primary biliary cholangitis and autoimmune hepatitis are common autoimmune diseases of the liver. Both have typical clinical presentations, including certain autoantibodies on serologic testing. Histologic features are also often typical: primary biliary cholangitis shows bile duct destruction (sometimes with granulomas), and autoimmune hepatitis shows prominent portal and lobular lymphoplasmacytic inflammation. Both have a wide differential diagnosis, including one another; they may also simultaneously occur within the same patient. Careful use of clinical and histologic criteria may be necessary for diagnosis. First-line therapy is immunosuppression for autoimmune hepatitis and ursodeoxycholic acid for primary biliary cholangitis. Both diseases may progress to cirrhosis.

OVERVIEW

Primary biliary cholangitis (PBC) and autoimmune hepatitis (AIH) are the 2 most common autoimmune diseases that primarily involve the liver. They are distinct entities but have some clinicopathologic overlap, and 1 patient can be afflicted with both diseases. Although primary sclerosing cholangitis (PSC) is often placed alongside these diagnoses, its etiology remains unknown.[1]

Disclosure Statement: Neither author has any financial interests to disclose.
a Department of Pathology and Laboratory Medicine, University of Rochester Medical Center, 601 Elmwood Avenue, Box 626, Rochester, NY 14642, USA; b Department of Pathology, Microbiology, and Immunology, Vanderbilt University Medical Center, 1161 21st Avenue South, C-3316 MCN, Nashville, TN 37232-2561, USA
* Corresponding author.
E-mail address: raul_gonzalez@urmc.rochester.edu

surgpath.theclinics.com

PRIMARY BILIARY CHOLANGITIS

OVERVIEW OF PRIMARY BILIARY CHOLANGITIS

"Primary biliary cirrhosis" has recently been renamed primary biliary cholangitis, because not all patients develop cirrhosis.[2] This autoimmune disease, which targets the canals of Hering and the interlobular bile ducts within portal tracts, is also the most common intrinsic biliary disorder of the liver.[3] Its incidence is rising and is highly variable among different countries[4] and among different regions within countries[5]; it has previously been reported as 4.5 per 100,000 people per year in the United States.[6] Patients are most often middle-aged women, and the male:female ratio is 1:9 or greater.[4] The disease rarely if ever affects children. More than a dozen risk loci have been identified by genome-wide association studies,[7] and relatives of patients with PBC have an increased risk of developing the disease.[8]

CLINICAL FEATURES OF PRIMARY BILIARY CHOLANGITIS

Patients with PBC may present with typical biliary-pattern symptoms (jaundice, pruritus, abdominal pain, and fatigue), although up to half of patients are asymptomatic.[9] Alkaline phosphatase levels are increased to 2 or more times the upper limit of normal, and this increase is sustained for 6 months or longer; similarly, γ-glutamyl transferase levels are increased to 5 or more times the upper limit of normal.[10] Bilirubin levels may vary, and aspartate aminotransferase (AST) and alanine aminotransferase (ALT) levels may increase slightly from PBC but not to an impressive degree. Patients may demonstrate an increase in serum IgM.

Pathologic Key Features
OF PRIMARY BILIARY CHOLANGITIS

1. Bile ducts experience nonsuppurative cholangitis (infiltration by lymphocytes), surrounded by mild to moderate chronic portal inflammation.

2. Florid duct lesions (granulomatous destruction of bile ducts) effectively clinch the diagnosis when present.

3. Duct loss and lobular cholestasis are seen later in the disease process and should not be observed early.

4. Lobular necroinflammatory activity should be minimal or absent, unless another disease process (such as AIH) is simultaneously occurring.

Patients with PBC often have antimitochondrial antibodies (AMAs) by serology,[11] as do their first-degree relatives.[8] Of the various types (M1 through M9), M2 is considered the most specific for the disease. Serologic testing is currently performed by enzyme-linked immunosorbent assay. AMAs are sometimes considered pathognomonic for PBC, although their sensitivity and specificity are only approximately 90%. Patients with all the features of PBC but who are serologically negative for AMAs may be diagnosed with AMA-negative PBC, also termed, *autoimmune cholangitis*.[12] Most patients with AMAs but no other evidence of disease do not go on to develop PBC.[13] Other serologic findings in PBC patient include anti–smooth muscle antibodies (ASMAs) (up to 67%),[14] antinuclear antibodies (up to 50%),[15] and rheumatoid factor (70%).[16]

Radiology and cholangiography are of little direct value in diagnosing PBC, because the extrahepatic bile ducts are not affected and there are no specific findings. The tests serve more to exclude other possible biliary abnormalities.

Patients with PBC may develop other autoimmune diseases, including scleroderma and Sjögren syndrome.[16] They may also develop AIH, a situation known as *AIH-PBC overlap*, that requires careful clinical and pathologic examination for proper diagnosis.[17]

MICROSCOPIC FEATURES OF PRIMARY BILIARY CHOLANGITIS

The typical findings of PBC on hematoxylin-eosin stain include mild to moderate lymphoplasmacytic portal inflammation with variable interface hepatitis, distorted interlobular bile ducts involved by lymphocytes (nonsuppurative cholangitis), and bile ductular reaction along the periphery of the portal tracts in early disease stages (**Figs. 1 and 2**).[18,19] These findings may be patchy and may vary in severity from one portal area to the next; in some cases, the biopsy changes may be minimal, making a histologic diagnosis difficult. Nodular regenerative hyperplasia has also been described as a common early finding in PBC.[20] CD1a-positive Langerhans cells may be present within the biliary epithelium of PBC patients.[21]

As the disease progresses, the inflamed bile ducts are destroyed, leading to bile duct loss and eventually ductopenia. If necessary, this can be quantified by an immunohistochemical stain for CK19, which highlights biliary epithelium (**Fig. 3**).[22] Lobular cholestasis also manifests later in the disease, with visible bile appearing in canaliculi and in hepatocyte cytoplasm. Longstanding cholestasis elicits cholate stasis (feathery

Fig. 1. (*A*) Patchy chronic portal inflammation is visible at low power. Interlobular bile ducts are difficult to visualize. (*B*) The interlobular bile duct in this portal tract is distorted, and occasional lymphocytes invade the epithelial cells.

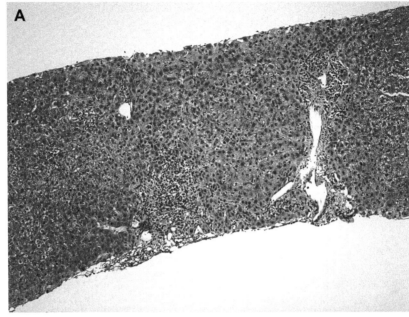

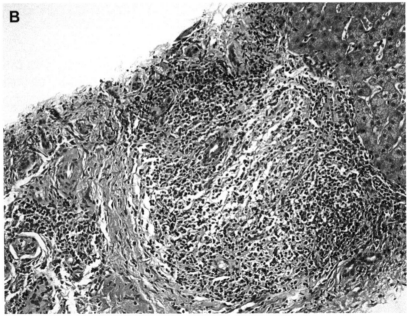

degeneration) of hepatocytes, which become enlarged and rounded, with rarefied cytoplasm and occasional Mallory hyaline (**Fig. 4**). Granulomatous destruction of the bile ducts is not always present but is an invaluable clue to the diagnosis of PBC when seen. These florid duct lesions generally arise in the center of the portal tract and may expand to nearly fill it. The affected bile duct may be partially visible or completely obscured (**Fig. 5**).

The lobules are relatively quiet in PBC, aside from the late cholestatic findings described previously. There may be mild, inconspicuous lymphocytic inflammation, and rare small epithelioid granulomas may be seen. Additionally, bile ducts larger than 100 μm are not affected by PBC and remain unremarkable histologically (**Fig. 6**).

PBC causes liver fibrosis that eventually results in cirrhosis, and several staging systems have been proposed for quantifying the progression of

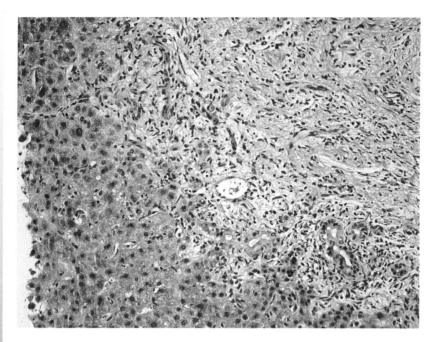

Fig. 2. The edge of this portal tract demonstrates bile ductular reaction, with occasional accompanying neutrophils.

the disease. The most commonly used are the Scheuer system and the Ludwig system (**Table 1**).[23–25] End-stage livers bear the typical findings of biliary-pattern cirrhosis, with haphazardly shaped regenerative hepatocyte nodules forming a jigsaw pattern as they interdigitate. Native bile ducts may be sparse or completely absent. The nodules may sometimes be surrounded by ductular reaction, which combine with cholate stasis to form a halo effect at low power (**Fig. 7**), although ductular reaction is often absent in PBC cirrhosis due to the disease's overall destruction of biliary epithelium.

DIAGNOSIS AND DIFFERENTIAL DIAGNOSIS OF PRIMARY BILIARY CHOLANGITIS

In many cases, clinical and pathologic features point to the diagnosis of PBC in a straightforward manner. The 3 criteria that need to be met are (1) elevated alkaline phosphatase for longer than 6 months, (2) serologic evidence of AMAs, and (3) histologic changes consistent with PBC.[26] Detailed clinical history, however, may not always be available, and some disease processes can mimic PBC histologically, particularly if florid duct lesions are not evident.

Pitfalls
IN DIAGNOSING PRIMARY BILIARY CHOLANGITIS

! Disease findings can be mild and/or patchy on biopsy.

! Florid duct lesions do not always occur in PBC. They can rarely occur in other liver diseases (such as chronic hepatitis C), and other granulomatous processes can mimic them.

! Not all patients with PBC have antimitochondrial antibodies (hence the term, *AMA-negative PBC*), and some patients with AIH develop AMAs.

! Prominent portal tract inflammation and interface hepatitis can occur in the absence of true overlap with AIH.

! Cholestasis early in the disease course is highly unlikely and should prompt consideration of other diagnoses.

Differential Diagnosis
OF PRIMARY BILIARY CHOLANGITIS

ΔΔ

PBC vs	Helpful Distinguishing Features
Autoimmune cholangitis	Negative for AMAs, otherwise essentially the same clinical and pathologic findings
AIH	Lobular necroinflammatory infiltrate Higher rate of ASMAs Duct inflammation but not destruction
PSC	Onion skin fibrosis around medium-sized bile ducts Milder inflammatory infiltrate No AMAs
Large duct obstruction	Cholestasis earlier in the disease course Prominent portal edema in acute phase No duct destruction/loss
Drug-induced liver injury	Ductular reaction and fibrosis less prominent No florid duct lesions May show early cholestasis

The European Association for the Study of the Liver recently released comprehensive guidelines on diagnosis and management of PBC.[27]

Autoimmune Cholangitis

The main difference between autoimmune cholangitis and PBC is that patients with the former lack AMAs on serology (Fig. 8).[12] This occurs in up to 10% of patients who fit all nonserologic criteria for PBC, and this may represent a false-negative result in some patients. These patients are more likely to have elevated IgM and other serologic findings (such as ASMAs). They may also show less inflammation on liver biopsy. Prognosis and clinical approach to treatment are essentially the same as for PBC.

Autoimmune Hepatitis

Clinically, patients with AIH have markedly increased AST and ALT levels, whereas alkaline phosphatase is normal to mildly elevated. A majority of patients have ASMAs, although these occur in up to 20% of PBC patients. Conversely, a minority of AIH patients may have AMAs. Patients with AIH have increased serum IgG rather than IgM.[19,28]

The most helpful clue for distinguishing AIH from PBC on biopsy is the presence of readily apparently lobular inflammation and acidophil bodies, because this is rare to absent in PBC. Additionally, AIH does not cause florid duct lesions. Beyond these 2 features, the diseases can mimic one another quite readily. Both diseases can show prominent portal inflammation with plasma cells as well as interface hepatitis (Fig. 9). Additionally, both diseases can show bile duct distortion and inflammation, accompanied by a ductular reaction, although this is more common in PBC (Fig. 10). Duct loss should not occur in AIH.

Approximately 10% of patients with PBC also have AIH. Diagnosing overlap between these 2 diseases can be difficult, for the reasons discussed previously. Clinical and microscopic criteria for both diseases must be met (Table 2).[29] Overlap should not be called lightly, because patients with PBC but not AIH do not benefit from treatment with immunosuppression.

Primary Sclerosing Cholangitis

Classic PBC (with serum AMAs and florid duct lesions) is easy to distinguish from classic PSC (with typical cholangiography findings and onion skin periductal fibrosis histologically) (Fig. 11). Both diseases, however, demonstrate a similar constellation of nonspecific biliary findings that may blur their distinction, including reactive duct changes early and ductular reaction, duct loss, and late cholestasis. PSC is often a relatively pauci-inflammatory process, so more than a minimal amount of portal inflammation should favor the diagnosis of PBC (or possibly PSC-AIH overlap). If a patient is young, male, and/or afflicted with inflammatory bowel disease, PSC is more likely.

Large Duct Obstruction

Large duct obstruction is rarely biopsied, because the diagnosis can usually be confirmed clinically. In acute obstruction, the main histologic finding is prominent portal tract edema, accompanied by a mixed inflammatory infiltrate and possibly ductular reaction (Fig. 12). Lobular cholestasis is also present, which essentially rules out PBC, given that cholestasis is a late finding in that disease (Fig. 13). Chronic duct obstruction shows portal fibrosis rather than edema; ducts are not lost, unlike in PBC.

Ascending Cholangitis

Ascending cholangitis causes similar biliary-type histologic changes as PBC. The key to the

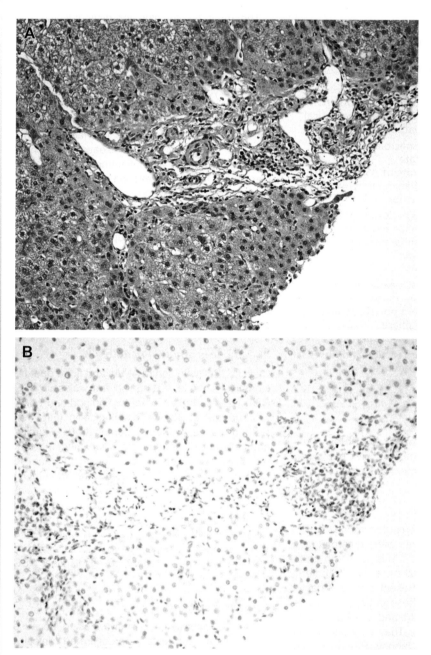

Fig. 3. (A) This portal tract lacks a visible interlobular bile duct. Duct loss is common in the later stages of PBC. (B) An immunostain for CK19, which highlights biliary epithelium, confirms the absence of a bile duct.

diagnosis is the presence of neutrophils in the lumen of a native interlobular bile duct. This must not be confused with neutrophils in and around bile ductular reaction in PBC and other biliary diseases; ductular reaction naturally produces chemokines, which benignly attract neutrophils. This process should not be mistaken for true acute inflammation within portal tracts.

Drug-Induced Liver Injury

Many drugs can cause cholestasis or cholestatic hepatitis, including sulfamethoxazole/ trimethoprim, amoxicillin/clavulanate, antiepileptic medication, and antituberculosis drugs (Fig. 14).[30] Histologic findings are variable but usually include mild portal inflammation, ductular reaction, and cholestasis. Clinical history is important, because a patient's medication list should be reviewed for

Fig. 4. Prolonged chole-stasis leads to cholate stasis, or feathery degen-eration of lobular hepa-tocytes. The cells are enlarged and rounded, with rarefied cytoplasm, intracytoplasmic chole-stasis, and focal Mallory hyaline.

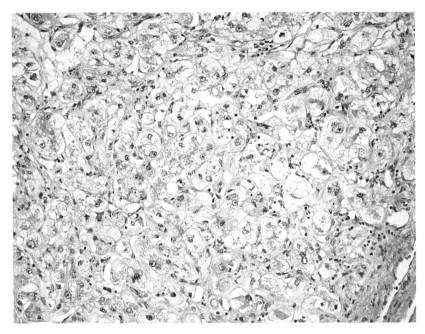

potentially offending substances, and the length of symptoms is important as well. Histologically, these drugs usually cause less ductular reaction than PBC, and they do not induce liver fibrosis. Early cholestasis also strongly suggests a non-PBC etiol-ogy for the findings. In rare instances, herbal sub-stances and some drugs can cause florid duct lesions identical to those in PBC. Drugs have been linked to the formation of M6 but not M2 AMAs.[31]

Various Causes of Granuloma Formation

Other diseases that elicit granuloma formation are unlikely to be confused for PBC, but in cases of a

Fig. 5. An ill-formed epithelioid granuloma populates the center of this inflamed portal tract, encroaching on and destroying the native bile duct.

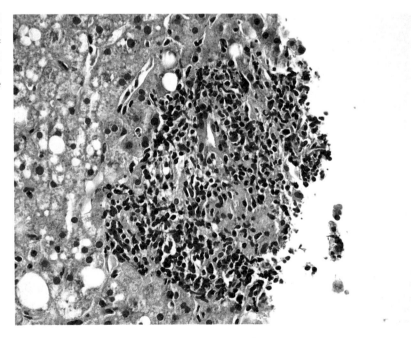

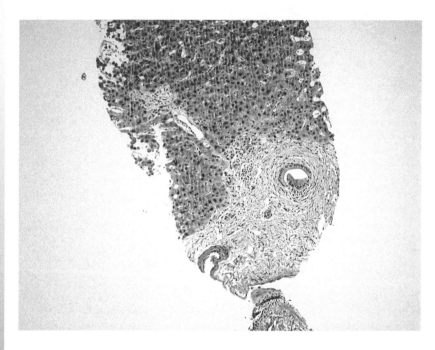

Fig. 6. Larger bile ducts are relatively unaffected in PBC, and lobular inflammation is scant as well.

diagnosis that is not particularly straightforward, the following diseases may need to be considered:

- Sarcoidosis (clinical history essential)
- Tuberculosis (granulomas may be caseating)
- Cytomegalovirus infection (clinical history essential; patients usually immunocompetent, and viral cytopathic effect is rare)

- Drug-induced liver injury (clinical history essential)
- Crohn disease (clinical history essential)

Rare patients have also been reported to have both PBC and idiopathic granulomatous hepatitis.[32]

Various Causes of Cholestasis

Cholestasis arises late in PBC, and the disease usually has had ample time to cause fibrosis and duct loss. The following diseases can cause cholestasis; they are unlikely to be confused for PBC, but the possibility does exist:

- Total parenteral nutrition (clinical history essential)
- Cholestasis of pregnancy (clinical history essential)
- Sepsis (cholestasis sometimes present within duct or ductule lumens)
- Fibrosing cholestatic hepatitis (patients are often immunosuppressed)
- Numerous pediatric liver diseases (patient age rules out PBC)

Various Causes of Duct Loss/Ductopenia

Many longstanding liver diseases can cause duct loss. By the time PBC has caused ductopenia,

Table 1
Scheuer system and Ludwig system for grading of primary biliary cholangitis

Stage	Scheuer Staging System	Ludwig Staging System
1	Florid duct lesions (or nonsuppurative cholangitis)	Portal hepatitis
2	Ductular proliferation	Periportal hepatitis
3	Scarring (or bridging fibrosis)	Bridging necrosis and/or septal fibrosis
4	Cirrhosis	Cirrhosis

Data from Scheuer PJ. Primary biliary cirrhosis. Proc R Soc Med 1967;60:1257–60; and *From* Ludwig J, Dickson ER, McDonald GS. Staging of chronic nonsuppurative destructive cholangitis (syndrome of primary biliary cirrhosis). Virchows Arch A Pathol Anat Histol 1978;379:103–12.

Fig. 7. Cirrhotic nodules in end-stage PBC show a peripheral halo at low power due to cholate stasis and sometimes ductular reaction.

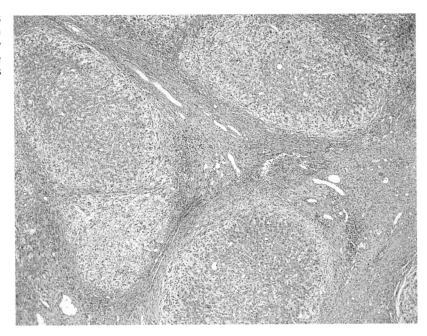

the liver is often quite fibrotic, if not cirrhotic. Still, other diseases may need to be considered:

- Iatrogenic adulthood ductopenia (no fibrosis)
- Chronic (ductopenic) rejection (no fibrosis; clinical history essential)
- Graft-versus-host disease (no fibrosis; clinical history essential)
- Long-term total parenteral nutrition (clinical history essential)

TREATMENT AND PROGNOSIS OF PRIMARY BILIARY CHOLANGITIS

There are no medical treatments for PBC that can halt disease progression, but ursodeoxycholic acid has been show to slow progression and also reduce symptoms.[27] Obeticholic acid recently received conditional approval by the European Medicines Agency as add-on treatment in patients failing treatment with ursodeoxycholic

Fig. 8. This biopsy shows findings identical to those seen in PBC. The patient was negative for AMAs clinically and, therefore, was diagnosed with autoimmune cholangitis.

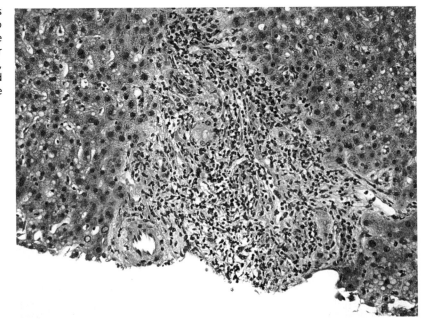

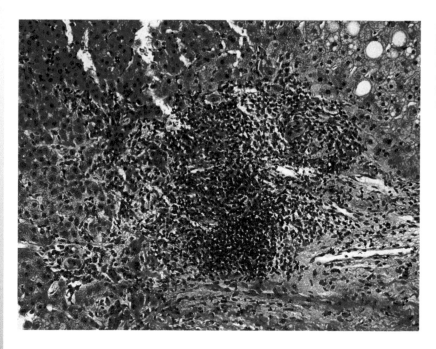

Fig. 9. This prominent portal inflammatory infiltrate in a case of PBC spills into the adjacent hepatocytes. This interface hepatitis can mimic that of AIH.

acid,[33] although serious adverse events may occur.[34] Off-label therapies, such as budesonide, are sometimes also used.[27] Steroids are not indicated unless a patient also has AIH. Ultimately, the only effective treatment is orthotopic liver transplantation; the disease recurs in up to 42% of grafts,[35] and overall survival after transplantation is approximately 75%. The UK-PBC Consortium recently released a laboratory value-based scoring system that appears to predict the risk of a patient dying or requiring liver transplant.[36]

Approximately 25% of symptomatic patients with PBC develop cirrhosis, whereas asymptomatic patients only develop cirrhosis in 5% of cases.[37,38] Symptomatic patients may also

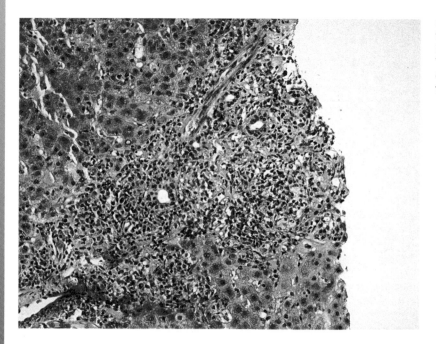

Fig. 10. Bile duct distortion and injury are prominent in this case of AIH. The patient had no clinical features suggestive of PBC.

Table 2
Criteria for diagnosing overlap of primary biliary cholangitis and autoimmune hepatitis

Diagnosis	Criteria
PBC	• Serum alkaline phosphatase ≥2× upper limit of normal or serum γ-glutamyl transpeptidase ≥5× upper limit of normal • AMAs • Liver biopsy showing florid duct lesions
AIH	• Alanine transaminase ≥5× upper limit of normal • IgG ≥2× upper limit of normal or ASMAs • Liver biopsy showing moderate/severe interface hepatitis

Scoring: At least 2 of the 3 criteria must be met for both diagnoses to diagnose PBC-AIH overlap.

Data from Chazouillères O, Wendum D, Serfaty L, et al. Primary biliary cirrhosis-autoimmune hepatitis overlap syndrome: clinical features and response to therapy. Hepatology 1998;28:296–301.

have a shorter disease course, although overall, the length from diagnosis to transplantation or death is approximately 15 to 20 years. Patients are at a slightly increased risk of developing hepatocellular carcinoma, in particular men and those with prolonged biochemical nonresponse to treatment.[39] There is little to no increased risk of developing cholangiocarcinoma, unlike in PSC.

AUTOIMMUNE HEPATITIS

OVERVIEW OF AUTOIMMUNE HEPATITIS

AIH is a common form of hepatitic injury with an incidence of up to 1 per 100,000 people per year in the United States.[40] As with many other autoimmune diseases, AIH affects primarily women, with a male:female ratio of 1:4.[41] Patients can be any age, with incidence peaks in adolescence and middle age.[42] There are technically 3 types of AIH, with the main differences being the type of detectable autoantibody (discussed later).[43] Additionally, type 2 is more common in children. Children with AIH may also have an increased risk of concurrent PSC.[44] Genetically, AIH has been linked to certain HLA DR3 and HLA DR4 alleles.[43]

CLINICAL FEATURES OF AUTOIMMUNE HEPATITIS

AIH is a chronic disease with acute exacerbation, and patients often present during such a flare. Symptoms include abdominal pain, pruritus, nausea, vomiting, and lethargy.[40] Laboratory work shows a marked increase in AST and ALT, accompanied by increased IgG. Mild hyperbilirubinemia may also occur, as well as a mild increase in alkaline phosphatase. Some patients may be

Fig. 11. Onion skin fibrosis surrounds an intermediate-sized bile duct in this case of PSC. Inflammation is mild.

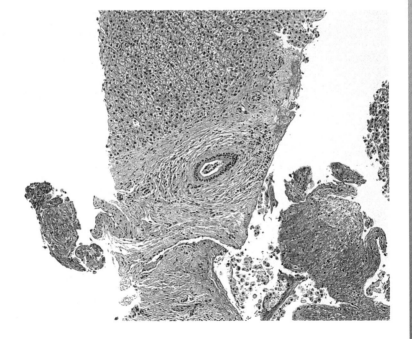

diagnosed during a subclinical moment in their disease course.

> ## Pathologic Key Features
> OF Autoimmune Hepatitis
>
> 1. Impressive portal and lobular chronic inflammation is typical of AIH, with interface hepatitis and acidophil bodies often present.
>
> 2. Severe acute disease may present with centrilobular and/or bridging necrosis.
>
> 3. Hepatocytes may undergo a variety of alterations, including giant multinucleated change, rosette formation, and emperipolesis.
>
> 4. Pediatric cases may show hyaline droplets within Kupffer cells.

AIH type 1 is the most common form of the disease, and patients are usually positive for antinuclear antibodies and ASMA, most often F-actin. A minority of patients are also positive for AMAs. AIH type 2 causes anti–liver/kidney microsomal type 1 antibodies; adults with this type have more severe disease than children. AIH type 3 causes antisoluble liver antigen or liver/pancreas antigen antibodies.[43]

Up to half of patients develop other autoimmune diseases, including but not limited to PBC.[42] Additional testing modalities (such as imaging) are of little help in establishing the diagnosis.

MICROSCOPIC FEATURES OF AUTOIMMUNE HEPATITIS

Liver biopsies from patients with active, untreated AIH show a moderate chronic inflammatory infiltrate in the portal tracts and lobules (**Fig. 15**).[19] Lymphocytes are always present; plasma cells are usually present and conspicuous but may sometimes be subtle or even absent (**Figs. 16** and **17**). The portal inflammation often spills into the surrounding parenchyma, causing interface hepatitis. The lobular activity may be subtle or striking, and acidophil bodies are readily identified (**Fig. 18**). In some patients, the inflammation is focused in zone 3, around the central veins (**Fig. 19**). Patients with severe disease may show either centrilobular zonal necrosis or bridging necrosis, with broad swaths of hepatocyte dropout stretching from portal tracts to central veins. Bridging necrosis may mimic bridging fibrosis on hematoxylin-eosin stain and even on a trichrome stain, but it shows areas of architectural collapse on reticulin stain.

A variety of additional uncommon findings have been reported in AIH as well. A minority of patients show biliary-type changes in the portal tract,[45] including duct inflammation and ductular reaction, and the lobules may sometimes contain cholestasis. Hepatocytes may form rosettes and may engulf inflammatory cells in a nondestructive manner (ie, emperipolesis); these 2 features have been touted as helpful in distinguishing AIH from chronic viral hepatitis.[46] AIH may also rarely cause giant cell change of hepatocytes, similar to that

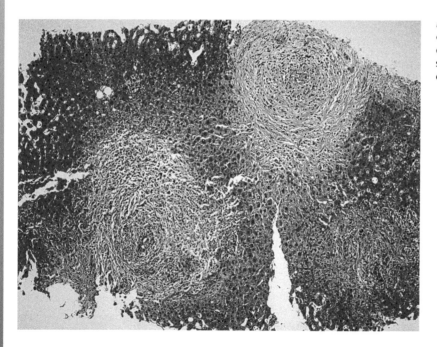

Fig. 12. Acute large duct obstruction is often easily recognized by striking portal tract edema.

Fig. 13. Cholestasis oc-curs very early in large duct obstruction, whereas it is a late finding in PBC.

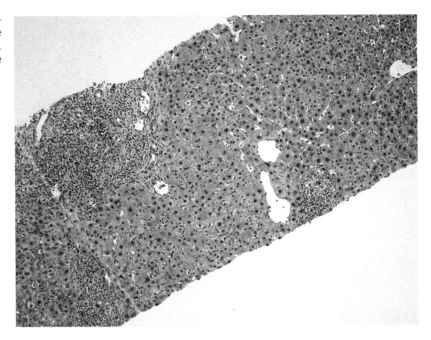

seen in many pediatric liver diseases (**Fig. 20**). Hy-aline droplets in Kupffer cells have recently been described in some pediatric patients with AIH.[47,48]

Because AIH is a chronic disease that may have spent years damaging a patient's liver prior to clin-ical presentation, well-developed fibrosis may be present on initial biopsy, even in patients who pre-sent acutely.[49] Up to one-third of patients may even be cirrhotic at presentation, and this risk is increased if the patient also has nonalcoholic stea-tohepatitis.[50] The disease follows the stereotypical pathway of portal fibrosis leading to periportal fibrosis, then bridging fibrosis, and ultimately cirrhosis. Once a liver is cirrhotic, it may be difficult or impossible to establish that AIH was the cause without clinical information or a prior diagnosis.

Fig. 14. This patient developed cholestatic hepatitis clinically after taking amoxicillin/clavu-lanate. Liver biopsy showed bile duct distor-tion, ductular reaction, and lobular cholestasis.

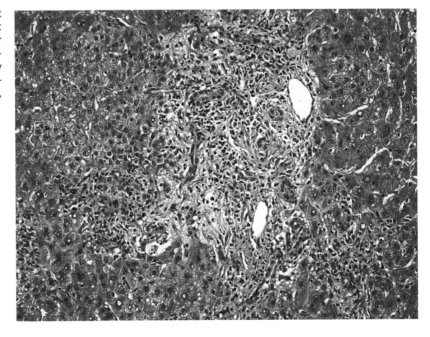

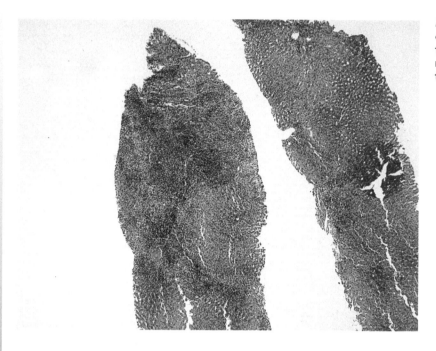

Fig. 15. Untreated AIH often shows moderate to severe chronic inflammation in the portal tracts and lobules.

Biopsies from patients receiving treatment for AIH may show a markedly reduced inflammatory infiltrate, with few or no lymphocytes or plasma cells in the portal tracts or lobules (**Fig. 21**). Similarly reduced inflammation can be seen in older patients.

Patients with striking clinical and pathologic features of biliary disease may have PBC or PSC in addition to AIH.

DIAGNOSIS AND DIFFERENTIAL DIAGNOSIS OF AUTOIMMUNE HEPATITIS

The International Autoimmune Hepatitis Group has issued a series of diagnostic criteria for AIH, along with a detailed scoring system with high sensitivity[51] and a simplified scoring system based on patient autoantibodies, IgG value, histology, and absence of viral hepatitis.[52] Other investigators have proposed purely histology-based scoring

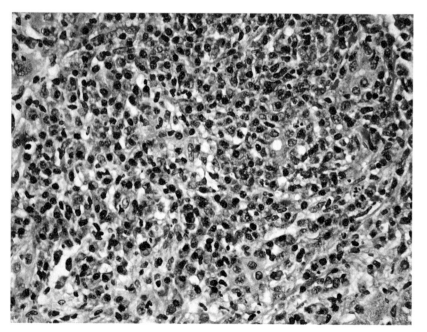

Fig. 16. Plasma cells are easily recognized as the predominant component of the portal inflammatory infiltrate in this case of AIH.

systems for AIH, some of which include ancillary staining.[53]

Pitfalls
IN DIAGNOSING
AUTOIMMUNE HEPATITIS

! Plasma cells do not have to be abundant to make a diagnosis of AIH; they are in fact sometimes absent.

! Patients receiving steroids may have little to no inflammation on liver biopsy.

! Bile duct distortion and inflammation may occur in AIH and do not necessarily indicate an overlap with PSC or PBC.

! Drug-induced AIH can mimic non–drug-induced disease both clinically and pathologically, although drug-induced cases should not show advanced fibrosis.

Differential Diagnosis
IN AUTOIMMUNE HEPATITIS

AIH vs	Helpful Distinguishing Features
PBC	No lobular necroinflammatory infiltrate Lower rate of ASMAs Duct destruction with florid duct lesions
Chronic viral hepatitis	Interface and lobular hepatitis often milder May show lymphoid follicles or ground-glass nuclei Viral serology/molecular testing is confirmatory
Wilson disease	Glycogenated nuclei and macrovesicular steatosis Rosettes and emperipolesis not seen Copper quantitation is confirmatory
IgG4-related sclerosing cholangitis	Clinical stricturing of bile ducts Perivenular inflammation with phlebitis Plasma cells are positive for IgG4 by immunohistochemistry
Drug-induced liver injury	May mimic AIH very closely Less fibrosis on biopsy Review of medication list is essential

The European Association for the Study of the Liver recently released comprehensive clinical practice guidelines for AIH.[42]

Primary Biliary Cholangitis

The finer points of distinguishing AIH from PBC are discussed previously. The 2 diagnoses can mimic one another both clinically and microscopically, meaning careful review of a patient's clinical information is warranted. Diagnosis of AIH-PBC overlap should be treated with care and not suggested without reasonable confidence.

Chronic Viral Hepatitis

Chronic infections with hepatitis B virus and hepatitis C virus are the main forms of chronic hepatitis aside from AIH. All 3 diseases can cause an increase in ALT and AST, although only AIH causes ASMA and increased IgG. Chronic viral hepatitis usually is diagnosed clinically based on serologic and molecular testing. Microscopically, chronic hepatitis C usually demonstrates lymphocytic inflammation neatly confined to the portal tracts, with little in the way of plasma cells, interface hepatitis, or lobular inflammation. Hepatitis B virus may show similar features to hepatitis C; the famed ground-glass hepatocytes of hepatitis B infection are not seen in all cases, and patients taking medications such as mycophoenolate mofetil and azathioprine for AIH may rarely develop glycogen pseudoinclusions that mimic ground-glass hepatocytes (**Fig. 22**).[54,55] As discussed previously, hepatocyte rosettes and emperipolesis favor AIH, although they can sometimes be seen in viral hepatitis.[46]

Wilson Disease

Wilson disease can cause a variety of histologic changes, including those that mimic AIH.[56] It can also present in acute or fulminant fashion. Tissue copper quantitation would be high in Wilson disease and normal in AIH, and patients with Wilson disease do not develop autoantibodies. Wilson disease can cause macrovesicular steatosis, although patients with AIH may also have nonalcoholic fatty liver disease.

IgG4-Related Sclerosing Cholangitis

IgG4-related sclerosing cholangitis clinically mimics PSC, with increased alkaline phosphatase and patchy stricturing of the intrahepatic and extrahepatic biliary tree.[57] Microscopically, the disease shows an abundant plasmacytic infiltrate

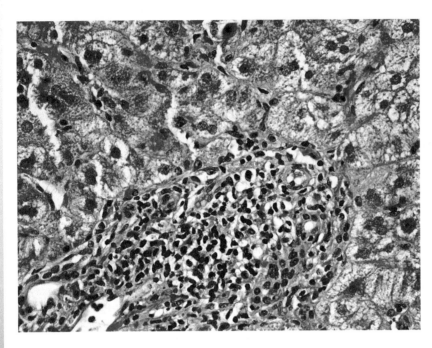

Fig. 17. In contrast to Fig. 16, lymphocytes predominate in this case of AIH; plasma cells are rare.

that can affect the liver, potentially mimicking AIH. The inflammation targets veins and can cause obliterative phlebitis, and storiform fibrosis may be seen in the background. Clinical history, combined with an immunohistochemical stain for IgG4, should quickly resolve the differential diagnosis.

Drug-Induced Liver Injury

Medications such as minocycline and nitrofurantoin can cause a hepatitic pattern of injury, sometimes with prominent lymphocytic inflammation that suggests the diagnosis of AIH.[30] The lack of fibrosis in these cases is a strong clue that a true chronic hepatitis is not at work. Rare patients

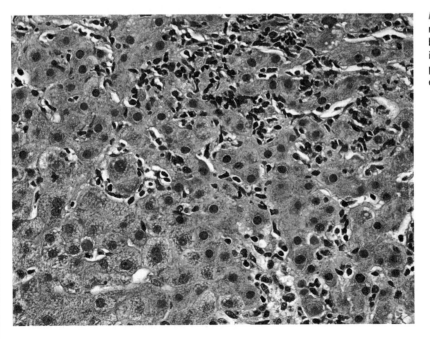

Fig. 18. Lobular inflammation and acidophil bodies are easily spotted in AIH; the presence of plasma cells supports the diagnosis.

Fig. 19. Centrilobular (zone 3) inflammation and hepatocyte dropout is not uncommon in AIH, especially in cases presenting acutely.

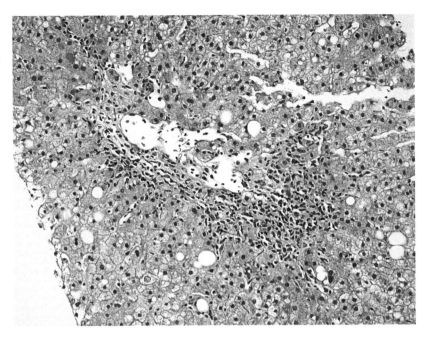

develop drug-induced AIH, where the biopsy findings are classic for AIH and clinical serology demonstrates ASMA or other autoantibodies (**Fig. 23**).[58] Thorough clinical work-up is essential to pinpoint a drug as the cause of these patients' disease. Patients with drug-induced AIH generally respond to immunosuppression, and the disease does not recur after withdrawal of treatment, unlike AIH.

Autoimmune Hepatitis–Like Disease in the Transplanted Liver

Patients transplanted for end-stage liver disease secondary to AIH can experience disease recurrence; this should be the favored diagnosis when encountering a necroinflammatory lymphoplasmacytic process that does not seem to represent acute cellular rejection and there is no evidence for viral infection.

Fig. 20. Focal giant multinucleated hepatocytes can be seen (*arrows*).

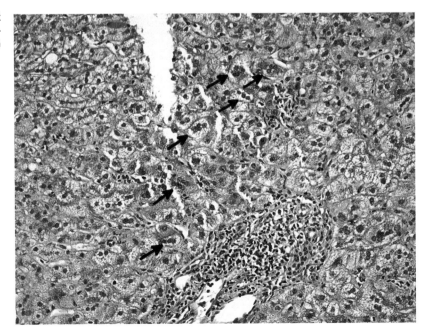

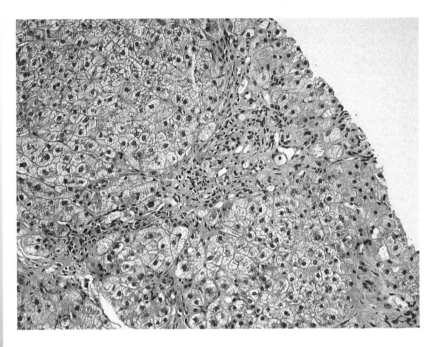

Fig. 21. If patients are receiving adequate treatment of their AIH (eg, steroids), their liver biopsies may show very mild inflammation.

Some patients transplanted for non-AIH reasons may develop AIH-like findings in their allograft. This is generally considered a variant of acute cellular rejection and has been given several names, including alloimmune hepatitis, de novo autoimmune hepatitis, and plasma cell hepatitis.[59]

PROGNOSIS OF AUTOIMMUNE HEPATITIS

AIH responds to prednisone in such a striking manner that if a patient with presumed AIH does not improve on such therapy, the diagnosis should be questioned.[60] This therapy both treats symptoms and prolongs patient survival. Patients with

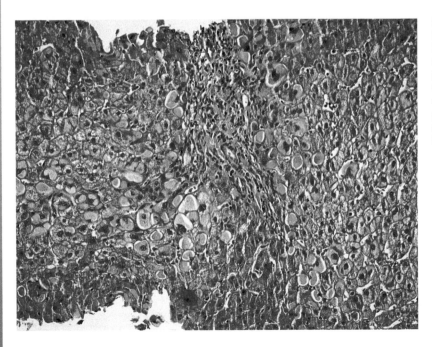

Fig. 22. This patient was taking azathioprine to treat AIH. Use of this medication resulted in glycogen accumulation within hepatocytes, which mimics the ground-glass cytoplasm characteristic of chronic hepatitis B infection.

Fig. 23. Shortly after beginning etanercept (a tumor necrosis factor inhibitor), this patient developed increased liver enzymes and anti–F-actin antibodies. Liver biopsy findings were indistinguishable from those of non–drug-induced AIH, save for a lack of fibrosis.

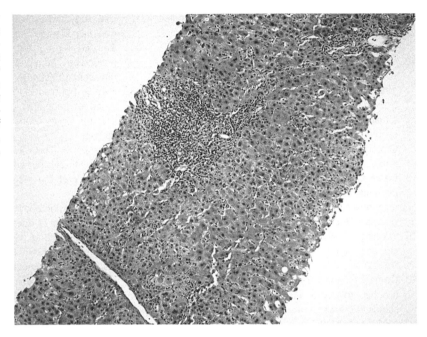

AIH and a concomitant liver disease, such as nonalcoholic steatohepatitis, often have a poorer prognosis.[61]

Untreated or poorly controlled AIH ultimately causes end-stage liver disease, requiring orthotopic liver transplantation. Such patients may be at increased risk for portal vein thrombosis.[62] The vast majority of patients do well after transplant, with a 5-year survival rate of 96%, although the disease recurs in up to 42% of patients.[35]

REFERENCES

1. Lindor KD, Kowdley KV, Harrison ME, American College of Gastroenterology. ACG clinical guideline: primary sclerosing cholangitis. Am J Gastroenterol 2015;110:646–59.
2. Beuers U, Gershwin ME, Gish RG, et al. Changing nomenclature for PBC: from 'cirrhosis' to 'cholangitis'. Hepatology 2015;62:1620–2.
3. Saxena R, Hytiroglou P, Thung SN, et al. Destruction of canals of Hering in primary biliary cirrhosis. Hum Pathol 2002;33:983–8.
4. Boonstra K, Beuers U, Ponsioen CY. Epidemiology of primary sclerosing cholangitis and primary biliary cirrhosis: a systematic review. J Hepatol 2012;56:1181–8.
5. Griffiths L, Dyson JK, Jones DE. The new epidemiology of primary biliary cirrhosis. Semin Liver Dis 2014;34:318–28.
6. Kim WR, Lindor KD, Locke GR 3rd, et al. Epidemiology and natural history of primary biliary cirrhosis in a US community. Gastroenterology 2000;119:1631–6.
7. Qiu F, Tang R, Zuo X, et al. A genome-wide association study identifies six novel risk loci for primary biliary cholangitis. Nat Commun 2017;8:14828.
8. Lazaridis KN, Juran BD, Boe GM, et al. Increased prevalence of antimitochondrial antibodies in first-degree relatives of patients with primary biliary cirrhosis. Hepatology 2007;46:785–92.
9. Kaplan MM, Gershwin ME. Primary biliary cirrhosis. N Engl J Med 2005;353:1261–73.
10. Matsuo I, Omagari K, Kinoshita H, et al. Elevation of serum gamma-glutamyl transpeptidase precedes that of alkaline phosphatase in the early stages of primary biliary cirrhosis. Hepatol Res 1999;3:223–32.
11. Gershwin ME, Rowley M, Davis PA, et al. Molecular biology of the 2-oxo-acid dehydrogenase complexes and anti-mitochondrial antibodies. Prog Liver Dis 1992;10:47–61.
12. Ozaslan E, Efe C, Gokbulut Ozaslan N. The diagnosis of antimitochondrial antibody-negative primary biliary cholangitis. Clin Res Hepatol Gastroenterol 2016;40:553–61.
13. Dahlqvist G, Gaouar F, Carrat F, et al. Large-scale characterization study of patients with antimitochondrial antibodies but nonestablished primary biliary cholangitis. Hepatology 2017;65:152–63.
14. Kurki P, Miettinen A, Linder E, et al. Different types of smooth muscle antibodies in chronic active hepatitis and primary biliary cirrhosis: their diagnostic and prognostic significance. Gut 1980;21:878–84.

15. Worman HJ, Courvalin JC. Antinuclear antibodies specific for primary biliary cirrhosis. Autoimmun Rev 2003;2:211–7.

16. Culp KS, Fleming CR, Duffy J, et al. Autoimmune associations in primary biliary cirrhosis. Mayo Clin Proc 1982;57:365–70.

17. Boberg KM, Chapman RW, Hirschfield GM, et al, International Autoimmune Hepatitis Group. Overlap syndromes: the International Autoimmune Hepatitis Group (IAIHG) position statement on a controversial issue. J Hepatol 2011;54:374–85.

18. Degott C, Zafrani ES, Callard P, et al. Histopathological study of primary biliary cirrhosis and the effect of ursodeoxycholic acid treatment on histology progression. Hepatology 1999;29:1007–12.

19. Washington MK. Autoimmune liver disease: overlap and outliers. Mod Pathol 2007;20(Suppl 1): S15–30.

20. Colina F, Pinedo F, Solís JA, et al. Nodular regenerative hyperplasia of the liver in early histological stages of primary biliary cirrhosis. Gastroenterology 1992;102:1319–24.

21. Graham RP, Smyrk TC, Zhang L. Evaluation of langerhans cell infiltrate by CD1a immunostain in liver biopsy for the diagnosis of primary biliary cirrhosis. Am J Surg Pathol 2012;36:732–6.

22. Bateman AC, Hübscher SG. Cytokeratin expression as an aid to diagnosis in medical liver biopsies. Histopathology 2010;56:415–25.

23. Scheuer P. Primary biliary cirrhosis. Proc R Soc Med 1967;60:1257–60.

24. Ludwig J, Dickson ER, McDonald GS. Staging of chronic nonsuppurative destructive cholangitis (syndrome of primary biliary cirrhosis). Virchows Arch A Pathol Anat Histol 1978;379:103–12.

25. Kakuda Y, Harada K, Sawada-Kitamura S, et al. Evaluation of a new histologic staging and grading system for primary biliary cirrhosis in comparison with classical systems. Hum Pathol 2013;44: 1107–17.

26. Nguyen DL, Juran BD, Lazaridis KN. Primary biliary cirrhosis. Best Pract Res Clin Gastroenterol 2010;24: 647–54.

27. European Association for the Study of the Liver. EASL clinical practice guidelines: the diagnosis and management of patients with primary biliary cholangitis. J Hepatol 2017;67:145–72.

28. Moreira RK, Revetta F, Koehler E, et al. Diagnostic utility of IgG and IgM immunohistochemistry in autoimmune liver disease. World J Gastroenterol 2010; 16:453–7.

29. Chazouillères O, Wendum D, Serfaty L, et al. Primary biliary cirrhosis-autoimmune hepatitis overlap syndrome: clinical features and response to therapy. Hepatology 1998;28:296–301.

30. Kleiner DE. Liver injury due to drugs and herbal agents. In: Saxil R, editor. Practical hepatic pathology: a diagnostic approach. 2nd edition. Philadelphia: Elsevier Saunders; 2018. p. 327–70.

31. Berg PA, Klein R. Mitochondrial antigens and autoantibodies: from anti-M1 to anti-M9. Klin Wochenschr 1986;64:897–909.

32. Paul S, Sepehr GJ, Weinstein B, et al. Co-occurrence of idiopathic granulomatous hepatitis and primary biliary cirrhosis. Dig Dis Sci 2014;59: 2831–5.

33. Invernizzi P, Floreani A, Carbone M, et al. Primary biliary cholangitis: advances in management and treatment of the disease. Dig Liver Dis 2017;49: 841–6.

34. Nevens F, Andreone P, Mazzella G, et al. A placebo-controlled trial of obeticholic acid in primary biliary cholangitis. N Engl J Med 2016;375:631–43.

35. Visseren T, Darwish Murad S. Recurrence of primary sclerosing cholangitis, primary biliary cholangitis and auto-immune hepatitis after liver transplantation. Best Pract Res Clin Gastroenterol 2017;31:187–98.

36. Carbone M, Sharp SJ, Flack S, et al. The UK-PBC risk scores: derivation and validation of a scoring system for long-term prediction of end-stage liver disease in primary biliary cholangitis. Hepatology 2016;63:930–50.

37. Prince M, Chetwynd A, Newman W, et al. Survival and symptom progression in a geographically based cohort of patients with primary biliary cirrhosis: follow-up for up to 28 years. Gastroenterology 2002;123:1044–51.

38. Prince MI, Chetwynd A, Craig WL, et al. Asymptomatic primary biliary cirrhosis: clinical features, prognosis, and symptom progression in a large population based cohort. Gut 2004;53:865–70.

39. Trivedi PJ, Lammers WJ, van Buuren HR, et al. Stratification of hepatocellular carcinoma risk in primary biliary cirrhosis: a multicentre international study. Gut 2016;65:321–9.

40. Gossard AA, Lindor KD. Autoimmune hepatitis: a review. J Gastroenterol 2012;47:498–503.

41. Francque S, Vonghia L, Ramon A, et al. Epidemiology and treatment of autoimmune hepatitis. Hepat Med 2012;4:1–10.

42. European Association for the Study of the Liver. EASL clinical practice guidelines: autoimmune hepatitis. J Hepatol 2015;63:971–1004.

43. Oo YH, Hubscher SG, Adams DH. Autoimmune hepatitis: new paradigms in the pathogenesis, diagnosis, and management. Hepatol Int 2010;4:475–93.

44. Gregorio GV, Portmann B, Karani J, et al. Autoimmune hepatitis/sclerosing cholangitis overlap syndrome in childhood: a 16-year prospective study. Hepatology 2001;33:544–53.

45. Czaja AJ, Carpenter HA. Autoimmune hepatitis with incidental histologic features of bile duct injury. Hepatology 2001;34:659–65.

46. de Boer YS, van Nieuwkerk CM, Witte BI, et al. Assessment of the histopathological key features in autoimmune hepatitis. Histopathology 2015;66: 351–62.

47. Tucker SM, Jonas MM, Perez-Atayde AR. Hyaline droplets in Kupffer cells: a novel diagnostic clue for autoimmune hepatitis. Am J Surg Pathol 2015; 39:772–8.

48. Lotowska JM, Sobaniec-Lotowska ME, Daniluk U, et al. Glassy droplet inclusions within the cytoplasm of Kupffer cells: a novel ultrastructural feature for the diagnosis of pediatric autoimmune hepatitis. Dig Liver Dis 2017;49:929–33.

49. Nguyen Canh H, Harada K, Ouchi H, et al. Acute presentation of autoimmune hepatitis: a multicentre study with detailed histological evaluation in a large cohort of patients. J Clin Pathol 2017;70:961–9, [Epub ahead of print].

50. De Luca-Johnson J, Wangensteen KJ, Hanson J, et al. Natural history of patients presenting with autoimmune hepatitis and coincident nonalcoholic fatty liver disease. Dig Dis Sci 2016;61:2710–20.

51. Alvarez F, Berg PA, Bianchi FB, et al. International autoimmune hepatitis group report: review of criteria for diagnosis of autoimmune hepatitis. J Hepatol 1999;31:929–38.

52. Hennes EM, Zeniya M, Czaja AJ, et al. Simplified criteria for the diagnosis of autoimmune hepatitis. Hepatology 2008;48:169–76.

53. Balitzer D, Shafizadeh N, Peters MG, et al. Autoimmune hepatitis: review of histologic features included in the simplified criteria proposed by the international autoimmune hepatitis group and proposal for new histologic criteria. Mod Pathol 2017;30:773–83.

54. Brunt EM, Di Bisceglie AM. Histological changes after the use of mycophenolate mofetil in autoimmune hepatitis. Hum Pathol 2004;35:509–12.

55. Chan AWH, Quaglia A, Haugk B, et al. Atlas of liver pathology. New York: Springer; 2014. p. 136.

56. Stromeyer FW, Ishak KG. Histology of the liver in Wilson's disease: a study of 34 cases. Am J Clin Pathol 1980;73:12–24.

57. Deshpande V, Sainani NI, Chung RT, et al. IgG4-associated cholangitis: a comparative histological and immunophenotypic study with primary sclerosing cholangitis on liver biopsy material. Mod Pathol 2009;22:1287–95.

58. Björnsson E, Talwalkar J, Treeprasertsuk S, et al. Drug-induced autoimmune hepatitis: clinical characteristics and prognosis. Hepatology 2010;51: 2040–8.

59. Fiel MI, Schiano TD. Plasma cell hepatitis (de-novo autoimmune hepatitis) developing post liver transplantation. Curr Opin Organ Transplant 2012;17: 287–92.

60. Czaja AJ. Difficult treatment decisions in autoimmune hepatitis. World J Gastroenterol 2010;16: 934–47.

61. Aizawa Y, Hokari A. Autoimmune hepatitis: current challenges and future prospects. Clin Exp Gastroenterol 2017;10:9–18.

62. Ruiz P, Sastre L, Crespo G, et al. Increased risk of portal vein thrombosis in patients with autoimmune hepatitis on the liver transplantation waiting list. Clin Transplant 2017;31:e13001.

Hepatic Adenomas
Classification, Controversies, and Consensus

Michael Torbenson, MD

KEYWORDS

- Hepatic adenoma • Heptaocellular adenoma • Histology • Pathology • Classification
- Inflammatory adenoma • HNF1 alpha inactivated adenoma • Beta-catenin activated adenoma
- Androgen adenoma • Pigmented adenoma • Myxoid adenoma • Malignant transformation

Key points

- Hepatocellular adenomas are classified using immunostains in order to identify tumors at greatest risk for malignant transformation and for hemorrhage.

- These three rare types of hepatocellular adenomas do not fit as well in the current classification system, but are also at high risk for malignancy: androgen related hepatocellular adenomas, pigmented hepatocellular adenomas, myxoid hepatocellular adenomas.

- Risk factors for malignant transformation include patient gender, patient age, adenoma size, cytological atypia, beta-catenin activation, adenoma subtype.

ABSTRACT

Rapid advances in molecular and anatomic pathology have greatly improved our understanding of hepatocellular adenomas. Principle among them is a clinically relevant, histology-based classification that identifies hepatic adenomas at greatest risk for malignant transformation. This new classification system has led to general consensus on the major subtypes of hepatic adenomas. However, controversy remains regarding how to incorporate less common types of hepatic adenomas into the classification system and how to incorporate adenoma subtyping into clinical care. This article provides an in-depth review of how adenomas are classified, with a focus on the current rationale, the consensus, and controversies.

OVERVIEW

There have been rapid advances in our understanding of hepatic adenomas over the past decade or so. Notable advances include a clinically relevant, histology based classification system, recognition that fatty liver disease is a risk factor for inflammatory adenomas, and further clarification of risk factors for malignant transformation. In terms of nomenclature, hepatic adenoma and hepatocellular adenoma are synonyms and can be used interchangeably. Liver adenoma or liver cell adenoma are sometimes used, but are less desirable terms, because a bile duct adenoma would in theory also be covered by these more generic terms.

DEFINITION

Hepatic adenomas are benign, clonal proliferations of phenotypically mature hepatocytes. By light microscopy, they have no or minimal cytologic or architectural atypia. By molecular analysis they are chromosomal stable, with few mutations compared with hepatocellular carcinomas. Hepatic adenomatosis is defined as the presence of 10 or more adenomas. Hepatic adenomas occur in livers without cirrhosis. In most cases, the background liver is histologically normal, but steatosis or steatohepatitis can be found and are recognized as risk factors for inflammatory adenomas.[1]

Department of Laboratory Medicine and Pathology, 100 1st SE, Rochester, MN 55905, USA
E-mail address: Torbenson.michael@mayo.edu

Surgical Pathology 11 (2018) 351–366
https://doi.org/10.1016/j.path.2018.02.007

HEPATIC ADENOMA-LIKE NODULES IN CIRRHOTIC LIVERS

Several studies[2–5] have described nodules in alcohol related cirrhotic livers that are positive for serum amyloid A (SAA) by immunohistochemistry, and some studies have suggested using the term *hepatic adenoma* for these lesions. Although the data are interesting and important, the suggestion to call these lesions adenomas is premature and not warranted by the currently available data. The argument for calling these nodules adenomas is essentially that they are not hepatocellular carcinomas, they look somewhat like adenomas by light microscopy, and a subset stain with SAA and/or C-reactive protein (CRP) by immunohistochemistry. However, the morphology is often not typical of inflammatory adenomas.[2] In addition, a subset of both ordinary cirrhotic nodules and of hepatocellular carcinomas stain with CRP and SAA, so the mere fact of staining for these proteins does not indicate their proper classification is hepatic adenoma. Put another way, shared dysregulation of a common cellular signaling pathway by 2 lesions does not mean they are the same tumor. For example, fibrolamellar carcinomas can show reduced or absent expression of liver fatty acid binding protein (LFABP),[6] but this does not make them HNF1-alpha–inactivated hepatic adenomas. Nor is it informative if these SAA-positive lesions are clonal, because macroregenerative nodules are frequently clonal in cirrhosis.[7]

There are plausible scenarios to explain rare lesions that morphologically resemble inflammatory adenomas in cirrhotic livers. For example, the hepatic adenomas could have developed first because of the alcoholic liver disease, with the subsequent development of cirrhosis, also secondary to the alcohol use. Even if this were the case, the biological behavior of these lesions is not known. In contrast, the natural history of hepatic adenomas is well-established—they are benign with a small risk of malignant transformation, a risk that is predicted by clinical, histologic, and molecular findings. Lumping these entities together is currently not supported by published literature and it is hard to see how such an approach is in the best interest of patients.

For these reasons, making a diagnosis of a hepatic adenoma in a needle biopsy of a nodule in a cirrhotic liver is very strongly discouraged. In a fully resected specimen, the distinction is perhaps more of academic interest than clinical relevance, but classifying these SAA-positive nodules as definite hepatic adenomas still erodes the well-established clinicopathologic entity known as hepatic adenoma. Perhaps the landscape will change in the future, but at this point it is best to not classify these lesions as hepatic adenomas.

CLINICAL FINDINGS

Overall, 80% to 90% hepatic adenomas occur in one of the following settings[8]: (1) young to middle-aged women with exogenous estrogen use and (2) young to middle-aged women with fatty liver disease, a risk factor that also is most likely acting through endogenous estrogen increases. Excess androgen exposure in either young men or young women is also a well-recognized risk factor for hepatic adenomas. Other risk factors for adenomas include mechanical diseases leading to abnormal hepatic blood inflow (eg, Abernathy syndrome) or abnormal blood outflow (eg, Budd–Chiari syndrome),[9,10] genetic metabolic diseases (eg, glycogen storage disease, principally but not exclusively type 1), and McCune–Albright syndrome.[11]

Serum levels of CRP can be increased in cases of inflammatory adenomas, but practically speaking there are no blood tests clinically helpful in diagnosing or managing hepatic adenomas. Serologic studies show normal levels of alpha-fetoprotein and normal or mild nonspecific increases in liver enzymes.

CLINICAL MANAGEMENT

Guidelines from both the European Association for Study of the Liver[12] and the American College of Gastroenterology[13] do not recommend a routine role for biopsy in the diagnosis of hepatic adenoma, or for histologic subtype determination, but instead recommend biopsies only if imaging findings are not typical for a hepatic adenoma. This clinical management approach is based on published papers that report a very high sensitivity and specificity for diagnosing hepatic adenomas using MRI—performance characteristics that do not always match the experience of many clinicians in their local practice, so biopsies for diagnosing hepatic adenomas are still fairly common. Once a hepatic adenoma is diagnosed by imaging or histology, most cases are managed by the risk factors of gender and lesion size and interval growth, with tumors referred for surgery when they are in men, greater than 5 cm, or show interval growth during follow-up. When available, histologic risk factors (atypical cytology, beta-catenin activation) can also be used to guide management.

DIAGNOSTIC APPROACH

Hepatic adenomas are well-differentiated tumors with little or no cytologic atypia. At high power, the tumor cells should look essentially like the hepatocytes in the background liver (**Fig. 1**A, B). Mild patchy nuclear enlargement is common in

Fig. 1. Hepatic adenoma. (*A*) This hepatic adenoma shows essentially no cytologic atypia, but there is a very subtle increase in the N:C ratio. (*B*) The background liver from the same case in A is shown. (*C*) This inflammatory adenoma shows mild patchy cytologic atypia, with rare tumor cells showing larger and hyperchromatic nuclei, but with a generally preserved N:C ratio.

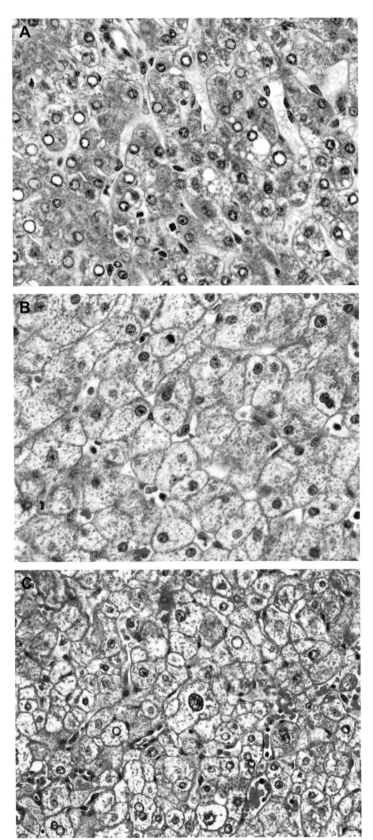

inflammatory adenomas (see **Fig. 1**C), but the cells retain a near normal N:C ratio, have nice round nuclei, and nuclear hyperchromasia is mild. More than minimal patchy cytologic atypia suggests hepatocellular carcinoma. Additional findings that can strongly suggest hepatocellular carcinoma include numerous Mallory–Denk bodies or eosinophilic inclusions in tumor cells, a macrotrabecular growth pattern, or small cell change. Outside of androgen-related adenomas, pseudoglands/hepatocellular rosettes and cholestasis are atypical findings. A nodule-in-nodule growth pattern almost always indicates malignant transformation to hepatocellular carcinoma. There should be no reticulin loss—remembering that focal reticulin loss is acceptable in areas of marked steatosis.[14]

Immunohistochemical stains are important in making a diagnosis of hepatic adenoma. A Ki-67 stain will show a proliferative rate of generally 2% or less. The best way to use the Ki-67 stain is to compare the tumor to the background liver—there should be no real difference detectable by visual examination. Glypican 3 should be negative, but remember that lipofuscin will often cross-react with glypican 3, so correlation of any positive staining with the hematoxylin and eosin (H&E) findings is necessary. Negative glypican 3 staining is not informative, because a large percent of well-differentiated hepatocellular carcinomas are negative. CD34 staining is advocated by some authors as a useful tool, with diffuse staining of the sinusoids favoring hepatocellular carcinoma and patchy staining favoring hepatic adenomas. However, this distinction is often not helpful, especially in biopsy specimens, because adenomas can show strong diffuse staining and some hepatocellular carcinomas will not. For these reasons, CD34 must be interpreted cautiously, and is not as useful as other stains. One study found that hepatic adenomas with diffuse CD34 staining were more likely to be beta-catenin activated or of the unclassified subtype.[15] Importantly, the immunostains used to subtype hepatic adenomas (LFABP, beta-catenin, glutamine synthetase, CRP, SAA) play no role in distinguishing an adenoma from hepatocellular carcinoma.[16]

GENERAL OVERVIEW OF HEPATIC ADENOMA SUBTYPES

There are several arguments for the importance of subtype determination. Hepatic adenoma subtypes have clinical relevance because they stratify for the risk of malignant transformation (beta-catenin–activated adenomas) and for the risk of tumor hemorrhage (beta-catenin–

activated adenomas, inflammatory adenomas, and potentially hedgehog-activated adenomas and adenomas positive for argininosuccinate synthase). Although size and clinical findings remain the foundation of current management strategies in most centers, histologic subclassification can help to guide management in several settings, including when there are ambiguous imaging characteristics, inadequate MRI access for follow-up, comorbidities that make surgical resection unadvisable, or patient reluctance for surgery in adenomas greater than 5 cm. HNF1-alpha–inactivated adenomas have a lower risk for malignant transformation, and identification of this subtype can give reassurance for continued monitoring instead of resection.

In a few percent of cases, the morphologic and immunohistochemical findings do not distinguish a hepatic adenoma from a well-differentiated hepatocellular carcinoma, principally because of cytologic atypia that is more than usual for an adenoma, but not enough for a firm diagnosis of well-differentiated hepatocellular carcinoma. In other cases, there may be equivocal reticulin loss or a Ki-67 proliferative rate that is clearly above the background liver. Difficulty in distinguishing a hepatic adenoma from a well-differentiated hepatocellular carcinoma occurs primarily in needle biopsies, but also sometimes even in fully resected specimens. Internal or external consultation with colleagues can be helpful on these cases. For those tumors that are unclassifiable as adenoma versus hepatocellular carcinoma, the diagnostic line in the surgical pathology report can vary depending on the case and the degree of suspicious for malignancy. Terms such as atypical hepatic adenoma, well-differentiated hepatic neoplasm of uncertain malignant potential,[17] or well-differentiated hepatic neoplasm, see note, are all appropriate on rare occasions. Regardless of the terminology in the diagnostic line, a comment should be included in the surgical pathology report that clearly states the reason(s) why the tumor is not readily classified. In these cases, rebiopsy can be very helpful, especially if the first biopsy was small or fragmented. Difficulty distinguishing a hepatic adenoma from a well-differentiated hepatocellular carcinoma histologically, despite an adequate biopsy, favors resection as the primary management, even if the tumor is less than 5 cm.

Although there are correlations between adenoma subtypes and radiologic imaging findings, proper subtyping can only be done using tissue for histology or molecular analysis; radiology alone is insufficient. When adenoma subtyping is deemed necessary for patient management, histologic and immunohistologic study are generally sufficient, although molecular analysis can be a helpful adjunct. Currently, most centers manage adenomas without relying on histologic subtyping for every case, instead relying on size, imaging, and clinical findings to guide treatment and follow-up decisions. If the clinical scenario and the imaging findings are typical for hepatic adenoma, and the imaging findings are stable over time, a biopsy will often not be performed. Biopsies are generally performed when there are atypical clinical or radiologic findings, or after interval growth of the tumor.

SUBTYPE DETERMINATION

It is important to make the diagnosis of hepatic adenoma and exclude hepatocellular carcinoma before using the immunostains to determine the adenoma subtype. Each of the immunostains used to define adenoma subtypes are also abnormal in a subset of hepatocellular carcinomas,[16] so these stains play no role in distinguishing an adenoma from a hepatocellular carcinoma (Table 1). They also play no role in determining whether a hepatocellular carcinoma arose from a preexisting hepatic adenoma.

A series of important papers showed that hepatic adenomas are genetically and histologically heterogeneous.[18–20] These genetic changes were then used to classify adenomas into 4 subtypes, and immunostain markers were developed that allowed their identification by routine surgical pathology: HNF1-alpha–inactivated adenoma, inflammatory adenoma, beta-catenin activated adenoma, and unclassified adenoma. Morphologic correlates were identified primarily for the HNF1-alpha–inactivated adenomas and inflammatory adenomas.

H&E morphology and genotype correlations were developed principally from estrogen-associated adenomas and they do not always fit as well for adenomas that develop in other settings. For example, hepatic adenomas arising in the setting of glycogen storage disease are almost always of the inflammatory or unclassified subtypes based on immunostains as well as genetic analysis,[21,22] but some of these adenomas do not look that much like the inflammatory adenomas that develop as a result of excess estrogen. As another example, HNF1-alpha–inactivated adenomas and inflammatory adenomas arising in the setting of excess androgen exposure often do not have the typical morphologically findings seen in adenomas arising from estrogen exposure. As a third more anecdotal observation, HNF1-alpha–inactivated adenomas that arise in individuals without a strong estrogen exposure risk often do not show the typical steatosis of HNF1-alpha–inactivated adenomas. These observations suggest that the morphologic findings of hepatic adenomas depend on their underlying risk factor plus their genetic profile. Thus, the morphology–genotype correlations described herein are primarily for adenomas that have excess estrogen as their underlying risk factor. The risk for each of the subtypes for bleeding and malignant transformation described elsewhere in this article are likewise based on estrogen-driven adenomas, but are not as clearly relevant to adenomas outside of estrogen exposure—they are presumed to be similar, but this remains less clearly proven.

HNF1-ALPHA–INACTIVATED ADENOMA

HNF1-alpha–inactivated adenomas subtype make up 35% of all hepatic adenomas (Fig. 2A). Less than 1% will also show beta-catenin activation by immunohistologic studies. The majority of tumors are sporadic, but rarely they occur in individuals with germline mutations in *HNF1A* (previously known as *TCF1*).[18] Individuals with germline *HNF1A* mutations also have an increased risk for mature onset diabetes of the young (MODY3). Although almost all adenomas in individuals with germline *HNF1A* mutations are HNF1alpha inactivated, inflammatory adenomas have also been reported.[8]

Most but not all HNF1-alpha–inactivated adenomas exhibit macrovesicular steatosis. It is important to keep in mind that some inflammatory adenomas also demonstrate significant steatosis, so fat alone is not a strong distinguishing feature of HNF1-alpha–inactivated adenomas. Resected specimens also commonly show microadenomas in the background liver. Microadenomas are small adenomas seen only on microscopic evaluation and not evident by gross examination. Biallelic inactivation of HNF1-alpha leads to loss of LFABP

Table 1
Immunostains used to subtype hepatic adenomas are frequently positive in hepatocellular carcinomas

Immunostain	Hepatocellular Carcinomas
LFABP	25% show LFABP loss
CRP	50% are positive
SAA	17% are positive
Beta-catenin	30% nuclear positive
Glutamine synthetase	50% show diffuse glutamine synthetase staining

Abbreviations: CRP, C-reactive protein; LFABP, liver fatty acid binding protein; SAA, serum amyloid A.

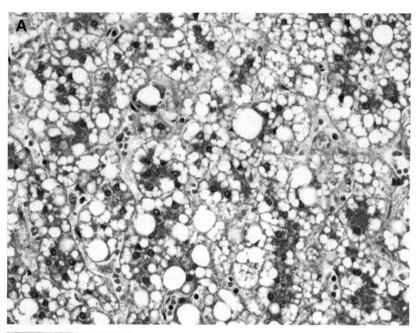

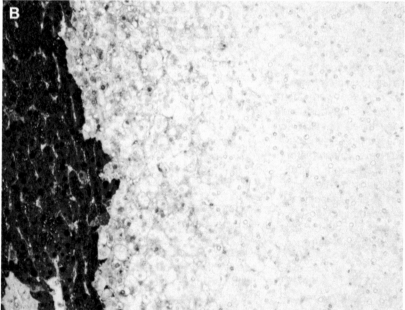

Fig. 2. HNF1A-inactivated hepatic adenoma. (A) The tumor shows fatty change. (B) An immunostain for liver fatty acid binding protein shows loss within the tumor (*right side of image*) and retained staining in the background liver.

expression and this findings is used as the defining feature of this adenoma subtype. The loss of LFABP can be readily detected by immunohistochemistry (see **Fig. 2**B). Whenever possible, choose a block for staining that has both normal liver and tumor and compare the two: there should be a clear distinction with absent or near absent staining within the tumor and strong expression within the nontumor liver.

The subcategory of HNF1-alpha–inactivated adenomas only rarely shows beta-catenin activation and, as a group, they have a lower risk of malignant transformation compared with inflammatory adenomas and to beta-catenin activated adenomas. However, hepatocellular carcinoma has been reported in sporadic HNF1-alpha–inactivated adenomas[8] as well those arising in the setting of MODY3.[18,23]

INFLAMMATORY ADENOMA

This subtype makes up 50% of all hepatic adenomas. About 10% will also show beta-catenin activation. Fatty liver disease is an important risk factor for inflammatory adenomas and can result from either the metabolic syndrome or alcohol use.[1,20] Because of these risk factors, both the tumor (Fig. 3A) and the background liver can be involved by fatty liver disease. Other morphologic findings include sinusoidal dilatation and congestion (see Fig. 3B), lymphocytic inflammation (generally mild and patchy; see Fig. 3C), and pseudoportal portal tracts (or *faux* portal tracts) composed of an artery, bile ductlike proliferation, and a sleeve of connective tissue (Fig. 3D). These pseudoportal tracts are very distinctive, but can at first glance be mistaken for a true portal tract. Although pseudoportal tracts are not present in all inflammatory adenomas, the majority of adenomas with them end up being classified as inflammatory adenomas by immunostains. Microadenomas can also be present in the background liver, although this finding is less common than with HNF1-alpha–inactivated adenomas.

Historically, before this entity was recognized as a subtype of hepatic adenoma,[19] the pseudoportal tracts were interpreted as favoring focal nodular hyperplasia. Thus, some of the earliest lesions were described under the term telangiectatic focal nodular hyperplasia.

Inflammatory hepatic adenomas are genetically heterogeneous, but most have mutations in *IL6ST*, *STAT3*, *FRK*, *JAK1*, or *GNAS*, all of which activate the JAK/STAT pathway. Adenomas are classified into the inflammatory subtype when they are strongly and diffusely positive for CRP and or SAA (Fig. 4). The CRP immunostain often is difficult to interpret owing to heavy background staining, so it is very helpful to stain a block that also has background liver for comparison. Essentially all hepatic adenomas with classic inflammatory adenoma morphology on H&E are positive for CRP/SAA, but some hepatic adenomas that lack the classic morphology are also positive and, therefore, immunostains are needed for proper subclassification. If the adenoma also shows beta-catenin activation, then a diagnosis of inflammatory adenoma with beta-catenin activation can be applied.

BETA-CATENIN–ACTIVATED ADENOMA

By definition, this subtype of adenoma shows beta-catenin activation, retained expression of LFABP, and negative staining for SAA and CRP.

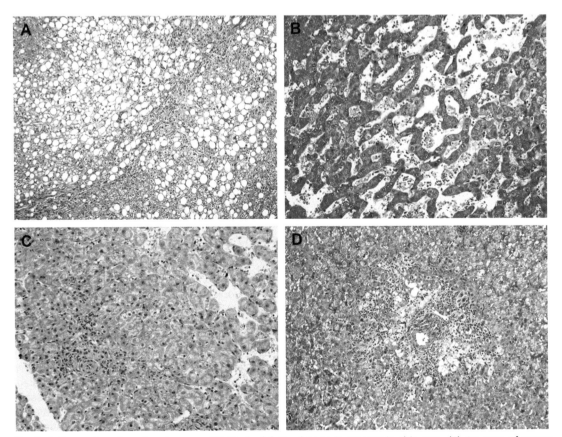

Fig. 3. Inflammatory hepatic adenoma. (*A*) Marked fatty change is present in this case. (*B*) An area of tumor congestion is seen. (*C*) There are rare foci of mild inflammation in this case. (*D*) A pseudoportal tract is seen.

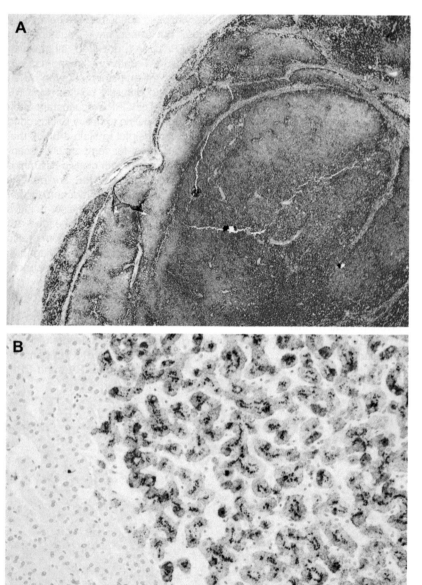

Fig. 4. Inflammatory hepatic adenoma, immunostains. (*A*) The adenoma (*right side of image*) is strongly and diffusely positive for C-reactive protein. The adjacent liver is negative. (*B*) The inflammatory adenoma is positive for serum amyloid A.

Morphologically, they are generally without distinguishing features.

Studies of this subtype have found a wide range in frequency, from 1% to 25% of all hepatic adenomas. The reasons for the wide range in frequency is unclear, but some case series reporting higher frequencies could be a result of selection bias (larger lesions and those with atypical imaging being selected for surgery), and/or varying criteria for the separation of well-differentiated hepatocellular carcinomas from hepatic adenomas. In addition, beta-catenin immunohistochemistry titrated for research laboratories can be ultrasensitive, even detecting staining in benign hepatocytes (beta-catenin is translocated to the nucleus during cell cycling as a normal physiologic finding, but protein levels are too weak to be detected by beta-catenin immunostains that are titrated for clinical diagnostic work). Use of these ultrasensitive assays in early studies sometimes led to higher rates of beta-catenin nuclear detection in hepatic adenomas.[24] Immunostains for glutamine synthetase staining can also be challenging to interpret because background staining can be an issue and many times tumors are not clearly negative or positive.

There are many different beta-catenin mutations reported in hepatic adenomas, but they tend to cluster into several major groups, each associated with different levels of Wnt signaling activation, which in turn correlates with the risk for malignant transformation (Table 2).[25] Recent studies have used the specific beta-catenin mutation to further subdivide both the beta-catenin–activated adenoma group and the group of inflammatory adenomas that are also beta-catenin activated.[8] This is easy to apply if your laboratory is routinely sequencing adenomas, but where this is not routinely applied it would be appropriate to stick with the traditional classification schema.

In clinical practice, beta-catenin activation is defined by strong and diffuse glutamine synthetase expression or by nuclear positivity for beta-catenin. When interpreting beta-catenin immunostains, a tumor is considered positive if even a single clearly positive lesional nucleus is identified (Fig. 5A). When reporting beta-catenin nuclear staining, it does help to indicate whether the nuclear staining is rare (<1% of tumor cells) or more than rare. Strong and diffuse glutamine synthetase staining also indicates beta-catenin activation (see Fig. 5B). Glutamine synthetase can exhibit considerable background staining, so it is important to compare the adenoma to the surrounding parenchyma whenever possible, using the staining intensity of the zone 3 hepatocytes in the background liver as a guide for what to call positive in the adenoma. The term diffuse for glutamine synthetase staining was defined early on as more than 50% of tumor cells, but most adenomas with strongly activating beta-catenin mutations will show strong glutamine synthetase staining in all or nearly all hepatocytes (>90%). Weaker activating beta-catenin mutations can lead to weaker and patchier glutamine synthetase reactivity—technically qualifying for beta-catenin activation, but these adenomas reportedly have a lower risk of malignant transformation than strong beta-catenin activators, and it is not clear if the risk is much above baseline. Negative cases include those exhibiting patchy weak staining of tumor cells, with more intense staining of a small rim of tumor cells surrounding draining veins (see Fig. 5C). An important pitfall to consider is that small biopsies of focal nodule hyperplasia can be mistaken as beta-catenin–activated adenomas when the biopsy samples an area of the focal nodular hyperplasia with strong diffuse glutamine synthetase staining (see Fig. 5D). Immunostains for beta-catenin nuclear accumulation and for glutamine synthetase do not capture all adenomas with beta-catenin mutations,[26] but they remain a useful tool for identifying cases with Wnt signaling activation.

UNCLASSIFIED ADENOMAS

This subtype makes up 10% of all hepatic adenomas. By definition, they cannot be classified into any other category of hepatic adenoma by immunohistologic or molecular methods. Morphologically, they are without any unifying or distinguishing features (Fig. 6A), although some can have fat and or glycogen accumulation in the tumor cells.

NEWLY REPORTED SUBTYPES

Recent studies have shown that the unclassified group of hepatic adenomas can be further

Table 2
Beta-catenin mutations in hepatic adenomas

Mutation	Activation of Wnt Pathway Downstream Targets	Beta-Catenin Nuclear Accumulation	Glutamine Synthetase	Risk of Hepatocellular Carcinoma
Large exon 3 deletions	Strong	>1% of nuclei	Strong and diffuse	High
Exon 3 deletion D32–37	Strong	>1% of nuclei	Strong and diffuse	high
Exon 3, T41	Moderate	>1% of nuclei	Strong and diffuse	High
Exon 3, S45	Weak	Absent to rare positive nuclei	Moderate to strong, patchy	Low
Exon 7, K335	Weak	Absent	Weak, patchy, or perivenular	Low
Exon 8, N387	Weak	Absent	Weak, patchy, or perivenular	Low

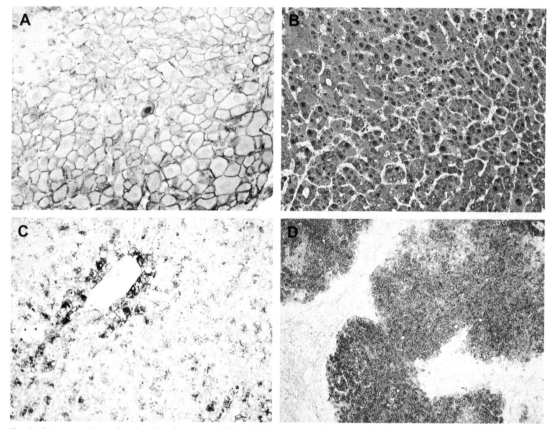

Fig. 5. Beta-catenin activation in adenomas. (*A*) An inflammatory hepatic adenoma shows a single tumor cell nucleus that is strongly positive for beta-catenin. (*B*) A glutamine synthetase stain is strongly positive in this androgen related adenoma that had numerous tumor cells with positive nuclear staining for beta-catenin. (*C*) This weak patchy staining for glutamine synthetase is considered negative. The more intense staining of tumor cells surrounding draining veins is common in adenomas that are negative for beta-catenin activation. (*D*) This focal nodular hyperplasia was mistaken for a beta-catenin active hepatic adenoma when a small biopsy showed strong diffuse glutamine synthetase staining.

subdivided, including a possible sonic hedgehog activated subtype[8] and a possible argininosuccinate synthase–positive subtype,[27] both of which have a high risk for bleeding. These new subtypes have not been independently validated, but the data are promising and it makes sense that clinically significant subgroups will be identified and removed from the unclassified group over time as our understanding of hepatic adenomas improves.

Adenomas with sonic hedgehog pathway activation make up 4% of all hepatic adenomas. The sonic hedgehog pathway is activated by a fusion of the *INHBE* and *GLI1* genes. This fusion gene was not identified in HNF1-alpha–inactivated adenomas or in inflammatory adenomas.[8] The morphologic correlates, if any, were not described, but they had the highest rate of clinically symptomatic bleeding. The proposed argininosuccinate synthase subtype is characterized by

increased expression of argininosuccinate synthase and arginosuccinate lyase, but overexpression of these proteins is not restricted to a morphologically or genetically distinct group of tumors,[27] so this may be a secondarily acquired phenotype.

OTHER SUBTYPES

Androgen adenomas arise in the setting of exogenous androgen use for recreational or medical purposes. The tumors exhibit more cytologic atypia than other adenomas (see **Fig. 6**B) and frequently demonstrate cholestasis and small pseudoglands (see **Fig. 6**C). By immunostain subtyping, they can be HNF1-alpha inactivated, inflammatory, or unclassified.[28] The majority also show beta-catenin activation.[28]

Pigmented adenomas are defined by the presence of heavy lipofuscin deposition within the

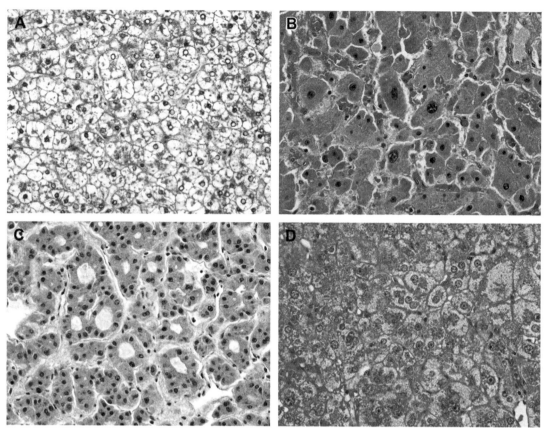

Fig. 6. Other types of hepatic adenoma. (*A*) This unclassified hepatic adenoma shows a mild glycogen accumulation. (*B*) This androgen-related hepatic adenoma shows nuclear hyperchromasia and enlargement. (*C*) Psuedoglands are prominent in this androgen-related adenoma. (*D*) A pigmented adenoma shows marked cytoplasmic lipofuscin.

adenoma (see **Fig. 6**D). These adenomas can be of any subtype but seem to be somewhat enriched for the HNF1-alpha subtype.[29] They frequently are associated with cytologic atypia, beta-catenin activation, and malignant transformation.[29–31] The background livers frequently show lipofuscin pigment deposition as well,[29] and these individuals may have germline alterations in autophagy or other pathways that contribute to lipofuscin accumulation.

Myxoid hepatic adenomas are characterized by abundant myxoid material dissecting through the tumor (**Fig. 7**A, B).[32] The myxoid material can be lightly Alcian blue and/or weakly mucicarmine positive, but it is not the true mucin of glandular neoplasms, but rather seems to be more similar to stromal mucin. Although the material seems to be within sinusoids on H&E staining, immunostains for CD34 suggest otherwise (**Fig. 7**C). Myxoid adenomas can be single or multiple. They have a high risk for malignant transformation (**Fig. 7**D).[32] These tumors are histologically very distinctive, but are also very rare

so the best way to fit them into the current classification system is not clear. To date, all have shown LFABP loss by immunostaining and unpublished observations indicate some but not all will have mutations (heterozygous) in *HNF1A*. However, their distinctive morphology and their high risk for malignant transformation suggest that classification as typical HNF1-alpha–inactivated adenomas is probably not the best approach. One of the earliest cases was described in the setting of the Carney complex,[33] so the activation of protein kinase A pathways may be a signature of these tumors, but data are insufficient to know the molecular findings that underlie this tumor's distinctive morphology and high risk for malignancy.

AN EXPANDED ADENOMA CLASSIFICATION SCHEMA

There are several types of hepatic adenomas that do not fit well into the current classification

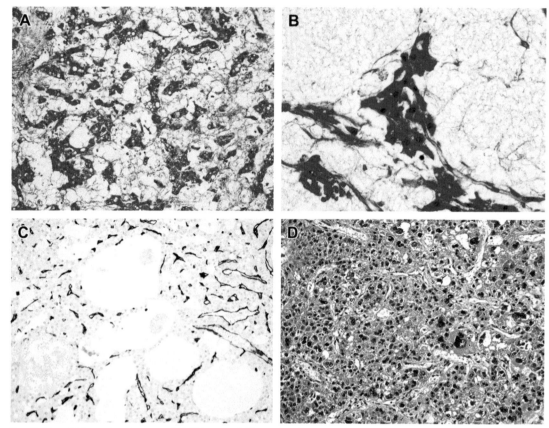

Fig. 7. Myxoid hepatic adenoma. (*A*) This myxoid hepatic adenoma shows abundant extracellular material dissecting throughout the tumor. (*B*) The myxoid material is loose and flocculent. The tumor cells are clearly hepatocellular, with no gland formation. (*C*) A CD34 stain suggest that the extracellular material is not in the sinusoids. (*D*) Transformation to hepatocellular carcinoma was evident in a central nodule.

schema, namely, androgen-associated adenomas, pigmented adenomas, and myxoid adenomas. As a group, they have an increased risk for malignant transformation, so they are important clinically. Because these adenomas do not fit well into the current classification schema, and for additional reasons outline herein, an alternative schema could be used that is based on the major underlying risk factor plus key genetic pathways (**Table 3**). This proposed classification approach considers beta-catenin–activated adenomas and pigmented adenomas to be secondary events along the pathway to malignant transformation of any adenoma. Importantly, using this approach, the classic morphology–genotypic correlation is manifested most strongly in estrogen-related adenomas. Myxoid adenomas are provisionally listed as being related to protein kinase A activation.

The approach of considering beta-catenin activation and heavy pigmentation as secondary events is supported by several lines of evidence. First, in cases of hepatic adenomatosis

(inflammatory or HNF1 inactivated), 1 or 2 of the adenomas may show beta-catenin activation or heavy pigmentation, whereas the others do not. This finding suggests that these changes are secondary events. Second, to date there have been no cases reported of adenomatosis composed exclusively or primarily of either beta-catenin–activated adenomas or pigmented adenomas. In contrast, cases of adenomatosis have been reported to be exclusively composed of HNF1-alpha,[8] inflammatory,[8] and myxoid hepatic adenomas.[32]

MALIGNANT TRANSFORMATION

Malignant transformation of hepatic adenomas is a rare but well-documented event. In the highly selected group of hepatic adenomas that undergo surgical resection, the malignant transformation frequency is about 5%.[34] The hepatocellular carcinomas that arise in hepatic adenomas show essentially the same morphologic features as hepatocellular carcinomas that arise in other

Table 3
An expanded system for classifying hepatic adenomas

	Estrogen-Related Adenomas		
Findings	**HNF1-Alpha Inactivated (40%)**	**Inflammatory Adenomas (50%)**	**Unclassified Adenomas (10%)**
Morphology	Diffuse steatosis	Sinusoidal dilation, inflammation, faux portal tracts	No distinct morphology
Key immunostain	Loss of LFABP	CRP and or SSA positive	Retained LFABP; CRP and SSA negative
Risk factors for malignancy	• Mostly undefined • Beta-catenin activation • Pigmented adenoma	• Beta-catenin activation • Pigmented adenoma	• Beta-catenin activation • Pigmented adenoma

	Androgen-Related Adenomas		
Findings	**HNF1-Alpha Inactivated (10%)**	**Inflammatory Adenomas (20%)**	**Unclassified Adenomas (70%)**
Morphology	Cholestasis, pseudoglands, mild atypia; little or no fat	Cholestasis, pseudoglands, mild atypia; may have features of estrogen-related inflammatory adenomas	Cholestasis, pseudoglands, mild atypia
Key immunostain	Loss of LFABP	CRP and or SSA positive	Retained LFABP; CRP and SSA negative
Risk factors for malignancy	• Beta-catenin activation • Pigmented adenoma	• Beta-catenin activation • Pigmented adenoma	• Beta-catenin activation • Pigmented adenoma

	Glycogen Storage Disease Adenomas		
Findings	**HNF1-Alpha Inactivated (0%)**	**Inflammatory Adenomas (70%)**	**Unclassified Adenomas (30%)**
Morphology	NA	May have features of estrogen related inflammatory adenomas	No distinct morphology, often have fat and glycogen
Key immunostain	NA	CRP and or SSA positive	Retained LFABP; CRP and SSA negative
Risk factors for malignancy	NA	• Beta-catenin activation	• Beta-catenin activation

	Adenomas with no Identifiable Risk Factors		
Findings	**HNF1-Alpha Inactivated (~20%)[a]**	**Inflammatory Adenomas (~20%)[a]**	**Unclassified Adenomas (~60%)[a]**
Morphology	No distinct morphology, mild steatosis sometimes	No distinct morphology; sometimes equivocal congestion, inflammation and faux portal tracts	No distinct morphology, often have fat and or glycogen
Key immunostain	Loss of LFABP	CRP and or SSA positive	Retained LFABP; CRP and SSA negative
Risk factors for malignancy	• Beta-catenin activation • Pigmented adenoma	• Beta-catenin activation • Pigmented adenoma	• Beta-catenin activation • Pigmented adenoma

(continued on next page)

Table 3
(continued)

| | Protein Kinase A–Associated Adenoma[b] | | |
	HNF1-Alpha Inactivated (100%)	Inflammatory Adenomas	Unclassified Adenomas
Morphology	Myxoid hepatic adenoma	NA	NA
Key immunostain	Loss of LFABP	NA	NA
Risk of malignancy	Undefined	NA	NA
Risk factors for malignancy	• Beta-catenin activation • Pigmented adenoma	NA	NA

Abbreviations: CRP, C-reactive protein; LFABP, liver fatty acid binding protein; NA, not applicable; SAA, serum amyloid A.
[a] Note: The frequencies are not well-described so these are broad estimates.
[b] Note: This is a provisional association that may need to change with better data.

settings.[35] There are 2 basic patterns of malignant transformation.[35] First, there can be a distinct nodule within the adenoma that has a higher grade cytology than the background adenoma, with reticulin loss, increased proliferation, and other features of malignancy. Second, there can be patchy but definite reticulin loss in a hepatic adenoma that overall has a homogenous morphologic appearance, without a distinctive subnodule of malignant transformation. The first pattern tends to be easier to diagnose than the second.

The risk factors for malignant transformation are not well-understood because of the difficulty of doing natural history studies on adenomas and

the relative rarity of both adenomas and malignant transformation. However, there are a handful of important and well-established risk factors (**Table 4**). Of these, data on beta-catenin are the best developed at the molecular level. Beta-catenin activation is primarily seen in androgen-associated adenomas, inflammatory adenomas, and unclassified adenomas, and is significantly less common in HNF1-alpha–inactivated adenomas. It is interesting to note that HNF1-alpha inactivation and Wnt signaling activation are largely mutually exclusive in both hepatic adenomas[36] and hepatocellular carcinomas.[16] The reasons for this finding are not clear, but this fact suggest distinct pathways of tumorigenesis. Heavy lipofuscin pigment deposition can also occur in any adenoma subtype and is an important risk factor for malignancy.[29] The molecular changes underlying this secondary event are currently unknown. However, lipofuscin accumulation suggests dysregulation of autophagy pathways and autophagy dysregulation has been linked to carcinogenesis in many organs, including the liver.[37]

Table 4
Risk factors for malignant transformation of hepatic adenomas

Risk Factor	Note
Size >5 cm	Rare cases have been reported in smaller adenomas.
Beta-catenin activation	Some mutations have greater risk than others for malignancy (see **Table 2**).
Heavy lipofuscin pigment in adenoma	These are called pigmented adenomas. The underlying biology is not clear, but may be related to dysregulation of autophagy.
Androgen-associated adenomas	Clinically aggressive tumors are uncommon despite the atypical histologic features that suggest malignancy in many of these tumors.
Myxoid morphology	
TERT promoter mutation	

REFERENCES

1. Paradis V, Champault A, Ronot M, et al. Telangiectatic adenoma: an entity associated with increased body mass index and inflammation. Hepatology 2007;46:140–6.
2. Calderaro J, Nault JC, Balabaud C, et al. Inflammatory hepatocellular adenomas developed in the setting of chronic liver disease and cirrhosis. Mod Pathol 2016;29:43–50.
3. Kumagawa M, Matsumoto N, Watanabe Y, et al. Contrast-enhanced ultrasonographic findings of serum amyloid A-positive hepatocellular neoplasm: does hepatocellular adenoma arise in cirrhotic liver? World J Hepatol 2016;8:1110–5.

4. Sasaki M, Yoneda N, Sawai Y, et al. Clinicopathological characteristics of serum amyloid A-positive hepatocellular neoplasms/nodules arising in alcoholic cirrhosis. Histopathology 2015;66:836–45.

5. Sasaki M, Yoneda N, Kitamura S, et al. A serum amyloid A-positive hepatocellular neoplasm arising in alcoholic cirrhosis: a previously unrecognized type of inflammatory hepatocellular tumor. Mod Pathol 2012;25:1584–93.

6. Graham RP, Terracciano LM, Meves A, et al. Hepatic adenomas with synchronous or metachronous fibrolamellar carcinomas: both are characterized by LFABP loss. Mod Pathol 2016;29(6):607–15.

7. Paradis V, Laurendeau I, Vidaud M, et al. Clonal analysis of macronodules in cirrhosis. Hepatology 1998;28:953–8.

8. Nault JC, Couchy G, Balabaud C, et al. Molecular classification of hepatocellular adenoma associates with risk factors, bleeding, and malignant transformation. Gastroenterology 2017;152:880–94.e6.

9. Sempoux C, Paradis V, Komuta M, et al. Hepatocellular nodules expressing markers of hepatocellular adenomas in Budd-Chiari syndrome and other rare hepatic vascular disorders. J Hepatol 2015;63:1173–80.

10. Chira RI, Calauz A, Manole S, et al. Unusual discovery after an examination for abdominal pain: Abernethy 1b malformation and liver adenomatosis. A case report. J Gastrointest Liver Dis 2017;26:85–8.

11. Nault JC, Fabre M, Couchy G, et al. GNAS-activating mutations define a rare subgroup of inflammatory liver tumors characterized by STAT3 activation. J Hepatol 2012;56:184–91.

12. European Association for the Study of the Liver (EASL). EASL clinical practice guidelines on the management of benign liver tumours. J Hepatol 2016;65:386–98.

13. Marrero JA, Ahn J, Rajender Reddy K, American College of Gastroenterology. ACG clinical guideline: the diagnosis and management of focal liver lesions. Am J Gastroenterol 2014;109:1328–47, [quiz: 48].

14. Singhi AD, Jain D, Kakar S, et al. Reticulin loss in benign fatty liver: an important diagnostic pitfall when considering a diagnosis of hepatocellular carcinoma. Am J Surg Pathol 2012;36:710–5.

15. Bellamy CO, Maxwell RS, Prost S, et al. The value of immunophenotyping hepatocellular adenomas: consecutive resections at one UK centre. Histopathology 2013;62:431–45.

16. Liu L, Shah SS, Naini BV, et al. Immunostains used to subtype hepatic adenomas do not distinguish hepatic adenomas from hepatocellular carcinomas. Am J Surg Pathol 2016;40:1062–9.

17. Bedossa P, Burt AD, Brunt EM, et al. Well-differentiated hepatocellular neoplasm of uncertain malignant potential: proposal for a new diagnostic category. Hum Pathol 2014;45:658–60.

18. Bluteau O, Jeannot E, Bioulac-Sage P, et al. Bi-allelic inactivation of TCF1 in hepatic adenomas. Nat Genet 2002;32:312–5.

19. Bioulac-Sage P, Rebouissou S, Sa Cunha A, et al. Clinical, morphologic, and molecular features defining so-called telangiectatic focal nodular hyperplasias of the liver. Gastroenterology 2005;128:1211–8.

20. Bioulac-Sage P, Rebouissou S, Thomas C, et al. Hepatocellular adenoma subtype classification using molecular markers and immunohistochemistry. Hepatology 2007;46:740–8.

21. Calderaro J, Labrune P, Morcrette G, et al. Molecular characterization of hepatocellular adenomas developed in patients with glycogen storage disease type I. J Hepatol 2013;58:350–7.

22. Sakellariou S, Al-Hussaini H, Scalori A, et al. Hepatocellular adenoma in glycogen storage disorder type I: a clinicopathological and molecular study. Histopathology 2012;60:E58–65.

23. Stueck AE, Qu Z, Huang MA, et al. Hepatocellular carcinoma arising in an HNF-1alpha-mutated adenoma in a 23-Year-Old woman with maturity-onset diabetes of the young: a case report. Semin Liver Dis 2015;35:444–9.

24. Torbenson M, Lee JH, Choti M, et al. Hepatic adenomas: analysis of sex steroid receptor status and the Wnt signaling pathway. Mod Pathol 2002;15:189–96.

25. Rebouissou S, Franconi A, Calderaro J, et al. Genotype-phenotype correlation of CTNNB1 mutations reveals different ss-catenin activity associated with liver tumor progression. Hepatology 2016;64:2047–61.

26. Hale G, Liu X, Hu J, et al. Correlation of exon 3 beta-catenin mutations with glutamine synthetase staining patterns in hepatocellular adenoma and hepatocellular carcinoma. Mod Pathol 2016;29:1370–80.

27. Henriet E, Hammoud AA, Dupuy JW, et al. Argininosuccinate synthase 1 (ASS1): a marker of unclassified hepatocellular adenoma and high bleeding risk. Hepatology 2017;66(6):2016–28.

28. Gupta S, Naini BV, Munoz R, et al. Hepatocellular neoplasms arising in association with androgen use. Am J Surg Pathol 2016;40:454–61.

29. Mounajjed T, Yasir S, Aleff PA, et al. Pigmented hepatocellular adenomas have a high risk of atypia and malignancy. Mod Pathol 2015;28:1265–74.

30. Souza LN, de Martino RB, Thompson R, et al. Pigmented well-differentiated hepatocellular neoplasm with beta-catenin mutation. Hepatobiliary Pancreat Dis Int 2015;14:660–4.

31. Hechtman JF, Raoufi M, Fiel MI, et al. Hepatocellular carcinoma arising in a pigmented telangiectatic adenoma with nuclear beta-catenin and glutamine synthetase positivity: case report and review of the literature. Am J Surg Pathol 2011; 35:927–32.

32. Salaria SN, Graham RP, Aishima S, et al. Primary hepatic tumors with myxoid change: morphologically unique hepatic adenomas and hepatocellular carcinomas. Am J Surg Pathol 2015;39:318–24.

33. Terracciano LM, Tornillo L, Avoledo P, et al. Fibrolamellar hepatocellular carcinoma occurring 5 years after hepatocellular adenoma in a 14-year-old girl: a case report with comparative genomic hybridization analysis. Arch Pathol Lab Med 2004;128:222–6.

34. Stoot JH, Coelen RJ, De Jong MC, et al. Malignant transformation of hepatocellular adenomas into hepatocellular carcinomas: a systematic review including more than 1600 adenoma cases. HPB (Oxford) 2010;12:509–22.

35. Micchelli ST, Vivekanandan P, Boitnott JK, et al. Malignant transformation of hepatic adenomas. Mod Pathol 2008;21:491–7.

36. Pilati C, Letouze E, Nault JC, et al. Genomic profiling of hepatocellular adenomas reveals recurrent FRK-activating mutations and the mechanisms of malignant transformation. Cancer Cell 2014;25:428–41.

37. Liu L, Liao JZ, He XX, et al. The role of autophagy in hepatocellular carcinoma: friend or foe. Oncotarget 2017;8:57707–22.

Update on Ancillary Testing in the Evaluation of High-Grade Liver Tumors

Anne Koehne de Gonzalez, MD, Stephen M. Lagana, MD*

KEYWORDS

- Liver • Hepatocellular carcinoma • Immunohistochemistry • Albumin in situ hybridization
- Liver biopsy

Key points

- Liver biopsies for mass lesions may contain limited material, confounding hematoxylin-eosin diagnosis; a panel of immunostains, including hepatocyte in paraffin 1, arginase-1, CD10, polyclonal carcinoembryonic antigen, bile salt export pump, and glypican-3, may be helpful.
- In situ hybridization for albumin may also be helpful and is positive in tumors of liver origin, including hepatocellular carcinoma and intrahepatic cholangiocarcinoma.
- Scirrhous and fibrolamellar variants may present special challenges, because, unlike classic hepatocellular carcinoma, these variants can be positive for cytokeratin 7 and exhibit a fibrous stromal reaction, suggestive of metastatic adenocarcinoma or cholangiocarcinoma.

ABSTRACT

Tissue diagnosis is the gold standard for mass lesions of the liver, but needle core biopsies may sometimes prove challenging. Presented here is a review of a panel of immunohistochemical stains, including hepatocyte in paraffin 1, arginase-1, polyclonal carcinoembryonic antigen, CD10, bile salt export pump, glypican-3, as well as in situ hybridization for albumin RNA, to establish hepatocellular origin in cases in which hepatocellular carcinoma is suspected but the sample is limited or the morphology is challenging, as it may be with cases of scirrhous, fibrolamellar carcinoma, intrahepatic cholangiocarcinoma, and combined hepatocellular-cholangiocarcinoma.

OVERVIEW

Hepatocellular carcinoma (HCC) is the fifth most common cancer in men, the ninth most common cancer in women, and the second leading cause of death due to cancer worldwide.[1] Because HCC most commonly arises in patients with underlying liver disease and cirrhosis, these patients are routinely screened by imaging at 6-month intervals for the detection of small (1–2 cm) lesions, in hopes of detecting cancer at an early and potentially curative stage.[2] Biopsy of such lesions for definitive histologic diagnosis is frequently performed. However, the liver is also a major site of metastatic disease. Therefore, although in some cases the evaluation of liver lesions may be accomplished by routine hematoxylin-eosin (H&E) staining, it is common to use ancillary tests to arrive at a definitive diagnosis. The situation in which the pathologist becomes most reliant on ancillary testing is when the lesion is at the extreme ends of the differentiation spectrum. In noncirrhotic liver, very well-differentiated or low-grade hepatocellular lesions evoke a differential diagnosis, which includes hepatocellular adenoma, focal nodular hyperplasia, cirrhotic/regenerative/dysplastic nodule, and well-differentiated HCC. This review deals with the opposite problem,

---

Disclosure Statement: The authors have nothing to disclose.
Department of Pathology and Cell Biology, Columbia University, 622 W 168th Street, Vanderbilt Clinic 14-209, New York, NY 10032, USA
* Corresponding author.
E-mail address: sml2179@cumc.columbia.edu

Surgical Pathology 11 (2018) 367–375
https://doi.org/10.1016/j.path.2018.02.004

wherein the pathologist encounters an obvious malignancy of uncertain histogenesis. The differential in this setting typically includes metastatic disease, poorly differentiated HCC, and intrahepatic cholangiocarcinoma (ChCa). Several ancillary tests have been added to the pathologists' armamentarium over the last several years. This review focuses on what is most novel and most useful in the authors' experience.

STAINS TO DETERMINE LIVER ORIGIN

Classic HCC most often occurs in patients with chronic liver disease and is composed of polygonal cells with abundant, eosinophilic, often granular cytoplasm and can be recognized on H&E stained sections (as well as on reticulin special stain) by its thickened hepatic plates (greater than 3 cells), formation of pseudoacinar structures, lack of portal tracts within nodules, and invasion of adjacent portal tracts at the leading edge of the tumor. Bile production by tumor cells may be noted and, if present, is highly specific for HCC. Mucin production, on the other hand, excludes classic HCC. Additional variants with distinctive histologic (and sometimes clinical) features include fibrolamellar, steatohepatitic (associated with underlying steatohepatitis and hepatitis C[3–5]), and clear cell variants. It is the authors' practice to use at least a minimal panel of immunostains in all but the most classic cases (in which it may be reasonable to rely strictly on H&E morphology and a reticulin stain). When encountering a case in which HCC is strongly suspected and a minimal workup is performed for confirmation, the authors typically use arginase-1 (ARG-1) immunostain, because of its high overall sensitivity and specificity.[6] Cases can become more challenging based on either clinical or pathologic characteristics. When the background liver is not cirrhotic, HCC is still an important differential, with 7% to 54% of hepatocellular carcinomas arising in noncirrhotic liver.[7] This cohort includes the fibrolamellar variant, which commonly arises in younger, noncirrhotic patients (see later discussion). In noncirrhotic patients, metastatic tumors are more common, however.[7] So, when either the histology or clinical setting are opaque, a panel of ancillary tests should be used. Although a discussion of all markers of carcinoma of unknown primary is beyond the scope of this review, the authors often use an immunohistochemical (IHC) panel consisting of cytokeratin 7 (CK7), CK20, TTF1, GATA3, CDX2, PAX8, CD31 (to exclude epithelioid hemangioendothelioma), and NKX3.1 (in male patients). If the tumor is not unequivocally epithelial by H&E, the authors include CD45, C-KIT, HMB45/Melan-A, and perhaps other markers based on morphology. The authors now discuss HCC markers in detail.

THE UREA CYCLE STAINS: ARGINASE-1 AND HEPATOCYTE IN PARAFFIN 1

Hepatocyte in paraffin 1 (HepPar-1) is an antibody that binds the urea cycle enzyme carbamoyl phosphate synthetase 1, expressed in hepatocellular mitochondria,[8] as well as small intestine[9] and Barrett metaplasia.[10,11] Staining is cytoplasmic and often granular in appearance. HepPar-1 is sensitive for well-differentiated tumors (91% to 100%)[12,13]; but its sensitivity drops with loss of differentiation (to 22%–81% in poorly differentiated HCC[13–16]), with an overall sensitivity of approximately 70%[12,17] to 85%.[18] HepPar-1 has also been reported to have less sensitivity in cases of scirrhous HCC.[19] In terms of specificity, as mentioned earlier, in addition to frequent staining of hepatoid tumors in other organs,[13,17,20,21] carbamoyl phosphate synthetase 1 is expressed in the small intestine; HepPar-1 staining has been reported in some small intestinal adenocarcinomas and intestinal-type ampullary adenocarcinomas.[22] Occasional strong HepPar-1 staining has also been reported in other tumor types, including melanomas and lung, gallbladder, pancreas, stomach, ovarian, and neuroendocrine tumors; but the overall specificity has still been reported as approximately 95%.[15,17] HepaPar-1 staining has also occasionally been reported in cholangiocarcinoma, at a rate from 0% to 16.7% in 3 different small series.[12,15,16] Furthermore, HepPar-1 staining in HCC can be patchy, which may be a pitfall in biopsy cases with limited tissue. Despite these caveats, HepPar1-is a relatively sensitive and specific marker with utility as a part of a panel of immunostains to characterize hepatocellular origin.

ARG-1 is an antibody that binds the urea cycle enzyme ARG-1, an isoform that is highly specific to the liver,[23] and exhibits cytoplasmic staining, generally with strong intensity. Several studies have shown it to be a highly sensitive and specific marker for liver tissue,[6,12,24,25] with sensitivities ranging from 83% to 100%, although Yan and colleagues[6] report that, similar to HepPar-1, the sensitivity may decrease somewhat as the degree of differentiation in the tumor decreases. Krings and colleagues[19] report that it is also sensitive for the scirrhous variant of HCC, for which HepPar-1 is significantly less likely to be positive.[26] In terms of specificity, ARG-1 has also been found to be positive in very rare cases of colonic, pancreatic, gastric, and prostatic adenocarcinoma[6,12,27] but is useful for distinguishing between HCC and intrahepatic cholangiocarcinoma, as it is typically negative in the latter[6,25] (though some series have reported very rare positive staining).[12,13,28] As with HepPar-1 and older markers, such as alpha-fetoprotein, ARG-1 also stains a minority of hepatoid tumors of other organs.[29] Fortunately, such tumors are rare and unlikely to be found in a liver mass biopsy.

STAINS WITH A CANALICULAR PATTERN: BILE SALT EXPORT PUMP, CLUSTER OF DIFFERENTIATION 10, AND POLYCLONAL CARCINOEMBRYONIC ANTIGEN

Some IHC stains recognize antigens found at the bile canaliculus. Such canalicular staining pattern supports a hepatocellular origin. In the authors' experience, these markers are most useful when performed as a part of a larger panel.

Bile salt export pump (BSEP) is a membrane-bound ATP-binding cassette transporter uniquely expressed by hepatocytes. As the name implies, it is involved in the export of bile from within the hepatocyte into the canaliculus. Two recent studies[13,30] reported approximately 90% sensitivity and close to 100% specificity for HCC, with a third study reporting slightly lower sensitivity and specificity for less well-differentiated tumors.[24] Because of its expression on the canalicular membrane, it is generally seen in the characteristic twiglike canalicular pattern, although this pattern is not required for hepatocellular specificity as it is for CD10 and polyclonal carcinoembryonic antigen (pCEA) (because BSEP is not expressed in other tissue types).

pCEA is a marker that stains the fetal glycoprotein CEA and cross-reacts with biliary glycoprotein 1. This marker is specific for cells of liver origin when it highlights the bile canaliculi in a twiglike branching pattern. The canalicular pattern has been reported at about 70% sensitive and 100% specific for hepatocellular differentiation.[16,31,32] The main drawback of this stain is that it may be patchy and may also produce nonspecific cytoplasmic reactivity in HCC as well as ChCa and metastatic carcinoma. Thus, distinguishing the truly specific canalicular pattern for HCC may be difficult.[15,16,33–35] As with the immunostains discussed earlier, HepPar-1 and ARG-1, canalicular staining may be present in better differentiated tumors and lost in more poorly differentiated lesions.[33,34]

CD10 is a membrane metalloendopeptidase expressed in many tissues, whose function is to remove the amino group of hydrophobic residues. A canalicular reactivity pattern with the CD10 IHC stain is reported by Borscheri and colleagues[36] to have a sensitivity of 68% and specificity of 100% for tissue of hepatocellular origin (both neoplastic and non-neoplastic). Although the specificity of the canalicular pattern is helpful, canalicular staining may be difficult to recognize, with the pitfall that nonspecific cytoplasmic, membranous, and apical staining may be seen in a variety of neoplastic and non-neoplastic tissues from other sites.[35,37]

Overall, the published literature cautions that sensitivity for both pCEA and CD10 decreases along with worsening differentiation. It also seems that in poorly differentiated HCC, it can be difficult to predict which of these two canalicular markers may be positive; therefore, it is prudent to perform both of them.

GLYPICAN-3

Glypican-3 (GPC-3) is an oncofetal proteoglycan found on the cell surface of malignant hepatocytes. Staining is cytoplasmic and membranous and can be patchy within a given lesion, which is a potential pitfall for biopsies with limited material.[38] Although usually not expressed in benign liver,[39–41] one caveat with this antibody is that staining has been reported in some cirrhotic nodules with active hepatitis C infection.[42] Overall, the sensitivity of this marker has been reported as variable, but generally in the range of 75%.[43,44] Unlike the previously discussed markers, the sensitivity of GPC-3 is reportedly better for more poorly differentiated HCCs and worse for well-differentiated tumors[43]; expression has been associated with a poorer prognosis.[45] The reported specificity, 86% to 88%,[43,44] is slightly lower than some of the markers discussed earlier, as GPC-3 staining has also been reported in some germ cell tumors, ovarian and endometrioid tumors, neuroendocrine tumors, squamous cell carcinomas of the lung, melanomas, and liposarcoma.[46–49] Nonetheless, this is the only relatively specific marker that is likely to be positive in HCC but not benign hepatocellular lesions. Many of the other tumors that express it are either not frequently in a histologic differential with HCC (eg, liposarcoma and Müllerian-type adenocarcinomas) or react only infrequently with the GPC-3 antibody (eg, neuroendocrine tumors). For these reasons, GPC-3 is an important element of IHC panels to evaluate the possibility of HCC.

IN SITU HYBRIDIZATION FOR ALBUMIN

In situ hybridization (ISH) for albumin RNA is a technique that capitalizes on the fact that the hepatocytes are the main site of albumin synthesis. Unfortunately, an immunostain for albumin is not practical because the high concentration of albumin in the serum results in heavy background staining. Albumin ISH has been reported as both sensitive and specific (**Fig.** 1A, B) for the identification of tissue of liver origin,[50–55] including malignant tumors, such as HCC[56] and intrahepatic chololangiocarcinoma[25] (see later discussion). For HCC, the reported sensitivity and specificity are greater than 95% in both well and poorly differentiated tumors.

As noted with previously discussed markers, albumin ISH has also been reported to produce reactivity in hepatoid carcinomas from other organs.[50,56] Another pitfall is that albumin ISH seems to be positive in approximately 25% of pancreatic acinar carcinomas.[57] Although these are rare tumors, they have significant morphologic overlap with HCC, making this an important caveat to keep in mind.

SPECIFIC SITUATIONS

The stains discussed earlier are quite useful, especially when used in a panel to distinguish metastatic adenocarcinoma from primary HCC, especially in core biopsies of the liver, where limited sampling may cause difficulty. However, there are a few special situations that deserve more detailed discussion.

SCIRRHOUS HEPATOCELLULAR CARCINOMA

Scirrhous HCC, a rare variant of HCC with extensive stromal fibrosis, may histologically closely resemble ChCa or metastatic adenocarcinoma. The cells are often nested, which again may suggest adenocarcinoma. Key histologic distinctions include lack of mucin production, bile production in some cases, and hepatoid cytology (ie, pink cells with centrally placed nuclei and prominent nucleoli). Contributing to the confusion, whereas classic HCC is generally negative for biliary

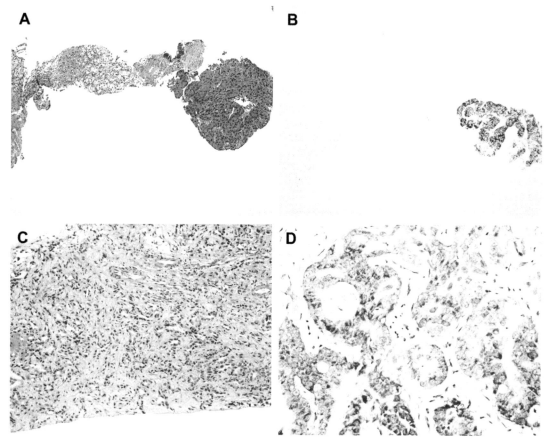

Fig. 1. HCC metastatic to adrenal gland (*A*, H&E, original magnification ×10) with diffuse positivity for albumin RNA in HCC and no background staining of adrenal tissue (*B*, albumin ISH-brown chromogen, original magnification ×10). Intrahepatic ChCa (*C*, H&E, original magnification ×20) also strongly positive for albumin RNA (*D*, albumin ISH-red chromogen, original magnification ×60).

cytokeratins CK7 and CK19, the scirrhous variant is often positive for CK7 and occasionally positive for CK19.[19] As mentioned earlier, the scirrhous variant may be less likely to be positive for HepPar-1; but the combined use of ARG-1 and GPC-3 has been reported to have 100% sensitivity for these tumors.[19]

FIBROLAMELLAR CARCINOMA

Fibrolamellar carcinoma (FLCC) is another variant of HCC in which there is stromal fibrosis; but the fibrosis has a characteristic lamellar appearance, surrounding cords or islands of tumor cells. The FLCC tumor cells also stain positively for CK7 and may be negative for GPC-3,[58] which may be a pitfall. However, they typically stain positively with HepPar-1, ARG-1, albumin ISH,[59,60] and CD68.[61] These tumors tend to arise in younger patients without underlying liver disease and have been linked to a specific fusion gene, *DNAJB1-PRKACA*.[62] Although it has been previously suggested that this variant may have a better prognosis than classic HCC, it is now thought that the improved prognosis is due to the lack of underlying chronic liver disease as well as the primarily young and healthy patient population in which it typically occurs.

CHOLANGIOCARCINOMA VERSUS HEPATOCELLULAR CARCINOMA

The distinction between well-differentiated HCC and well-differentiated ChCa is not typically a difficult undertaking. However, when one encounters a poorly differentiated tumor, and commonly used IHC markers of metastatic carcinoma are negative, then one may consider the differential of poorly differentiated HCC and ChCa. Besides the aforementioned scirrhous variant of HCC, one must also consider the possibility of combined HCC/ChCa. Typical combined HCC/ChCa should have recognizable areas of both hepatoid and adenocarcinomatous morphology, and these areas should have differing IHC characteristics.[63] Sampling can be a major pitfall in needle biopsies, but in resection or explant specimen it is typically a rather straightforward diagnosis (although collision tumors must be considered). One final special situation to consider before discussing the differential of typical poorly differentiated HCC versus ChCa is the category of combined HCC/ChCa with stem cell features (HCC/ChCa-SCF). The fourth edition of the *WHO Classification of Tumours of the Digestive System* has incorporated 3 subtypes of HCC/ChCa-SCF, though they caution that these are not currently

considered distinctive clinicopathologic entities.[63] Two of these 3 subtypes do not enter the histologic differential of the poorly differentiated liver tumor. The combined HCC/ChCa-SCF-typical subtype shows typical cells of HCC growing in nests with distinctive small blue hyperchromatic cells at the periphery of the nests. These primitive-appearing cells at the periphery mark immunohistochemically for stem cell markers (eg, CD117). Similarly, the cholangiocellular subtype of HCC/ChCa-SCF is not part of the differential of a poorly differentiated liver tumor. Rather, these tumors demonstrate low-grade ductular morphology. They are more likely to be considered as a well-differentiated ChCa (though they express stem cell markers) or even a benign process like a bile duct adenoma. The HCC/ChCa-SCF intermediate cell subtype is the only variant of HCC/ChCa-SCF that does enter the differential of poorly differentiated carcinoma in the liver. Tumor cells are small and hyperchromatic with scant cytoplasm. Cells cluster in nests and trabeculae and produce marked desmoplasia. They do not produce mucin; they coexpress markers of both hepatocyte and biliary differentiation, along with markers of stem-ness.[63] They can be distinguished from typical poorly differentiated HCC in that typical HCC does not demonstrate extensive desmoplasia and the neoplastic cells are not typically small. Rather, one often encounters anaplasia in poorly differentiated HCC. The distinction from a poorly differentiated ChCa may be more problematic. On biopsy, one may accept a lack of mucin as a sampling issue. If only a limited IHC workup consisting of biliary-type markers is performed, one would not be aware that the tumor expressed hepatoid markers and stem cell markers. To the extent that this distinction is important, it highlights the case for an expanded IHC panel.[64]

As may be inferred from the descriptions of the histologic features of these tumors, one difficult differential is the scirrhous variant of HCC (due to its desmoplastic stroma) and HCC/ChCa-SCF, intermediate cell type. Here, the cytology is likely the most important distinguishing feature, as the tumor cells of scirrhous HCC usually exhibit prominent pink cytoplasm and resemble hepatocytes; they are not small cells with hyperchromatic nuclei and limited cytoplasm. They also do not express markers of stem-ness frequently or robustly.[19]

The final differential is that of typical poorly differentiated HCC and typical poorly differentiated ChCa. In this setting, there is not extensive IHC overlap; however, there are a few pitfalls that should be kept in mind. Cholangiocarcinomas may very rarely express HepPar-1 and/or GPC-3

Table 1
Useful markers in hepatocellular carcinoma

Marker	Staining Pattern	Positive Staining	Reported Sensitivity in HCC (%)
HepPar-1	Cytoplasmic	Liver: normal and neoplastic	WD: 91–100 PD: 22–81[6,12,13,24,30,56]
ARG-1	Cytoplasmic/nuclear	Liver: normal and neoplastic	WD: 94–100 PD: 44–100[6,12,13,24,30,56]
BSEP	Any (predominantly canalicular)	Liver: normal and neoplastic	WD: 92–100 PD: 45–78[13,24,30]
pCEA	Canalicular	Liver: canalicular pattern is specific Nonliver: noncanalicular patterns	WD: 82–92 PD: 54–78[24,30]
CD10	Canalicular	Liver: canalicular pattern is specific Nonliver: noncanalicular patterns	WD: 72 PD: 67[30]
GPC-3	Cytoplasmic/ membranous	Benign liver: negative HCC: positive • Including scirrhous subtype • May be negative in fibrolamellar subtype	WD: 50–76 PD: 67–100[24,30,40,58,67]
Albumin ISH	Dotlike signal	Liver: normal and neoplastic • Often including intracellular cholangiocarcinoma	WD: 100 PD: 99[56]

Abbreviations: PD, poorly differentiated; WD, well differentiated.

(though almost never ARG-1), and they frequently express HSP70 and glutamine synthetase (markers useful in distinguishing HCC from precursor lesions).[19,56,65] The first 2 markers are certainly reasonable components of the assessment of a poorly differentiated tumor in a liver biopsy; therefore, even a pathologist using IHC appropriately may run into problems with occasional misleading staining. The last 2 markers (HSP70 and glutamine synthetase) can be quite useful in the assessment of low-grade hepatocellular lesions but are not part of the approach to poorly differentiated tumors, as they mark most malignancies one may encounter in the liver.[65–67]

ALBUMIN IN SITU HYBRIDIZATION IN CHOLANGIOCARCINOMA

An intriguing and controversial body of work is developing around the question of albumin ISH in intrahepatic cholangiocarcinoma. Before 2014, albumin RNA was detected in only a subset of intrahepatic ChCa.[68] In 2014, a multicenter study used an automated branched DNA ISH platform to identify albumin RNA in intrahepatic ChCa and determined that 82 of 83 intrahepatic ChCa were positive for albumin ISH, whereas none of the perihilar ChCa or distal common bile duct ChCa expressed albumin RNA (n = 24 and n = 22, respectively).[25] This study also found that all metastatic carcinomas of other sites were albumin negative. This finding was a major advance in liver tumor diagnostics, because intrahepatic ChCa is essentially a diagnosis of exclusion and there is no specific ancillary test for it. The topic received considerable interest at the 2017 annual meeting of the United States and Canadian Academy of Pathology. Unfortunately, several studies (published only in abstract form as of this writing) did not show equally robust results. One study showed positivity in only 14 of 31 intrahepatic ChCa.[69] Another group reported positivity in 14 of 22 intrahepatic ChCa.[70] A third group found positivity in 22 of 27 cases of intrahepatic ChCa but also detected staining in 5 of 13 gallbladder adenocarcinomas, 3 of 13 lung adenocarcinomas, and rare positivity in other cancers from other sites.[71] Thus, although these studies have not yet been published as peer-reviewed articles, it certainly seems as if the sensitivity and specificity of albumin ISH in ChCa is imperfect. Given this evolving literature, and the authors' own (unpublished, Stephen M. Lagana, 2017) experience with this marker, certain conclusions seem reasonable for the time being. First, albumin ISH cannot distinguish between poorly differentiated HCC and ChCa, as it will mark a fair to very high percentage of both. As to its value in determining if an adenocarcinoma in the liver is a primary intrahepatic ChCa, it would seem that the positive predictive value is high, whereas the negative predictive value is unclear. The authors do use this test for this purpose in their practice (**Fig.** 1C, D); when it is positive, the authors make a statement to the effect of *suggestive of primary intrahepatic cholangiocarcinoma*.

SUMMARY

Correct diagnosis of liver lesions is vital, as it determines the staging and the course of treatment of patients. Distinguishing primary tumors from secondary tumors, and subtyping primary tumors, is often a challenge; but with the addition of newer IHC tests and ISH for albumin RNA, our surgical pathology tool kit has improved significantly (**Table 1**). Given the drastic therapeutic implications of proper classification, and the frequently astronomical costs of said treatments, especially when compared with the costs of IHC and ISH, the authors consider it appropriate to have a low threshold for ancillary testing, particularly in biopsy material.

REFERENCES

1. Ferlay J, Soerjomataram I, Dikshit R, et al. Cancer incidence and mortality worldwide: sources, methods and major patterns in GLOBOCAN 2012. Int J Cancer 2015;136(5):E359–86.
2. Sherman M, Colombo M. Hepatocellular carcinoma screening and diagnosis. Semin Liver Dis 2014; 34(4):389–97.
3. Salomao M, Yu WM, Brown RS Jr, et al. Steatohepatitic hepatocellular carcinoma (SH-HCC): a distinctive histological variant of HCC in hepatitis C virus-related cirrhosis with associated NAFLD/NASH. Am J Surg Pathol 2010;34(11):1630–6.
4. Yeh MM, Liu Y, Torbenson M. Steatohepatitic variant of hepatocellular carcinoma in the absence of metabolic syndrome or background steatosis: a clinical, pathological, and genetic study. Hum Pathol 2015; 46(11):1769–75.
5. Salomao M, Remotti H, Vaughan R, et al. The steatohepatitic variant of hepatocellular carcinoma and its association with underlying steatohepatitis. Hum Pathol 2012;43(5):737–46.
6. Yan BC, Gong C, Song J, et al. Arginase-1: a new immunohistochemical marker of hepatocytes and hepatocellular neoplasms. Am J Surg Pathol 2010; 34(8):1147–54.
7. Trevisani F, Frigerio M, Santi V, et al. Hepatocellular carcinoma in non-cirrhotic liver: a reappraisal. Dig Liver Dis 2010;42(5):341–7.
8. Butler SL, Dong H, Cardona D, et al. The antigen for Hep Par 1 antibody is the urea cycle enzyme carbamoyl phosphate synthetase 1. Lab Invest 2008;88(1): 78–88.
9. Mac MT, Chung F, Lin F, et al. Expression of hepatocyte antigen in small intestinal epithelium and adenocarcinoma. Am J Clin Pathol 2009;132(1):80–5.
10. Chu PG, Jiang Z, Weiss LM. Hepatocyte antigen as a marker of intestinal metaplasia. Am J Surg Pathol 2003;27(7):952–9.
11. Shah SS, Chandan VS. Hepatocyte antigen expression in Barrett esophagus and associated neoplasia. Appl Immunohistochem Mol Morphol 2017, [Epub ahead of print].
12. Radwan NA, Ahmed NS. The diagnostic value of arginase-1 immunostaining in differentiating hepatocellular carcinoma from metastatic carcinoma and cholangiocarcinoma as compared to HepPar-1. Diagn Pathol 2012;7:149.
13. Fujikura K, Yamasaki T, Otani K, et al. BSEP and MDR3: useful immunohistochemical markers to discriminate hepatocellular carcinomas from intrahepatic cholangiocarcinomas and hepatoid carcinomas. Am J Surg Pathol 2016;40(5):689–96.
14. Wennerberg AE, Nalesnik MA, Coleman WB. Hepatocyte paraffin 1: a monoclonal antibody that reacts with hepatocytes and can be used for differential diagnosis of hepatic tumors. Am J Pathol 1993;143(4):1050–4.
15. Chu PG, Ishizawa S, Wu E, et al. Hepatocyte antigen as a marker of hepatocellular carcinoma: an immunohistochemical comparison to carcinoembryonic antigen, CD10, and alpha-fetoprotein. Am J Surg Pathol 2002;26(8):978–88.
16. Lau SK, Prakash S, Geller SA, et al. Comparative immunohistochemical profile of hepatocellular carcinoma, cholangiocarcinoma, and metastatic adenocarcinoma. Hum Pathol 2002;33(12):1175–81.
17. Lugli A, Tornillo L, Mirlacher M, et al. Hepatocyte paraffin 1 expression in human normal and neoplastic tissues: tissue microarray analysis on 3,940 tissue samples. Am J Clin Pathol 2004;122(5):721–7.
18. Ordonez NG. Arginase-1 is a novel immunohistochemical marker of hepatocellular differentiation. Adv Anat Pathol 2014;21(4):285–90.
19. Krings G, Ramachandran R, Jain D, et al. Immunohistochemical pitfalls and the importance of glypican 3 and arginase in the diagnosis of scirrhous hepatocellular carcinoma. Mod Pathol 2013;26(6):782–91.
20. Maitra A, Murakata LA, Albores-Saavedra J. Immunoreactivity for hepatocyte paraffin 1 antibody in hepatoid adenocarcinomas of the gastrointestinal tract. Am J Clin Pathol 2001;115(5):689–94.
21. Fan Z, van de Rijn M, Montgomery K, et al. Hep par 1 antibody stain for the differential diagnosis of hepatocellular carcinoma: 676 tumors tested using tissue microarrays and conventional tissue sections. Mod Pathol 2003;16(2):137–44.
22. Lagana S, Hsiao S, Bao F, et al. HepPar-1 and Arginase-1 Immunohistochemistry in Adenocarcinoma of the Small Intestine and Ampullary Region. Arch Pathol Lab Med 2015;139(6):791–5.

23. Multhaupt H, Fritz P, Schumacher K. Immunohisto-chemical localisation of arginase in human liver using monoclonal antibodies against human liver arginase. Histochemistry 1987;87(5):465–70.

24. Nguyen T, Phillips D, Jain D, et al. Comparison of 5 immunohistochemical markers of hepatocellular differentiation for the diagnosis of hepatocellular carcinoma. Arch Pathol Lab Med 2015;139(8):1028–34.

25. Ferrone CR, Ting DT, Shahid M, et al. The ability to diagnose intrahepatic cholangiocarcinoma definitively using novel branched DNA-enhanced albumin RNA in situ hybridization technology. Ann Surg Oncol 2016;23(1):290–6.

26. Matsuura S, Aishima S, Taguchi K, et al. 'Scirrhous' type hepatocellular carcinomas: a special reference to expression of cytokeratin 7 and hepatocyte paraffin 1. Histopathology 2005;47(4):382–90.

27. Geramizadeh B, Seirfar N. Diagnostic value of arginase-1 and glypican-3 in differential diagnosis of hepatocellular carcinoma, cholangiocarcinoma and metastatic carcinoma of liver. Hepat Mon 2015;15(7):e30336.

28. Shiran MS, Isa MR, Sherina MS, et al. The utility of hepatocyte paraffin 1 antibody in the immunohisto-logical distinction of hepatocellular carcinoma from cholangiocarcinoma and metastatic carcinoma. Malays J Pathol 2006;28(2):87–92.

29. Chandan VS, Shah SS, Torbenson MS, et al. Arginase-1 is frequently positive in hepatoid adenocarcinomas. Hum Pathol 2016;55(Supplement C):11–6.

30. Lagana SM, Salomao M, Remotti HE, et al. Bile salt export pump: a sensitive and specific immunohisto-chemical marker of hepatocellular carcinoma. Histopathology 2015;66(4):598–602.

31. Pan CC, Chen PC, Tsay SH, et al. Differential immunoprofiles of hepatocellular carcinoma, renal cell carcinoma, and adrenocortical carcinoma: a systemic immunohistochemical survey using tissue array technique. Appl Immunohistochem Mol Morphol 2005;13(4):347–52.

32. Ma CK, Zarbo RJ, Frierson HF Jr, et al. Comparative immunohistochemical study of primary and metastatic carcinomas of the liver. Am J Clin Pathol 1993; 99(5):551–7.

33. Wee A. Diagnostic utility of immunohistochemistry in hepatocellular carcinoma, its variants and their mimics. Appl Immunohistochem Mol Morphol 2006; 14(3):266–72.

34. Porcell AI, De Young BR, Proca DM, et al. Immuno-histochemical analysis of hepatocellular and adeno-carcinoma in the liver: MOC31 compares favorably with other putative markers. Mod Pathol 2000; 13(7):773–8.

35. Morrison C, Marsh W Jr, Frankel WL. A comparison of CD10 to pCEA, MOC-31, and hepatocyte for the distinction of malignant tumors in the liver. Mod Pathol 2002;15(12):1279–87.

36. Borscheri N, Roessner A, Rocken C. Canalicular immunostaining of neprilysin (CD10) as a diagnostic marker for hepatocellular carcinomas. Am J Surg Pathol 2001;25(10):1297–303.

37. Chu P, Arber DA. Paraffin-section detection of CD10 in 505 nonhematopoietic neoplasms. Frequent expression in renal cell carcinoma and endometrial stromal sarcoma. Am J Clin Pathol 2000;113(3): 374–82.

38. Anatelli F, Chuang ST, Yang XJ, et al. Value of glypican 3 immunostaining in the diagnosis of hepatocellular carcinoma on needle biopsy. Am J Clin Pathol 2008;130(2):219–23.

39. Capurro M, Wanless IR, Sherman M, et al. Glypican-3: a novel serum and histochemical marker for hepatocellular carcinoma. Gastroenterology 2003;125(1): 89–97.

40. Yamauchi N, Watanabe A, Hishinuma M, et al. The glypican 3 oncofetal protein is a promising diagnostic marker for hepatocellular carcinoma. Mod Pathol 2005;18(12):1591–8.

41. Libbrecht L, Severi T, Cassiman D, et al. Glypican-3 expression distinguishes small hepatocellular carcinomas from cirrhosis, dysplastic nodules, and focal nodular hyperplasia-like nodules. Am J Surg Pathol 2006;30(11):1405–11.

42. Abdul-Al HM, Makhlouf HR, Wang G, et al. Glypican-3 expression in benign liver tissue with active hepatitis C: implications for the diagnosis of hepatocellular carcinoma. Hum Pathol 2008;39(2): 209–12.

43. Mounajjed T, Zhang L, Wu TT. Glypican-3 expression in gastrointestinal and pancreatic epithelial neoplasms. Hum Pathol 2013;44(4):542–50.

44. Vasuri F, Malvi D, Bonora S, et al. From large to small: the immunohistochemical panel in the diagnosis of early hepatocellular carcinoma. Histopathology 2017;72(3):414–22.

45. Shirakawa H, Suzuki H, Shimomura M, et al. Glypican-3 expression is correlated with poor prognosis in hepatocellular carcinoma. Cancer Sci 2009; 100(8):1403–7.

46. Coston WM, Loera S, Lau SK, et al. Distinction of hepatocellular carcinoma from benign hepatic mimickers using glypican-3 and CD34 immunohistochemistry. Am J Surg Pathol 2008;32(3):433–44.

47. Stadlmann S, Gueth U, Baumhoer D, et al. Glypican-3 expression in primary and recurrent ovarian carcinomas. Int J Gynecol Pathol 2007;26(3):341–4.

48. Baumhoer D, Tornillo L, Stadlmann S, et al. Glypican 3 expression in human nonneoplastic, preneoplastic, and neoplastic tissues: a tissue microarray analysis of 4,387 tissue samples. Am J Clin Pathol 2008; 129(6):899–906.

49. Nakatsura T, Kageshita T, Ito S, et al. Identification of glypican-3 as a novel tumor marker for melanoma. Clin Cancer Res 2004;10(19):6612–21.

50. Krishna M, Lloyd RV, Batts KP. Detection of albumin messenger RNA in hepatic and extrahepatic neoplasms. A marker of hepatocellular differentiation. Am J Surg Pathol 1997;21(2):147–52.

51. Papotti M, Pacchioni D, Negro F, et al. Albumin gene expression in liver tumors: diagnostic interest in fine needle aspiration biopsies. Mod Pathol 1994;7(3): 271–5.

52. Murray GI, Paterson PJ, Ewen SW, et al. In situ hybridisation of albumin mRNA in normal liver and hepatocellular carcinoma with a digoxigenin labelled oligonucleotide probe. J Clin Pathol 1992;45(1): 21–4.

53. Kakar S, Muir T, Murphy LM, et al. Immunoreactivity of Hep Par 1 in hepatic and extrahepatic tumors and its correlation with albumin in situ hybridization in hepatocellular carcinoma. Am J Clin Pathol 2003; 119(3):361–6.

54. Yamaguchi K, Nalesnik MA, Carr BI. In situ hybridization of albumin mRNA in normal liver and liver tumors: identification of hepatocellular origin. Virchows Arch B Cell Pathol Incl Mol Pathol 1993;64(6): 361–5.

55. Oliveira AM, Erickson LA, Burgart LJ, et al. Differentiation of primary and metastatic clear cell tumors in the liver by in situ hybridization for albumin messenger RNA. Am J Surg Pathol 2000;24(2):177–82.

56. Shahid M, Mubeen A, Tse J, et al. Branched chain in situ hybridization for albumin as a marker of hepatocellular differentiation: evaluation of manual and automated in situ hybridization platforms. Am J Surg Pathol 2015;39(1):25–34.

57. Askan G, Deshpande V, Klimstra DS, et al. Expression of markers of hepatocellular differentiation in pancreatic acinar cell neoplasms: a potential diagnostic pitfall. Am J Clin Pathol 2016; 146(2):163–9.

58. Shafizadeh N, Ferrell LD, Kakar S. Utility and limitations of glypican-3 expression for the diagnosis of hepatocellular carcinoma at both ends of the differentiation spectrum. Mod Pathol 2008;21(8): 1011–8.

59. Ward SC, Huang J, Tickoo SK, et al. Fibrolamellar carcinoma of the liver exhibits immunohistochemical evidence of both hepatocyte and bile duct differentiation. Mod Pathol 2010;23(9):1180–90.

60. Koehne de Gonzalez A, Fazlollahi L, Coffey A, et al. In-situ hybridization for albumin RNA in pediatric liver cancers compared to common immunohistochemical markers. Mod Pathol 2016;29(2s):422A.

61. Ross HM, Daniel HD, Vivekanandan P, et al. Fibrolamellar carcinomas are positive for CD68. Mod Pathol 2011;24(3):390–5.

62. Graham RP, Torbenson MS. Fibrolamellar carcinoma: a histologically unique tumor with unique molecular findings. Semin Diagn Pathol 2017;34(2):146–52.

63. Bosman F, Carneiro F, Hruban R, et al, editors. WHO classification of tumours of the digestive system, vol 3, 4th edition. Lyon (France): International Agency for Research on Cancer (IARC); 2010.

64. Akiba J, Nakashima O, Hattori S, et al. The expression of arginase-1, keratin (K) 8 and K18 in combined hepatocellular-cholangiocarcinoma, subtypes with stem-cell features, intermediate-cell type. J Clin Pathol 2016;69(10):846–51.

65. Lagana SM, Moreira RK, Remotti HE, et al. Glutamine synthetase, heat shock protein-70, and glypican-3 in intrahepatic cholangiocarcinoma and tumors metastatic to liver. Appl Immunohistochem Mol Morphol 2013;21(3):254–7.

66. Di Tommaso L, Franchi G, Park YN, et al. Diagnostic value of HSP70, glypican 3, and glutamine synthetase in hepatocellular nodules in cirrhosis. Hepatology 2007;45(3):725–34.

67. Di Tommaso L, Destro A, Seok JY, et al. The application of markers (HSP70 GPC3 and GS) in liver biopsies is useful for detection of hepatocellular carcinoma. J Hepatol 2009;50(4):746–54.

68. Coulouarn C, Cavard C, Rubbia-Brandt L, et al. Combined hepatocellular-cholangiocarcinomas exhibit progenitor features and activation of Wnt and TGFbeta signaling pathways. Carcinogenesis 2012; 33(9):1791–6.

69. Avadhani V, Siddiqui M, Lawson D, et al. Is albumin RNA in situ hybridization (RISH) a reliable marker for intrahepatic cholangiocarcinomas? Mod Pathol 2017;30(2s):413A.

70. Lin F, Shi J, Wang H, et al. Detection of albumin expression by RNA in situ hybridization is a sensitive and specific method for identification of hepatocellular carcinomas and intrahepatic cholangiocarcinomas. Mod Pathol 2017;30(2s):420A.

71. Lehrke H, Boland J, Mounajjed T, et al. Albumin in-situ hybridization may be positive in adenocarcinomas and other tumors from diverse sites. Mod Pathol 2017;30(2s):419A.

Fibrolamellar Carcinoma
What Is New and Why It Matters

Rondell P. Graham, MBBS[a,b,*]

KEYWORDS

- Fibrolamellar carcinoma • PRKACA • Protein kinase A • Hepatocellular carcinoma • Pale bodies
- Fibrolamellar hepatocellular carcinoma • Carney complex • Central scar

---

Key points

- Fibrolamellar carcinoma is a unique primary liver carcinoma with a distinct predilection for young individuals, a characteristic morphology, immunophenotype and recurrent genomic abnormalities typically involving *PRKACA*.
- The diagnosis is made by recognition of the compatible morphology with the appropriate immunphenotype or detection of the key genomic event.
- Fibrolamellar carcinoma should be considered a different entity from conventional hepatocellular carcinoma on clinical, histologic, and biologic grounds. Fibrolamellar carcinoma also merits its own staging system.

ABSTRACT

Fibrolamellar carcinoma is distinctive at clinical and histologic levels. A novel *DNAJB1-PRKACA* fusion gene characterizes almost all cases, distinguishes it from other hepatocellular neoplasms, and drives the pathogenesis of this unique tumor. A subset of cases of fibrolamellar carcinoma is associated with alternate mechanisms of protein kinase A activation. This review article discusses common and unusual histologic features of fibrolamellar carcinoma, its differential diagnoses, and how to make the diagnosis while avoiding key pitfalls. The impact of the discovery of the fusion gene on the understanding of the tumor and the prognosis of fibrolamellar carcinoma are also discussed.

deepened understanding of FLC, posed some new questions about the tumor's biology, and challenged some prior perceptions. This review summarizes the recent literature on the frequency and origins of FLC, its clinical presentation, the characteristic gross and microscopic findings, the molecular pathology, and prognosis.

OVERVIEW

Fibrolamellar carcinoma (FLC) is a unique primary liver carcinoma. The recent discovery of the *DNAJB1-PRKACA* fusion gene in FLC[1] reenergized the study of this distinctive neoplasm, leading to important contributions that have

Key Points
EPIDEMIOLOGY OF FIBROLAMELLAR CARCINOMA

1. FLC is rare.
2. Available data indicate a frequency of approximately 1% to 5% of primary liver carcinomas with hepatocellular differentiation.
3. The etiology of FLC is unknown.
4. The earliest reported FLC is from 1915.
5. It has been reported that there is a slight predilection for FLC to affect patients of European descent.
6. FLC has a global distribution. It has been reported from every continent.

Disclosure Statement: No conflicts of interest to disclose.
[a] Division of Anatomic Pathology, Mayo Clinic, 200 First Street Southwest, Rochester, MN 55905, USA;
[b] Division of Laboratory Genetics and Genomics, Mayo Clinic, 200 First Street Southwest, Rochester, MN 55905, USA
* Mayo Clinic, 200 First Street Southwest, Rochester, MN 55905.
E-mail address: Graham.rondell@mayo.edu

Surgical Pathology 11 (2018) 377–387
https://doi.org/10.1016/j.path.2018.02.006

Key Points
CLINICAL FEATURES OF FIBROLAMELLAR CARCINOMA

1. FLC affects young patients.

2. In the largest published series to date, there was a single case (1 of 95 with available data) in a patient over 50 years of age and 3 patients (3%) over 40 years of age at first diagnosis.

3. FLCs frequently present with late recurrences; 5-year recurrence-free survival is approximately 10% to 20%.

4. Patients with FLC typically do not have underlying chronic liver disease

5. The diagnosis of FLC on a background of cirrhosis should be met with skepticism and thoughtful review.

6. The most common presentation of FLC is as an abdominal mass. Features of the mass effect include hepatomegaly, abdominal pain, and biliary obstruction (either from intraluminal growth or from extrinsic compression of the biliary tree).

7. Vena caval obstruction has also been reported, but this is less common.

8. FLC may uncommonly present with paraneoplastic manifestations. for example, gynecomastia, increased serum neurotensin, and increased serum transcobalamin I (haptocorrin).

9. FLC often presents with regional lymph node metastases and shows a propensity to spread along the peritoneum. Ovarian metastases have been reported.

10. FLC is not associated with serum α-fetoprotein (AFP) elevation.

11. FLC may show a central scar on imaging. This is nonspecific.

Key Points
PROTEIN KINASE A DRIVES FIBROLAMELLAR CARCINOMA

1. *DNAJB1-PRKACA* drives FLC tumorigenesis in greater than 95% of cases.

2. A rare subset of FLC is characterized by loss of function of PRKAR1A (instead of the fusion gene). Most of these patients have the Carney complex.

3. *PRKAR1A* is the gene mutated in most cases of the Carney complex.

4. FLC is likely to be a part of the Carney complex; a notion shared by J. Aidan Carney, MD (personal communication 2017), who continues to follow families with the complex.

5. A single case of histologically typical FLC showing *PRKACA* amplification and without the *DNAJB1-PRKACA* fusion gene has been identified.

6. The discovery of the fusion gene has, therefore, also catalyzed the discovery of 2 alternate genomic events that underlie a subset of FLC.

7. Gynecomastia, increased serum neurotensin, and serum transcobalamin I in FLC have now been linked to increased PRKACA and protein kinase A activity; for example, protein kinase A increases CYP19A1, a metabolic enzyme responsible for the production of aromatase. This leads to the increased synthesis of estrogen from androgen in adipose tissue and gynecomastia.

Pitfalls

! FLC has a predilection for young patients but conventional hepatocellular carcinoma is still the most common primary liver malignancy.

! Conventional hepatocellular carcinoma, scirrhous hepatocellular carcinoma, cholangiocarcinoma, and FLC all may express keratin 7 and keratin 19.

! Pale bodies are seen in both conventional hepatocellular carcinoma and FLC.

GROSS FEATURES

FLC forms multinodular large tan-colored masses on macroscopic examination. A green hue may be noted against the tan backdrop due to bile production by the neoplastic cells (Fig. 1). A central scar is noted in approximately 70% of cases (see Fig. 1) and tumor thrombi may be seen.[2] The adjacent non-neoplastic liver is noncirrhotic.

MICROSCOPIC FEATURES

FLC is histologically distinctive and on scanning magnification the neoplastic cells appear monotonous (Fig. 2A). FLC is characterized by eosinophilic neoplastic cells with abundant granular cytoplasm, a reflection of abundant mitochondria (Fig. 2B). The nuclei exhibit open chromatin and prominent macronucleoli and this is a distinctive diagnostic feature. Binucleate or multinucleated tumor cells can be seen in many cases on careful

inspection (see Fig. 2B). FLC almost never shows diffuse marked pleomorphism, and a tumor with such an appearance is unlikely to be an example of FLC. The tumor cells are typically arranged in trabecular cords that are separated by intervening ribbons of fibrosis (Fig. 2C). Classically, the fibrous bands are arranged in parallel arrays but in many cases the arrangement of the fibrous bands is somewhat random (see Fig. 2C).

Pale bodies are found in approximately 50% of FLCs (Fig. 2D) but they are not specific for the diagnosis. The available data indicate that cytoplasmic pale bodies are composed of fibrinogen, but whether fibrinogen is the sole constituent or 1 of several components of pale bodies has not been examined. Hyaline bodies may be seen as well but they too are not necessary for or specific for the diagnosis of FLC.

Other common morphologic features include intracellular and canalicular cholestasis and calcifications that may be within tumor cells or in the fibrous bands. These histologic findings are not specific and also do not usually give pathologists pause in making the diagnosis of FLC. A common finding that frequently prompts careful inspection, however, is the presence of pseudoglands. Pseudoglands (Fig. 2E) contain luminal mucin, and intracytoplasmic mucin in these areas has also been described. The neoplastic cells show the same cytologic features as typically seen in FLC, and classic areas of FLC are often seen in other histologic sections. Cytologic specimens usually show the classic findings (Fig. 2F) and the diagnosis is readily suggested by expert cytopathologists.

Some cases of FLC display unusual histologic features that can be a source of diagnostic challenge, particularly in needle biopsies. These features include solid growth without intervening

Fig. 1. Gross photograph of an FLC forming a multinodular mass with a central scar.

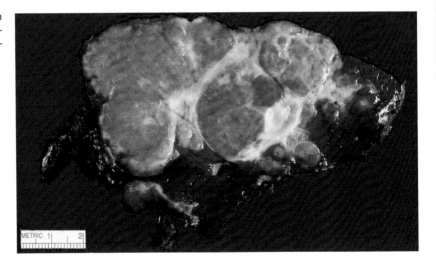

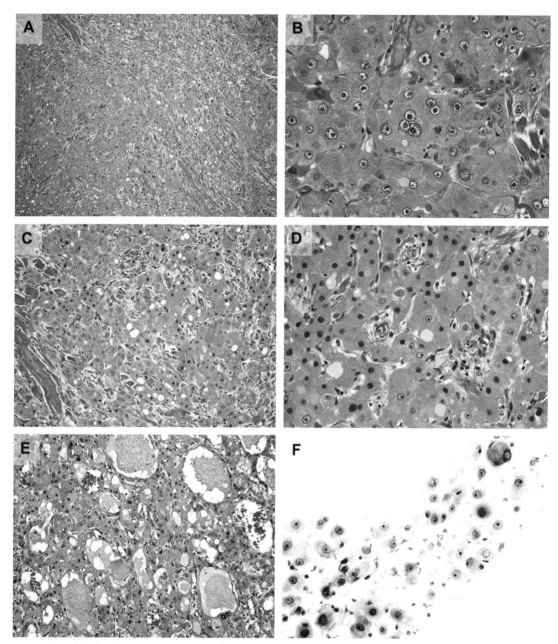

Fig. 2. Typical FLC. (*A*) Low-magnification photomicrograph of FLC. Bands of fibrosis intersect tumor trabecula (original magnification ×40). (*B*) The tumor cells of FLC characteristically bear nuclei with open chromatin and prominent macronucleoli. Binucleate cells are not infrequently seen (original magnification ×400 original magnification). (*C*) Occasional cases of FLC show mild macrovesicular steatosis (original magnification ×100 original magnification). (*D*) Pale bodies characterized by pale eosinophilic intracytoplasmic gobules are a well-recognized but nonspecific histologic feature of FLC (original magnification ×200). (*E*) FLC may form pseudoglands as shown in this image. The pseudogland lumina are filled with pink secretions that are often positive for alcian blue (original magnification ×100). (*F*) This fine-needle aspiration smear shows that the characteristic nuclear and cytoplasmic features of FLC are seen in cytology preparations as well (original magnification ×200).

bands of fibrosis in the tumor, a peliotic pattern, and the presence of non-necrotizing granulomatous inflammation. Examples of these unusual features are shown in **Fig. 3**. For the diagnostician, it is useful to note that in all these unusual patterns, the classic cytologic features of FLC are also evident. In addition, identification of more typical areas of FLC elsewhere in the specimen is helpful

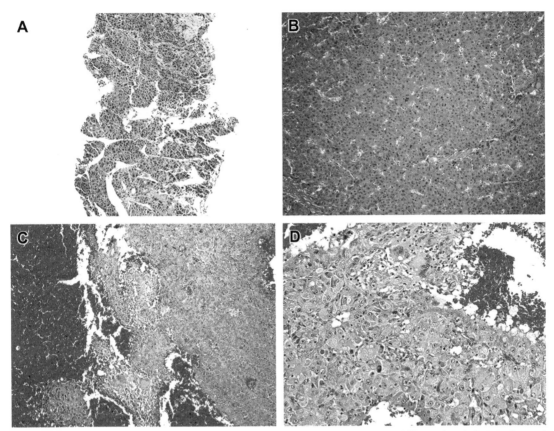

Fig. 3. Less common patterns of FLC. (*A*) Some cases of FLC do not have the typical fibrous bands (original magnification ×100). (*B*) Another example of FLC with limited intratumoral fibrosis (original magnification ×200). (*C*) In some cases, peliotic areas may be seen (original magnification ×200). (*D*) On high magnification, the cells still show the classic granular eosinophilic cytoplasm and prominent macronuceoli. In this case without prior treatment, foreign body–type giant cells were seen within the tumor (original magnification ×400).

in arriving at an accurate final diagnosis. Ancillary studies are most useful in these unusual cases and are discussed in detail later.

DIFFERENTIAL DIAGNOSIS

The chief morphologic mimics of FLC are scirrhous hepatocellular carcinoma, conventional hepatocellular carcinoma (**Fig. 4**A, B), poorly differentiated cholangiocarcinoma, and metastatic pancreatic neuroendocrine tumors. Both conventional hepatocellular carcinoma and the scirrhous variant of hepatocellular carcinoma arise in a background of cirrhosis. They are characterized by serum AFP elevation[3] and usually show an extent and severity of pleomorphism that is beyond what is expected in FLC. Scirrhous hepatocellular carcinoma may express keratin 7 and keratin 19[4] like FLC but may be negative for hepatocellular markers.[5] Cholangiocarcinoma may also be confused with FLC. Useful clues to remember

are that both cholangiocarcinoma and FLC are associated with prominent fibrosis but the former does not produce bile, does not have the characteristic cytomorphology of FLC, and frequently shows true gland formation. Pancreatic neuroendocrine tumor may also closely mimic FLC as noted initially by Craig and colleagues[6] (**Fig. 4**C, D). The key distinguishing features for each of these entities are summarized in **Table 1**.

DIAGNOSIS

Ancillary diagnostic studies are useful in the diagnosis of FLC. Despite the well-described typical morphology, cases of FLC are still misdiagnosed. Several published series of cases diagnosed as FLC from large academic centers include tumors with clinical features (cirrhosis and elevated AFP) that are inconsistent with the diagnosis of FLC.[7,8] For example, a Surveillance, Epidemiology, and End Results program database study (1986–2000)

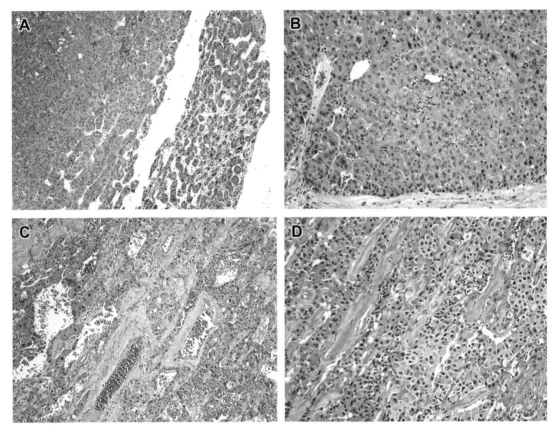

Fig. 4. Histologic mimics of FLC. (*A*) This conventional hepatocellular carcinoma mimics FLC in some ways. It is characterized by eosinophilic cells with macronucleoli and a monotonous appearance. The pattern of growth and nuclear pleomorphism, however, on the right of the image are not features associated with FLC (original magnification ×100). (*B*) Conventional hepatocellular carcinoma showing a degree of nuclear pleomorphism not seen in FLC (200× original magnification). (*C*) Metastatic pancreatic neuroendocrine tumor with a richly vascular stroma and tumor cells with abundant granular cytoplasm mimicking FLC (×100 original magnification). (*D*) Another pancreatic neuroendocrine tumor characterized by monotonous cells with granular cytoplasm and intratumoral fibrosis resembling FLC superficially (×200 original magnification).

reported 14 of 68 newly diagnosed cases (21%) of FLC in patients over 60 years of age strongly suggesting misdiagnosis.[9] Indeed, a subset of cases of FLC challenge even expert pathologists with significant experience in the area.[10]

Immunohistochemistry can be used to aid experienced pathologists in challenging cases and colleagues who rarely encounter liver neoplasms. As expected, FLC consistently expresses markers of hepatocellular differentiation[11] (HepPar1, Arginase 1, and albumin mRNA as detected by in situ hybridization). FLC is often positive for keratin 7[12] and most cases are also positive for CD68 due to abundant cytoplasmic lysosomes[13] (**Fig. 5**). Expression of both markers provides greater support for the diagnosis because up to 30% of conventional hepatocellular carcinoma can be positive for keratin 7[14,15] and 10% to 20% of conventional hepatocellular carcinomas may be positive for CD68.[13] In a

large series of cases initially diagnosed as FLC, 1 of 8 cases ultimately reclassified as conventional hepatocellular carcinomas (mimicking FLC) was positive for both keratin 7 and CD68.[10] FLC is typically diffusely positive but patchy expression for either marker or both markers can be seen. In addition, rare examples (1%) of otherwise typical FLC may be negative for keratin 7 or CD68.[10] The reasons for patchy or absent expression are unknown. Nonetheless, keratin 7 and CD68 are useful affirmative markers for the diagnosis of FLC in 85% to 90% of cases.[10]

There are some additional IHC markers that show consistent findings in FLC but are not routinely used in routine diagnostic practice.

Liver fatty acid–binding protein (LFABP) is a cytoplasmic protein highly expressed in the liver and involved in the transport and metabolism of long-chain fatty acids.[16] LFABP is negative or

Table 1
Key distinguishing features of morphologic mimics of fibrolamellar carcinoma

Diagnosis	Key Features
Conventional hepatocellular carcinoma	Frequent cirrhosis Morphologically heterogeneous *DNAJB1-PRKACA* absent
Scirrhous hepatocellular carcinoma	Hypercalcemia and elevated serum AFP Conspicuous nuclear pleomorphism Typically no macronucleoli KRT7 positive *DNAJB1-PRKACA* absent
Metastatic pancreatic NET	Typically multiple masses Monotonous oncocytic neoplastic cells No bile production Synaptophysin and chromogranin are typically positive Islet 1 positive in 85%-90%
Cholangiocarcinoma	Tumor cells lack the cytologic features of FLC No bile production HepPar1, arginase1 typically negative
Focal nodular hyperplasia	Abnormal vessels within the central scar Bile ductular proliferation Lesional cells lack the cytologic features of FLC Map-like glutamine synthetase

Abbreviation: NET, neuroendocrine tumor.

very weakly positive in all cases of FLC tested to date.[17] LFABP is lost in conventional hepatocellular carcinomas[18] and in type 1 hepatocellular adenomas,[19] suggesting that loss of this protein is not specific to any type of hepatocellular neoplasm. Instead, LFABP may be a part of an important tumor suppressor mechanism in hepatocellular neoplasia.

Anterior gradient 2 is a protein expressed in mucin-secreting tissues and endocrine organs.[20] It is believed to function as an oncogenic protein in several tumors but the oncogenic mechanism remains unclear.[20] Interestingly, 75% of FLCs express anterior gradient 2 in contrast to only 1 of 44 conventional hepatocellular carcinomas, suggesting that anterior gradient 2 may have some usefulness in distinguishing these 2 tumor types.[21] It is important to point out that biliary and pancreatic adenocarcinomas are typically positive for anterior gradient 2.[22]

MOLECULAR PATHOLOGY OF FIBROLAMELLAR CARCINOMA

Honeyman and colleagues[1] initially identified a recurrent intrachromosomal deletion on chromosome 19 leading to fusion of *DNAJB1-PRKACA* in 10 cases of FLC. This catalyzed further advances in the field. First, the somatic fusion gene, *DNAJB1-PRKACA* was validated as a specific recurrent genomic event in a subsequent larger series of FLC and a novel clinical diagnostic fluorescence in situ hybridization (FISH) test was developed[23] (see **Fig. 5**D).

A break-apart FISH probe has been validated clinically and offers a sensitivity of 97% and a specificity of 100% in the context of primary hepatocellular neoplasms.[10,23] Polymerase chain reaction–based detection of *DNAJB1-PRKACA* is also available and is theoretically more specific, but the very low requirement of 50 neoplastic cells for *PRKACA* break-apart FISH makes it the preferred test. Both of these newly available clinical tests have allowed for improved accuracy in the diagnosis of FLC. Detection of *DNAJB1-PRKACA* or *PRKACA* rearrangement is the most accurate ancillary test for the diagnosis of FLC. Review of cases diagnosed as hepatocellular carcinoma as part of The Cancer Genome Atlas confirms this point.[24] Three cases of FLC were misclassified as hepatocellular carcinoma during vetting and curation of cases by experienced pathologists, but subsequent transcriptome analysis uncovered the FLC fusion transcript prompting re-review.[24] It is also noteworthy that the *DNAJB1-PRKACA* fusion transcript was sufficient to induce the development of liver tumors morphologically similar to FLC in mice.[25] This consolidates the significance of the fusion transcript and PRKACA activity in the pathogenesis of FLC.

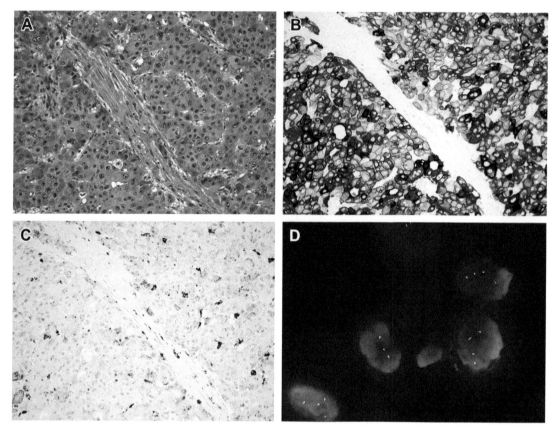

Fig. 5. Ancillary studies in the diagnosis of FLC. (*A*) Classic histology of FLC with a ribbon of fibrosis separating tumor cells with the classic histologic features of FLC (200× original magnification). (*B*) Keratin 7 is strongly and diffusely positive in most cases as is shown here (×200 original magnification). (*C*) CD68 shows granular dotlike cytoplasmic staining in most cases. The intensity and extent of staining can be variable, as shown in this example (×200 original magnification). (*D*) *PRKACA* break-apart FISH is the single most useful ancillary test for diagnosis of FLC. Separate green signals in each of the nuclei confirm *PRKACA* rearrangement and the diagnosis of FLC (×1000 original magnification).

ARE THERE MIXED FIBROLAMELLAR-HEPATOCELLULAR CARCINOMAS?

Several publications[26–30] have described tumors with features of typical FLC that include areas that were deemed more likely to be conventional hepatocellular carcinoma. Careful review of the images from 2 of these case reports[27,28] and 1 case series[26] reveals that histologically the entire lesion (so-called mixed FLC–hepatocellular carcinoma) shows the same cytologic features, whereas a portion shows the typical architecture (fibrous bands) and another shows solid and or pseudoacinar growth. The latter areas may also bear cells that have less cytoplasm but again harbor granular eosinophilic cytoplasm and the characteristic FLC nuclear features. One study purporting to report differing natural history between pure FLC and mixed FLC did not include any photomicrographs and so independent evaluation of the morphology was not possible.[29] A

follow-up study by some of the same group did not include any hematoxylin-eosin–stained images.[31] Importantly, 1 of the case reports identified the same fusion transcript in both the typical areas of FLC and the other less typical areas.[27] The author's experience with this has been the same.[10,17,23,32,33] Some cases of FLC harbor areas with the classic morphology and areas with unusual features as illustrated previously in this review. Craig and colleagues,[6] in their seminal article, noted that a proportion of FLC cases displayed areas without fibrous bands and with pseudoacinar growth. The reasonable interpretation of these data is that these tumors are all just FLC, inclusive of areas without the classic morphology. Nevertheless, intriguing questions remain. What is the meaning of these areas of solid growth or unusual morphology in FLC? Are they a feature of clonal evolution/progression? Are they a manifestation of degeneration? These questions await further study.

Table 2
Key differences between fibrolamellar carcinoma and conventional hepatocellular carcinoma

Characteristic	Fibrolamellar Carcinoma	Conventional Hepatocellular Carcinoma
Patient age	Young patients	Typically middle-aged adults
Cirrhosis	No cirrhosis	Frequent cirrhosis
AFP	Normal serum AFP	Typically elevated serum AFP
Regional lymph nodes	Frequently involved	Uncommonly involved
Peritoneal spread	Frequent	Uncommon
Late recurrence (>1 year)	Frequent	Uncommon
Histology	Characteristic, oft monotonous cells with abundant granular cytoplasm and intratumoral fibrosis	Usually regional heterogeneity Conspicuous nuclear pleomorphism
Immunophenotype	Frequent KRT7 and CD68 coexpression	Rare KRT7 and CD68 coexpression
Anterior gradient 2	Often expressed	Rarely expressed
DNAJB1-PRKACA	Present	Absent
Association with Carney complex and PRKAR1A loss	Present, rare	Absent
PRKACA amplification	Very rare	Absent

FIBROLAMELLAR CARCINOMA IS DISTINCT FROM CONVENTIONAL HEPATOCELLULAR CARCINOMA

Discoveries fueled by molecular techniques have advanced knowledge of FLC. **Table 2** summarizes how FLC differs clinically, histologically, and molecularly from conventional hepatocellular carcinoma. In view of these differences, it seems reasonable to consider FLC distinct from hepatocellular carcinoma and not just as a variant of the same. This has implications for biologic studies of FLC and the staging schema for FLC, as discussed later.

PROGNOSIS

Perhaps the most controversial issue in the literature on FLC is prognosis. Some early studies reported an improved survival in FLC compared with conventional hepatocellular carcinoma,[6,34–36] whereas others did not.[37,38] A study by Kakar and colleagues,[8] however, showed that the overall survival in FLC compared with hepatocellular carcinoma in noncirrhotic patients was similar. In short, the improved survival initially reported was a reflection of patient age and a lack of underlying cirrhosis. A subsequent large single-institution study and a large systemic meta-analysis have affirmed the similar prognoses of FLC and conventional hepatocellular carcinoma.[39,40] Features associated with adverse outcome in FLC include

vascular invasion, number of tumors, and surgical resectability.

In the current AJCC Cancer Staging Manual, FLC is handled in the same way as conventional hepatocellular carcinoma.[41] This AJCC staging system, however, does not stratify FLC well. In a large single-institution series of 65 consecutive patients treated with resection, there was no statistical difference between the outcomes of patients across stages.[39] Furthermore, regional lymph node metastases, which are an adverse prognostic feature in conventional hepatocellular carcinoma, were not significantly associated with adverse outcome.[39] Another large series of FLC did not find the presence of regional lymph node metastases a significant adverse prognostic factor.[42] It is apparent, therefore, that regional lymph node metastases do not warrant designation as stage IV in FLC. Prolonged survival can be achieved in FLC with surgical excision of involved regional lymph nodes.[43] The propensity for FLC to invade the hilum of the liver may explain the frequency of regional lymph node metastases. Taken together, these data also indicate that FLC merits its own staging schema.

REFERENCES

1. Honeyman JN, Simon EP, Robine N, et al. Detection of a recurrent DNAJB1-PRKACA chimeric transcript in fibrolamellar hepatocellular carcinoma. Science 2014;343(6174):1010–4.

2. Ichikawa T, Federle MP, Grazioli L, et al. Fibrolamellar hepatocellular carcinoma: imaging and pathologic findings in 31 recent cases. Radiology 1999; 213(2):352–61.

3. Lee JH, Choi MS, Gwak GY, et al. Clinicopathologic characteristics and long-term prognosis of scirrhous hepatocellular carcinoma. Dig Dis Sci 2012;57(6): 1698–707.

4. Kim YJ, Rhee H, Yoo JE, et al. Tumour epithelial and stromal characteristics of hepatocellular carcinomas with abundant fibrous stroma: fibrolamellar versus scirrhous hepatocellular carcinoma. Histopathology 2017;71(2):217–26.

5. Matsuura S, Aishima S, Taguchi K, et al. 'Scirrhous' type hepatocellular carcinomas: a special reference to expression of cytokeratin 7 and hepatocyte paraffin 1. Histopathology 2005;47(4):382–90.

6. Craig JR, Peters RL, Edmondson HA, et al. Fibrolamellar carcinoma of the liver: a tumor of adolescents and young adults with distinctive clinico-pathologic features. Cancer 1980;46(2):372–9.

7. Mavros MN, Mayo SC, Hyder O, et al. A systematic review: treatment and prognosis of patients with fibrolamellar hepatocellular carcinoma. J Am Coll Surg 2012;215(6):820–30.

8. Kakar S, Burgart LJ, Batts KP, et al. Clinicopathologic features and survival in fibrolamellar carcinoma: comparison with conventional hepatocellular carcinoma with and without cirrhosis. Mod Pathol 2005;18(11):1417–23.

9. El-Serag HB, Davila JA. Is fibrolamellar carcinoma different from hepatocellular carcinoma? A US population-based study. Hepatology 2004;39(3): 798–803.

10. Graham RP, Yeh MM, Lam-Himlin D, et al. Molecular testing for the clinical diagnosis of fibrolamellar carcinoma. Mod Pathol 2018;31(1):141–9.

11. Ward SC, Huang J, Tickoo SK, et al. Fibrolamellar carcinoma of the liver exhibits immunohistochemical evidence of both hepatocyte and bile duct differentiation. Mod Pathol 2010;23(9):1180–90.

12. Van Eyken P, Sciot R, Brock P, et al. Abundant expression of cytokeratin 7 in fibrolamellar carcinoma of the liver. Histopathology 1990;17(2):101–7.

13. Ross HM, Daniel HD, Vivekanandan P, et al. Fibrolamellar carcinomas are positive for CD68. Mod Pathol 2011;24(3):390–5.

14. Klein WM, Molmenti EP, Colombani PM, et al. Primary liver carcinoma arising in people younger than 30 years. Am J Clin Pathol 2005;124(4): 512–8.

15. Chu P, Wu E, Weiss LM. Cytokeratin 7 and cytokeratin 20 expression in epithelial neoplasms: a survey of 435 cases. Mod Pathol 2000;13(9):962–72.

16. Smathers RL, Petersen DR. The human fatty acid-binding protein family: evolutionary divergences and functions. Hum Genomics 2011;5(3):170–91.

17. Graham RP, Terracciano LM, Meves A, et al. Hepatic adenomas with synchronous or metachronous fibrolamellar carcinomas: both are characterized by LFABP loss. Mod Pathol 2016;29(6):607–15.

18. Cho SJ, Ferrell LD, Gill RM. Expression of liver fatty acid binding protein in hepatocellular carcinoma. Hum Pathol 2016;50:135–9.

19. Bioulac-Sage P, Rebouissou S, Thomas C, et al. Hepatocellular adenoma subtype classification using molecular markers and immunohistochemistry. Hepatology 2007;46(3):740–8.

20. Chevet E, Fessart D, Delom F, et al. Emerging roles for the pro-oncogenic anterior gradient-2 in cancer development. Oncogene 2013;32(20):2499–509.

21. Vivekanandan P, Micchelli ST, Torbenson M. Anterior gradient-2 is overexpressed by fibrolamellar carcinomas. Hum Pathol 2009;40(3):293–9.

22. Lepreux S, Bioulac-Sage P, Chevet E. Differential expression of the anterior gradient protein-2 is a conserved feature during morphogenesis and carcinogenesis of the biliary tree. Liver Int 2011;31(3): 322–8.

23. Graham RP, Jin L, Knutson DL, et al. DNAJB1-PRKACA is specific for fibrolamellar carcinoma. Mod Pathol 2015;28(6):822–9.

24. Dinh TA, Vitucci EC, Wauthier E, et al. Comprehensive analysis of the cancer genome atlas reveals a unique gene and non-coding RNA signature of fibrolamellar carcinoma. Sci Rep 2017;7:44653.

25. Engelholm LH, Riaz A, Serra D, et al. CRISPR/Cas9 engineering of adult mouse liver demonstrates that the dnajb1-prkaca gene fusion is sufficient to induce tumors resembling fibrolamellar hepatocellular carcinoma. Gastroenterology 2017;153(6): 1662–73.e10.

26. Chagas AL, Kikuchi L, Herman P, et al. Clinical and pathological evaluation of fibrolamellar hepatocellular carcinoma: a single center study of 21 cases. Clinics (Sao Paulo) 2015;70(3):207–13.

27. Griffith OL, Griffith M, Krysiak K, et al. A genomic case study of mixed fibrolamellar hepatocellular carcinoma. Ann Oncol 2016;27(6):1148–54.

28. Castro-Villabon D, Barrera-Herrera LE, Rodriguez-Urrego PA, et al. Hepatocellular carcinoma with both fibrolamellar and classical components: an unusual morphological pattern. Case Rep Pathol 2015; 2015:609780.

29. Malouf GG, Brugieres L, Le Deley MC, et al. Pure and mixed fibrolamellar hepatocellular carcinomas differ in natural history and prognosis after complete surgical resection. Cancer 2012;118(20):4981–90.

30. Okano A, Hajiro K, Takakuwa H, et al. Fibrolamellar carcinoma of the liver with a mixture of ordinary hepatocellular carcinoma: a case report. Am J Gastroenterol 1998;93(7):1144–5.

31. Malouf GG, Job S, Paradis V, et al. Transcriptional profiling of pure fibrolamellar hepatocellular carcinoma

reveals an endocrine signature. Hepatology 2014; 59(6):2228–37.

32. Graham RP, Garcia JJ, Greipp PT, et al. FGFR1 and FGFR2 in fibrolamellar carcinoma. Histopathology 2016;68(5):686–92.

33. Graham RP, Craig JR, Jin L, et al. Environmental exposures as a risk factor for fibrolamellar carcinoma. Mod Pathol 2017;30(6):892–6.

34. Epstein BE, Pajak TF, Haulk TL, et al. Metastatic non-resectable fibrolamellar hepatoma: prognostic features and natural history. Am J Clin Oncol 1999; 22(1):22–8.

35. Farhi DC, Shikes RH, Murari PJ, et al. Hepatocellular carcinoma in young people. Cancer 1983;52(8): 1516–25.

36. Nagorney DM, Adson MA, Weiland LH, et al. Fibro-lamellar hepatoma. Am J Surg 1985;149(1):113–9.

37. Haas JE, Muczynski KA, Krailo M, et al. Histopathology and prognosis in childhood hepatoblastoma and hepatocarcinoma. Cancer 1989;64(5): 1082–95.

38. Katzenstein HM, Krailo MD, Malogolowkin MH, et al. Fibrolamellar hepatocellular carcinoma in children and adolescents. Cancer 2003;97(8):2006–12.

39. Yamashita S, Vauthey JN, Kaseb AO, et al. Prognosis of fibrolamellar carcinoma compared to non-cirrhotic conventional hepatocellular carcinoma. J Gastrointest Surg 2016;20(10):1725–31.

40. Njei B, Konjeti VR, Ditah I. Prognosis of patients with fibrolamellar hepatocellular carcinoma versus conventional hepatocellular carcinoma: a systematic review and meta-analysis. Gastrointest Cancer Res 2014;7(2):49–54.

41. AJCC cancer staging manual. 7th edition. New York: Springer; 2010.

42. Stipa F, Yoon SS, Liau KH, et al. Outcome of patients with fibrolamellar hepatocellular carcinoma. Cancer 2006;106(6):1331–8.

43. Kaseb AO, Shama M, Sahin IH, et al. Prognostic indicators and treatment outcome in 94 cases of fibro-lamellar hepatocellular carcinoma. Oncology 2013; 85(4):197–203.

Hepatic Lymphoma Diagnosis

Won-Tak Choi, MD, PhD*, Ryan M. Gill, MD, PhD

KEYWORDS

- Aggressive NK-cell leukemia • B-lymphoblastic leukemia/lymphoma • Burkitt lymphoma
- Chronic lymphocytic leukemia/small lymphocytic lymphoma • Classic Hodgkin lymphoma
- Diffuse large B-cell lymphoma • Follicular lymphoma • Hairy cell leukemia

Key points

- Although hepatic involvement by systemic lymphoma is common, rare cases of primary hepatic lymphoma (PHL) may be first encountered on liver biopsy.
- Epstein-Barr virus (EBV) typically infects B-cells through the EBV receptor (CD21). In EBV hepatitis, a liver biopsy most commonly shows a mild sinusoidal lymphohistiocytic infiltrate with only rare EBV-positive B-cells, which are best demonstrated by comparing a Pax-5 immunostain with an EBV *in situ* hybridization stain.
- Diffuse large B-cell lymphoma and extranodal marginal zone lymphoma of mucosa-associated lymphoid tissue are the most common PHLs.
- T-cell or natural killer (NK)-cell lymphomas are less commonly diagnosed on liver biopsy; specific considerations include peripheral T-cell lymphoma, not otherwise specified; hepatosplenic T-cell lymphoma; and aggressive NK-cell leukemia.
- Classic Hodgkin lymphoma (CHL) and nodular lymphocyte–predominant Hodgkin lymphoma can rarely involve the liver; ductopenia may be associated with CHL.

ABSTRACT

Systemic hematopoietic disorders may present on liver biopsy, and rare cases of primary hepatic lymphoma (PHL) may be encountered. Hepatopathologists must be familiar with the full spectrum of hematopoietic disorders involving the liver and be prepared to exclude benign mimics. PHL, which is confined to the liver without extrahepatic involvement, can present as solitary or multiple nodules, raising consideration for carcinoma on imaging, or may mimic benign inflammatory conditions, posing a diagnostic challenge. This article describes clinical, morphologic, and immunophenotypic features of some of the most common hematopoietic neoplasms involving the liver, along with differential diagnosis and recommended ancillary testing.

OVERVIEW

Although systemic hematopoietic neoplasms commonly involve the liver, hepatopathologists may encounter rare cases of primary hepatic lymphoma (PHL), which can often mimic benign conditions. PHL is defined as a liver-confined lymphoma without extrahepatic involvement,[1,2] and it constitutes approximately 0.4% of all primary extranodal non-Hodgkin lymphomas (NHLs).[3–5] It most commonly affects middle-aged men, with a mean age of 50 years to 62 years

Disclosure Statement: The authors have nothing to disclose.
Department of Pathology, University of California at San Francisco, 505 Parnassus Avenue, M552, Box 0102, San Francisco, CA 94143, USA
* Corresponding author.
E-mail address: Won-Tak.Choi@ucsf.edu

surgpath.theclinics.com

(range: 21–86 years), who present with nonspecific symptoms (fever, night sweats, and/or weight loss) and elevated lactate dehydrogenase in the setting of normal levels of α-fetoprotein and carcinoembryonic antigen.[4–8] The exact etiology of PHL is unknown, but chronic viral infection (ie, hepatitis B virus [HBV], hepatitis C virus [HCV], HIV, or Epstein-Barr virus [EBV]) and/or immune dysfunction (ie, autoimmune diseases or immunosuppression) may play a role in pathogenesis.[5,8,9] Although initially considered an aggressive disease,[2] recent studies indicate that PHL patients may have a more favorable prognosis than previously believed, with a reported 5-year survival rate of 77% to 83%.[4,5,8]

A majority of PHLs are B-cell lymphomas with diffuse large B-cell lymphoma (DLBCL) the most common subtype.[4,5,8] Although many cases of PHL efface the hepatic parenchyma and form solitary or multiple nodules, some cases may have more subtle morphologic findings in which neoplastic cells are small or intermediate in size with predominant portal and/or sinusoidal involvement.[4,5,8] For this reason, hepatopathologists must be familiar with clinical (ie, lactate dehydrogenase elevation, viral infection status, and transplant history), morphologic (ie, architectural pattern and atypical cytologic features [**Box 1**]), and immunophenotypic features of lymphoma on liver biopsies to distinguish between reactive and neoplastic lymphoid infiltrates. Assessment of an overall architectural pattern of injury (ie,

> **Box 1**
> **Atypical cytologic features of a hepatic lymphoid infiltrate that suggest a need for further work-up**
>
> Large cells
>
> Piling up in the sinusoids
>
> Increased or atypical mitotic figures
>
> Prominent nucleoli
>
> Hemophagocytosis
>
> Ductopenia
>
> Extramedullary hematopoiesis
>
> Geographic necrosis
>
> Granulomas
>
> Marked portal expansion/parenchymal effacement

portal/effacing vs sinusoidal) and cell size can be helpful in narrowing the differential diagnosis (**Fig. 1**, **Table 1**). Immunophenotyping is always required for classification of lymphoma, and an initial panel of B-cell and T-cell markers (including CD20, Pax-5, CD3, and CD5 immunohistochemical stains as well as Epstein-Barr encoding region [EBER] *in situ* hybridization [ISH] stain) is indicated when lymphoma is a consideration. A second round of stains targeted to a more

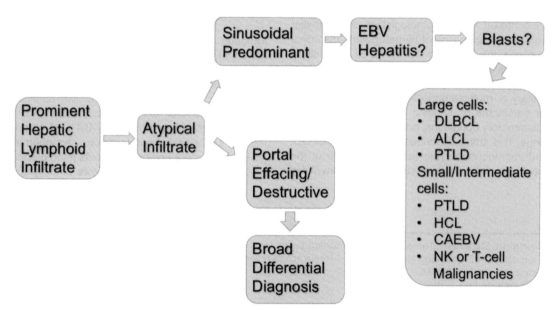

Fig. 1. Differential diagnosis of an atypical hepatic lymphoid infiltrate by architecture. CAEBV, chronic active EBV.

Table 1
Non-Hodgkin B-cell lymphomas classified by cell size

Small Lymphoid Cells	Intermediate-Sized Lymphyoid Cells	Large Lymphoid Cells
B-cell prolymphocytic leukemia CLL/SLL Extranodal MZL of MALT FL HCL LPL MCL PTLD	BL High-grade B-cell lymphoma with *MYC* and *BCL2* and/or *BCL6* rearrangements (some cases have large cells) High-grade B-cell lymphoma, NOS (including cases of blastoid large cells) PTLD	DLBCL, NOS (germinal center or activated/nongerminal center type) EBV-positive DLBCL, NOS Intravascular large B-cell lymphoma Lymphomatoid granulomatosis Plasmablastic lymphoma T-cell histiocyte-rich large B-cell lymphoma PTLD

specific differential diagnosis (**Box 2**) can then be used. Immunophenotypic variation is expected and must be interpreted in the context of morphology and clinical presentation. Clonality assessment can be helpful in selected cases, but clonality cannot be used in isolation for diagnosis of malignancy. In this review, the most common primary and secondary lymphomas involving the liver are reviewed, including the salient clinical, morphologic, and immunophenotypic features.

NON-HODGKIN B-CELL LYMPHOMAS

Most lymphomas involving the liver are of B-cell type, and they include DLBCL, Burkitt lymphoma (BL), B-lymphoblastic leukemia/lymphoma (B-LBL), chronic lymphocytic leukemia/small lymphocytic lymphoma (CLL/SLL), hairy cell leukemia (HCL), follicular lymphoma (FL), mantle cell lymphoma (MCL), and extranodal marginal zone lymphoma (MZL) of mucosa-associated lymphoid tissue (MALT).[4,5,8] Although high-grade B-cell lymphomas (including DLBCL, BL, and B-LBL) are aggressive and can occur over a wide age range, most small B-cell neoplasms (such as CLL/SLL, low-grade FL, and MZL) occur mainly in older patients and are indolent.[10] Despite a typical composition of small cells, MCL has a poor prognosis and can present with blastoid or pleomorphic large cells.[10]

DIFFUSE LARGE B-CELL LYMPHOMA

DLBCL is the most common subtype of PHL, accounting for 46% to 96% of cases.[2,4,5,8] It usually occurs in older patients (mean age 64 years; range: 55–73 years) and is often associated with chronic viral infection (ie, HBV, HCV, HIV, or EBV) and immunosuppression.[9,11–13] Most cases present as 1 or more discrete nodules demonstrating a diffuse infiltrate of CD20+ large lymphoid cells effacing the hepatic parenchyma (some patients may even present with acute liver failure) (**Fig. 2**A–C).[11,12,14,15] DLBCL can mimic active hepatitis histologically, with subtle portal, periportal, or sinusoidal infiltration.[7,11,16,17] Rare cases of reversible methotrexate-associated primary hepatic

Box 2
Example of immunophenotypic and *in situ* evaluation of an atypical hepatic lymphoid infiltrate

First round

- CD20, Pax-5, CD3, CD5, CD21, Cyclin D1, CD56, and EBER ISH (TdT if lymphoblastic morphology)

Second round

- If MCL, then SOX-11 to subclassify

- If a small B-lymphoid neoplasm is a consideration, then CD10, Bcl-6, CD23, CD43, Bcl-2, and Ki-67

- If ALCL is a consideration, then CD4, CD30, EMA, and ALK

- If DLBCL, then CD10, Bcl-6, MUM-1, Ki-67, cMyc, Bcl-2 and FISH for *MYC*, *BCL2*, and *BCL6*

- If a mature T-cell neoplasm is a consideration, then work-up may include additional T-cell markers (ie, CD2, CD4, CD7, CD8, TCRBF1, TCR gamma, TIA-1, granzyme B) and/or TCR clonality testing

- If Hodgkin lymphoma is a consideration, then for CHL: CD30, CD15, and MUM-1, and for NLPHL: OCT2 and PD-1

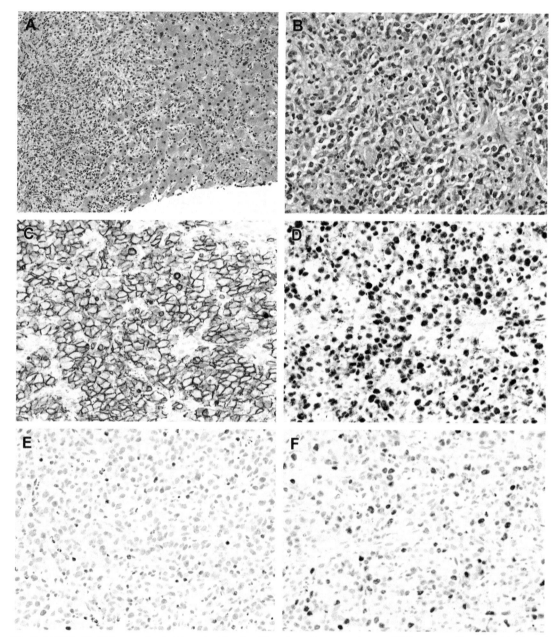

Fig. 2. DLBCL. (*A, B*) Large atypical lymphoid cells efface hepatic parenchyma; (*A*) hematoxylin-eosin (20×) and (*B*) hematoxylin-eosin (40×). (*C*) Positive CD20 (40×). (*D, E*) A GC DLBCL supported by positive Bcl-6 staining in greater than 30% of tumor cells ([*D*] 40×) whereas MUM-1 stain highlights less than 30% of cells ([*E*] 40×), (*F*) Immunostaining for cMyc is positive in greater than 40% of lymphoma cells (40×).

DLBCL in patients with rheumatoid arthritis have been reported.[9,12] DLBCL must be subclassified into a germinal center B-cell type (GC) or activated/non-germinal center B-cell type (non-GC) category, typically by using a panel of CD10, Bcl-6, and MUM-1 immunostains, because this designation may affect therapy.[18] GC type has either CD10 immunostaining in greater than or equal to 30% of malignant cells or Bcl-6 immunostaining in greater than or equal to 30% of malignant cells with MUM-1 staining less than 30% of cells (negative) (**Fig. 2**D, E). All other cases are considered non-GC type. Coexpression of cMyc (>40%) (**Fig. 2**F) and Bcl-2

(>50%) by immunostaining (ie, double-expressor lymphoma)[19] and EBV positivity[20] are adverse prognostic findings. Classification as double-hit (or triple-hit) lymphoma (which most often occurs in GC-type DLBCL) requires fluorescence ISH testing for *MYC*, *BCL2*, and *BCL6* rearrangements.

BURKITT LYMPHOMA

Primary hepatic BL is a rare but aggressive form of extranodal lymphoma.[21] It typically presents as solitary or multiple nodules in young men (mean age 32 years)[21,22] and forms a diffuse sheet of intermediate-sized neoplastic cells with distinct nucleoli, scant cytoplasm, and increased mitotic figures.[16,22,23] Numerous tingible-body macrophages are scattered among malignant cells, displaying the characteristic starry-sky appearance.[23] Widespread portal infiltrates of varying size have also been reported.[16] The tumor cells are usually positive for CD10, Bcl-6, CD43, and pan–B-cell markers (such as CD20) and show a high Ki-67 proliferative index (>95%). The etiology of primary hepatic BL is unknown, but recent reports describe several cases in patients with HBV, HCV, EBV, HIV, or immune suppression.[21,22] Specific *TCF3* or *ID3* (negative regulator of *TCF3*) mutations are present in 70% of sporadic and endemic BL and in 40% of immunodeficiency-related BL.[20]

B-LYMPHOBLASTIC LEUKEMIA/LYMPHOMA

Secondary hepatic involvement is more common in B-LBL patients, and this lymphoma may demonstrate a sinusoidal predominant pattern of infiltration.[24] Primary hepatic B-LBL is extremely rare.[25,26] Blasts show finely dispersed chromatin with scant cytoplasm and strongly express terminal deoxynucleotidyl transferase (TdT), which distinguishes this entity from mature B-cell neoplasms. In rare cases, diffuse hepatic parenchymal infiltration may result in fulminant liver failure.[27] Note that the presence of a few TdT-positive immature B-cells is not specific for hepatic involvement by B-LBL, because scattered TdT-positive cells have been detected in non-neoplastic hepatic infiltrates, in particular in pediatric liver biopsies with extramedullary hematopoiesis.[28]

CHRONIC LYMPHOCYTIC LEUKEMIA/SMALL LYMPHOCYTIC LYMPHOMA

CLL/SLL usually presents in leukemic phase with secondary involvement of the liver. Although sinusoidal infiltration can occur, CLL/SLL usually manifests as prominent and monotonous appearing portal lymphocytic infiltrates.[16] Tumor cells are small with round nuclear contours and express CD5 and CD23, in addition to typical B-cell markers. Cyclin D1 and SOX-11 stains are negative, excluding MCL. LEF1 expression is relatively specific for CLL/SLL. Although a majority of cases are indolent, some cases may result in fulminant acute liver failure due to extensive parenchymal infiltration.[29]

HAIRY CELL LEUKEMIA

Similar to B-LBL and CLL/SLL, HCL usually involves the liver as a leukemia, in the form of portal and sinusoidal infiltration.[30] It can rarely form discrete nodules, however.[31] Tumor cells are small to medium in size with abundant cytoplasm surrounding oval to indented nuclei. They are usually negative for both CD10 and CD5. Flow cytometric evaluation (to include CD25, CD11c, and CD103) can be helpful for diagnosis. *BRAF* V600E or *MAP2K1* mutations are identified in most cases.[20]

FOLLICULAR LYMPHOMA

Primary hepatic FL is rare and represents only 1% to 4% of PHLs.[2,5,13,32] It typically presents as solitary or multiple nodules in older males (mean age 63 years; range: 47–82 years).[32] Small to medium-sized centrocytes form either distinct follicles[16] or diffuse areas of lymphoma cells (with germinal center differentiation [ie, CD10+ and Bcl-6+ but also Bcl-2+]), which may efface the hepatic parenchyma.[32] An important feature of FL is the presence of follicular meshworks (which can be highlighted on CD21 and CD23 immunostains). A confluence of large cells outside of follicular meshworks should be considered evidence of transformation to DLBCL, whereas increased large cells within meshworks (ie, >15 centroblasts in a high-power field) are considered high-grade FL (ie, grade 3A or 3B, scale 1–3). The rate of HBV or HCV infection is not significantly increased in primary hepatic FL compared with that of general NHLs.[32]

MANTLE CELL LYMPHOMA

Primary hepatic MCL is rare, representing less than 5% of PHLs.[2,8] Most cases are composed of small to medium-sized lymphoid cells that express CD20, CD5, and Bcl-1/cyclin D1. Based on SOX-11 staining, MCL can be divided into 2 variants.[20] The SOX11-positive variant is composed of *IGVH*-unmutated, or minimally mutated, B-cells that involve lymph nodes and extranodal sites. With acquisition of additional molecular/cytogenetic abnormalities, this classic variant of MCL can change into an aggressive blastoid or pleomorphic form. The SOX11-negative variant is composed of *IGVH*-mutated B-cells and usually presents as an indolent leukemia without lymph node involvement; however, secondary mutations (such as *TP53*) can lead to aggressive disease.[20] *CCND2* is rearranged in a significant proportion of Bcl-1/cyclin D1-negative MCL.[20]

EXTRANODAL MARGINAL ZONE LYMPHOMA OF MUCOSA-ASSOCIATED LYMPHOID TISSUE

Primary hepatic MALT lymphoma is the second most common subtype of PHL.[2,13,33]

Chronic viral infection or inflammatory liver disease seems to contribute to its pathogenesis, because several MALT lymphoma cases have been reported in association with chronic HBV,[33,34] HCV,[34] and primary biliary cholangitis.[35,36] Primary hepatic MALT lymphoma tends to form solitary or multiple nodules in older patients (mean age 62 years; range: 36–85 years)[33,37–40] and often presents as dense monotonous portal infiltrates surrounding reactive B-cell follicles (**Fig. 3**A, B) with occasional infiltration of interlobular bile duct epithelium (lymphoepithelial lesions).[34,36,37,40,41] Rarely, it can efface large portions of hepatic parenchyma.[33] Tumor cells are mainly small, with slightly irregular nuclear contour, dense chromatin, and scant cytoplasm, without evidence of germinal center differentiation. Neoplastic B-cells aberrantly coexpress CD43 in a subset of MALT lymphomas. In the setting of plasmacytic differentiation, which can be extreme,

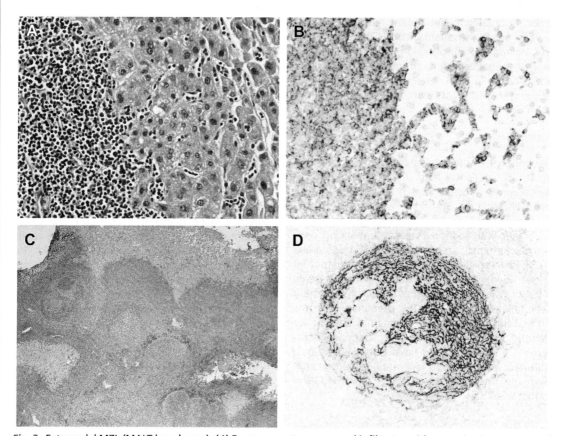

Fig. 3. Extranodal MZL (MALT lymphoma). (*A*) Dense monotonous portal infiltrates with extension into periportal sinusoids (hematoxylin-eosin, 40×). (*B*) Positive CD20 (40×). (*C*) Effacement of hepatic parenchyma by a diffuse infiltrate of small centrocyte-like cells with remnants of reactive follicles (hematoxylin-eosin, 4×). (*D*) CD21 stain highlights disrupted follicular meshworks with colonization by neoplastic cells (20×).

ISH staining for kappa and lambda light chains can establish the presence of a monotypic cell population and support diagnosis of lymphoma. Scattered reactive follicles are common in MALT lymphoma,[37] which may demonstrate follicular colonization by the lymphoma cells (Fig. 3C, D). Presence of diffuse sheets of small B-cells in interfollicular areas, where small T-cells predominate in a reactive process, argues for MALT lymphoma over a reactive infiltrate. In some cases, B-cell receptor clonality testing can be helpful in distinguishing MALT lymphoma from reactive infiltrates. Lymphoplasmacytic lymphoma (LPL) may be morphologically indistinguishable from MALT lymphoma, but LPL involves lymph nodes and bone marrow and is unlikely to present on liver biopsy. Based on recently revised criteria,[20] LPL should consist of a monotonous lymphoplasmacytic proliferation, in which there may be complete architectural effacement or follicular colonization.[20] Dutcher bodies may further suggest the diagnosis, but are not entirely specific for LPL. Neoplastic cells are positive for B-cell markers and monotypic on light chain ISH. Many LPL patients have systemic disease with clinical features of Waldenström macroglobulinemia (including IgM paraproteinemia and hyperviscosity), which can be helpful in distinguishing LPL from MALT lymphoma with extensive plasmacytic differentiation.[42,43] MYD88 L265P mutation is identified in most cases of LPL, although it is not entirely specific for LPL.[20]

MATURE T-CELL NEOPLASMS

T-cell lymphomas are much less common than B-cell lymphomas and more commonly involve the liver as part of a systemic disease.[4,8,13,44] Primary hepatic T-cell lymphoma is exceedingly rare, representing only 5% to 10% of PHLs, and usually follows an aggressive clinical course.[4,6,8,44–47] Nearly all cases are peripheral T-cell lymphoma (PTCL), not otherwise specified (NOS), or hepatosplenic T-cell lymphoma (HSTCL).[4]

PERIPHERAL T-CELL LYMPHOMA, NOT OTHERWISE SPECIFIED

PTCL, NOS usually occurs in middle-aged men with or without discrete lesions.[13,44,46] Malignant lymphoid infiltrate morphology varies from bland small lymphoid cells, mimicking hepatitis, to a mixture of small to large cells, to diffuse sheets of large cells.[44] PTCL, NOS may

completely obliterate the hepatic parenchyma, but a liver biopsy may also show only scattered malignant T-cells in portal, periportal, and/or sinusoidal regions, which can make diagnosis and immunophenotyping challenging.[44,46] Gene rearrangement studies may be necessary to confirm the presence of a clonal T-cell population.[44] Although EBV-associated lymphoproliferative disorders are mostly B-cell lymphomas, a rare case of primary hepatic PTCL associated with EBV infection has been reported.[46]

HEPATOSPLENIC T-CELL LYMPHOMA

HSTCL is a rare mature T-cell neoplasm derived from cytotoxic T-cells, which manifests as an extranodal systemic lymphoma.[48] It usually occurs in young patients who present with nonspecific systemic symptoms and hepatosplenomegaly but without lymphadenopathy.[47–49] Rare cases may be associated with inflammatory bowel disease treatment (such as infliximab).[50] The hallmark of liver involvement is marked sinusoidal dilatation by medium-sized malignant cells (often with 3 or 4 cells piling up) (Fig. 4A).[47,49,51] Usually, there is little to no infiltration in portal tracts, but a cytologically bland infiltrate can predominantly, or exclusively, involve portal tracts.[52,53] Malignant cells are usually gamma/delta T-cells with a nonactivated cytotoxic phenotype (ie, TIA-1$^+$, granzyme B$^-$) (Fig. 4B), and they characteristically do not express CD5, CD4, or CD8.[49] CD56 immunostain may be positive in neoplastic cells, but EBV-encoded small RNA (EBER) ISH stain is most often negative (Fig. 4C, D).[49] The lack of EBV and granzyme B staining is useful in distinguishing HSTCL from aggressive natural killer (NK)-cell leukemia. In challenging cases, molecular and cytogenetic testing can be helpful, because HSTCL shows a recurrent cytogenetic abnormality (isochromosome arm 7q10 and, possibly, trisomy 8)[49,54] and clonal T-cell receptor (TCR) gene rearrangement.[48]

IMMUNODEFICIENCY-ASSOCIATED LYMPHOPROLIFERATIVE DISORDERS: POST-TRANSPLANT LYMPHOPROLIFERATIVE DISORDERS

Transplant patients may develop abnormal, mostly EBV-driven, B-cell (or rarely T/NK-cell) proliferations in the liver, known as post-transplant lymphoproliferative disorders (PTLDs).[55–57] Nondestructive lesions of PTLD resemble reactive

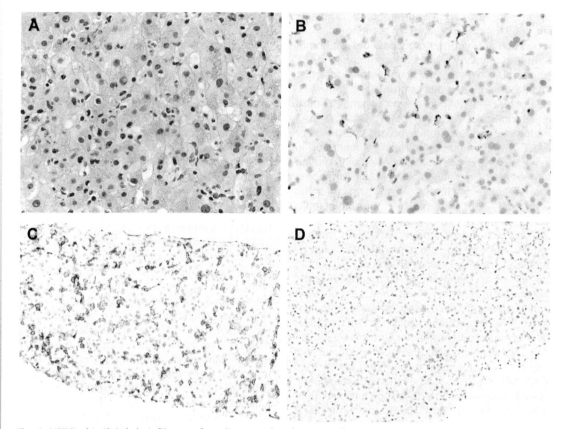

Fig. 4. HSTCL. (*A*, *B*) Subtle infiltrate of medium-sized malignant cells in sinusoids ([*A*] hematoxylin-eosin, 40×), which are positive for TIA-1 ([*B*], 40×). (*C*) Positive CD56 can be seen in a subset of HSTCL, as in this case (2×). (*D*) Negative EBER (20×).

lymphoid hyperplasia or chronic inflammation (ie, infectious mononucleosis) and do not efface the hepatic parenchyma, whereas polymorphic and monomorphic forms can resemble malignant lymphomas and efface the normal architecture.[56,57] Polymorphic PTLD consists of a polymorphic mixture of small and large cells (including plasma cells) and can mimic MZL.[56,57] Monomorphic sheets of large lymphoid cells, resembling DLBCL, is characteristic of monomorphic PTLD (**Fig. 5**), which can be of B- or T/NK-cell type.[56,57] Although many polymorphic, and almost all monomorphic, PTLDs are clonal, they may regress spontaneously (or following reduction of immunosuppression).[56,57] Classic Hodgkin lymphoma (CHL) may also occur as a PTLD.

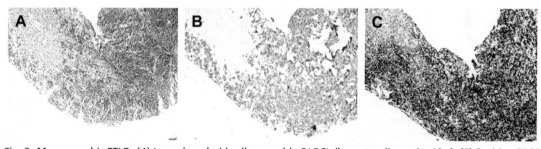

Fig. 5. Monomorphic PTLD. (*A*) Large lymphoid cells resemble DLBCL (hematoxylin-eosin, 10×). (*B*) Positive CD20 (10×). (*C*) Positive EBER (10×).

HODGKIN LYMPHOMAS

CLASSIC HODGKIN LYMPHOMA

Hepatic involvement by CHL is uncommon, but rare cases of primary CHL have been reported.[58] CHL usually forms discrete nodules with variable numbers of Hodgkin/Reed-Sternberg (HRS) cells in a background of mixed inflammatory cells, often involving or surrounding portal tracts (Fig. 6A, B).[16,58] CHL can rarely present as acute liver failure with extensive hepatic involvement.[59] Although CHL is of B-cell origin, most B-cell markers (including CD20) are negative. One B-cell antigen consistently expressed by the malignant cells is Pax-5, although the staining can be weak and focal. The HRS cells are also positive for CD15 and CD30, in most cases (Fig. 6C, D), sometimes with Golgi accentuation, and MUM-1 is also usually positive. Although some large B-cell NHLs and anaplastic large cell lymphoma (ALCL) can mimic CHL, both morphologically and immunohistochemically, large B-cell NHLs are positive for multiple B-cell markers, and ALCL does not express Pax-5.

NODULAR LYMPHOCYTE–PREDOMINANT HODGKIN LYMPHOMA

Only rare cases of secondary hepatic involvement by nodular lymphocyte–predominant Hodgkin lymphoma (NLPHL) have been reported, including 1 case presenting as fulminant hepatic failure due to extensive hepatic infiltration.[60] NLPHL is usually nodular (with associated follicular dendritic cell aggregates on CD21 stain) and can be distinguished from CHL by demonstrating staining of large lymphocyte-predominant cells with B-cell markers (ie, CD20, Bcl-6, CD79a, and OCT2), usually without coexpression of CD15 and CD30. Follicular T-cells (ie, PD-1–positive T-cells) may be noted to rosette around the large B-cells, which can aid in distinction from T-cell histiocyte-rich large B-cell lymphoma (a form of DLBCL), although it may not be possible to always distinguish

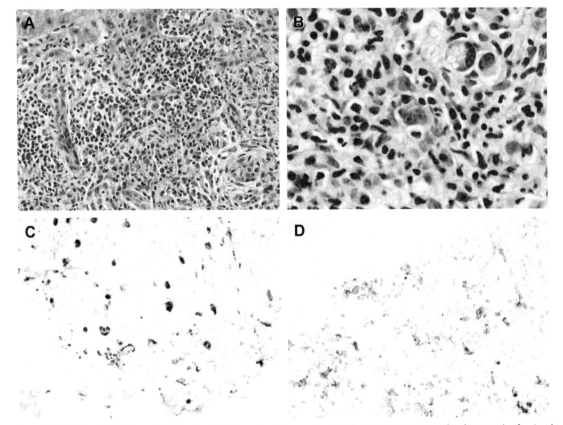

Fig. 6. CHL. (A, B) Scattered HRS cells ([B] hematoxylin-eosin, 100×) are present in a background of mixed inflammatory cells ([A] hematoxylin-eosin, 40×). (C, D) The HRS cells are positive for (C) CD15 (40×) and (D) CD30 (40×).

NLPHL from T-cell histiocyte-rich large B-cell lymphoma.

LYMPHOMA MIMICS: NODULAR LYMPHOID LESION

Hepatic nodular lymphoid lesion (NLL) (also known as reactive lymphoid hyperplasia) can mimic lymphoma by displacing the surrounding hepatic parenchyma and forming a discrete mass.[61,62] It is a benign lesion, however, consisting entirely of polyclonal B-cells and T-cells forming reactive follicles.[61,62] Unlike MALT lymphoma, no diffuse sheets of B-cells outside benign reactive follicles are seen on CD20 stain.[61,62] Rather, the interfollicular areas show a mixed population of CD3+ T-cells and few CD20+ B-cells.[61,62] B-cell clonality testing can be helpful in some cases. Many patients with NLLs have hepatic chronic inflammatory conditions, such as HBV, HCV, primary biliary cholangitis, or autoimmune disorders, suggesting that NLL represents an immune-mediated benign reactive hyperplasia.[61,62] NLL is treated by local excision.[61,62]

EPSTEIN-BARR VIRUS-POSITIVE HEPATIC LYMPHOID INFILTRATES

EBV typically infects B cells, through the EBV receptor (CD21). In EBV hepatitis, a liver biopsy most commonly shows a mild sinusoidal lymphohistiocytic infiltrate without piling up of the cells, hemophagocytosis, or overt atypia (Fig. 7A, B). There is usually no hepatocyte injury or necrosis, but non-necrotizing granulomas (and rarely fibrin ring granulomas) can be present. Lineage markers are helpful in excluding an EBV-driven malignancy or chronic active EBV infection (which may involve B-cells, T-cells, or NK-cells). In EBV hepatitis, there is a predominant population of T-cells (ie, CD3+ and

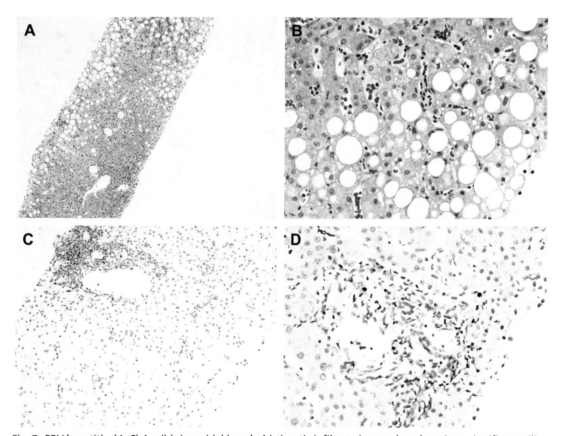

Fig. 7. EBV hepatitis. (A, B) A mild sinusoidal lymphohistiocytic infiltrate is seen, but there is no significant piling up of the cells, hemophagocytosis, or overt atypia. ([A] hematoxylin-eosin, 10×, and [B] hematoxylin-eosin, 40×). (C) Pax-5 stain highlights scattered B-cells (20×). (D) EBER highlights a similar distribution of scattered positive B cells (40×).

CD5+ small mature lymphocytes) with only occasional scattered B-cells (ie, Pax-5+ small mature lymphocytes) (**Fig. 7**C). The EBER ISH highlights a similar distribution of occasional positive cells (as seen on the Pax-5 stain) (**Fig. 7**D). If a majority of cells, out of proportion to the number of Pax-5+ B-cells, are EBER positive, then a typical EBV hepatitis is excluded. Note that NK-cells express cytoplasmic CD3 (ie, CD3ε), so CD3 immunohistochemical staining of paraffin sections labels NK-cells (in addition to T-cells, which are more specifically identified by surface CD3 labeling in flow cytometric evaluation), and thus the EBER positive population in this scenario could be either T-lineage or NK-lineage (or NK/T-lineage) and further evaluation is needed (NK-cells are CD5 negative, but so are some T-cell lymphomas, such as HSTCL, as discussed previously). Also, if a majority of cells are B-cell lineage and EBER positive, then an EBV-driven B-cell lymphoproliferative disorder should be considered, in particular in the post-transplant setting, as discussed previously. Aggressive NK-cell leukemia (ANKL) is an NK-cell neoplasm with a leukemic component that usually presents in young Asian men and has a fulminant course. ANKL has the same immunophenotype as NK/T-cell lymphoma (CD2+, cCD3+, CD56+, TIA-1+, granzyme B+, sCD3−, CD5−) with evidence of EBV infection of the neoplastic cells (ie, EBER ISH positive), and there is extensive hemophagocytosis (**Fig. 8**). TCR genes are not rearranged. ANKL can be readily distinguished from HSTCL on bone marrow evaluation, because the latter has a sinusoidal growth pattern (whereas ANKL shows diffuse/interstitial infiltration). Distinction from large granular lymphocytic leukemia (LGLL) is aided by EBER ISH, because LGLL is negative (and T cell-LGLL demonstrates surface CD3, on flow cytometric evaluation, with TCR clonality on molecular testing) (**Fig. 9**).

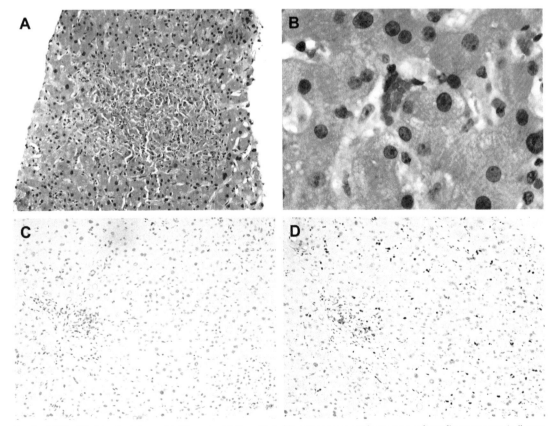

Fig. 8. ANKL. (*A*) Atypical sinusoidal lymphohistiocytic infiltrate is seen with an area of confluent necrosis (hematoxylin-eosin, 20×). (*B*) Hemophagocytosis is common (hematoxylin-eosin, 100×). (*C*) Negative Pax-5 (20×). (*D*) Positive EBER (20×).

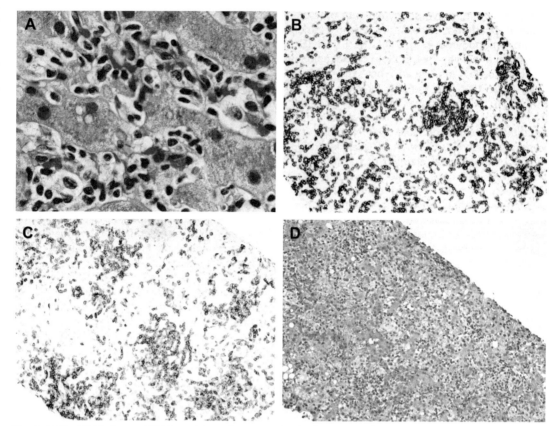

Fig. 9. LGLL. (*A*) Similar to EBV hepatitis and ANKL, LGLL is characterized by a sinusoidal pattern of atypical lymphoid infiltration (hematoxylin-eosin, 100×). (*B*) Positive CD3 (20×). (*C*) Positive CD5 (20×). (*D*) Negative EBER (20×).

REFERENCES

1. Caccamo D, Pervez NK, Marchevsky A. Primary lymphoma of the liver in the acquired immunodeficiency syndrome. Arch Pathol Lab Med 1986;110:553–5.
2. Lei KI. Primary non-Hodgkin's lymphoma of the liver. Leuk Lymphoma 1998;29:293–9.
3. Freeman C, Berg JW, Cutler SJ. Occurrence and prognosis of extranodal lymphomas. Cancer 1972; 29:252–60.
4. Peng Y, Qing AC, Cai J, et al. Lymphoma of the liver: clinicopathological features of 19 patients. Exp Mol Pathol 2016;100:276–80.
5. Page RD, Romaguera JE, Osborne B, et al. Primary hepatic lymphoma: favorable outcome after combination chemotherapy. Cancer 2001;92:2023–9.
6. Mishra S, Shukla A, Tripathi AK, et al. Primary T-cell lymphoma of liver. BMJ Case Rep 2013;22:1–3.
7. Lee JA, Jeong WK, Min JH, et al. Primary hepatic lymphoma mimicking acute hepatitis. Clin Mol Hepatol 2013;19:320–3.
8. Ugurluer G, Miller RC, Li Y, et al. Primary hepatic lymphoma: a retrospective, multicenter rare cancer network study. Rare Tumors 2016;8:6502.
9. Kikuma K, Watanabe J, Oshiro Y, et al. Etiological factors in primary hepatic B-cell lymphoma. Virchows Arch 2012;460:379–87.
10. A clinical evaluation of the International Lymphoma Study Group classification of non-Hodgkin's lymphoma. The non-hodgkin's lymphoma classification project. Blood 1997;89:3909–18.
11. Zheng J, Hou Y, Zhou R, et al. Clinicopathological features of primary hepatic diffuse large B-cell lymphoma: a report of seven cases and a literature review. Int J Clin Exp Pathol 2015;8:12955–60.
12. Kawahara A, Tsukada J, Yamaguchi T, et al. Reversible methotrexate-associated lymphoma of the liver in rheumatoid arthritis: a unique case of primary hepatic lymphoma. Biomark Res 2015;6:10.
13. Bronowicki JP, Bineau C, Feugier P, et al. Primary lymphoma of the liver: clinical-pathological features and relationship with HCV infection in French patients. Hepatology 2003;37:781–7.
14. Takeuchi N, Naba K. Primary hepatic lymphoma is difficult to discriminate from a liver abscess. Case Rep Gastrointest Med 2014;2014:925307.
15. Romacho López L, León Díaz FJ, Sánchez Pérez B, et al. Acute liver failure caused by primary

non-hodgkin's lymphoma of the liver. Transplant Proc 2016;48:3000–2.

16. Jaffe ES. Malignant lymphomas: pathology of hepatic involvement. Semin Liver Dis 1987;7:257–68.

17. Scheimberg IB, Pollock DJ, Collins PW, et al. Pathology of the liver in leukaemia and lymphoma. A study of 110 autopsies. Histopathology 1995;26:311–21.

18. Hans CP, Weisenburger DD, Greiner TC, et al. Confirmation of the molecular classification of diffuse large B-cell lymphoma by immunohistochemistry using a tissue microarray. Blood 2004; 103:275–82.

19. Galati G, Rampa L, Vespasiani-Gentilucci U, et al. Hepatitis C and double-hit B cell lymphoma successfully treated by antiviral therapy. World J Hepatol 2016;8:1244–50.

20. Swerdlow SH, Campo E, Pileri SA, et al. The 2016 revision of the World Health Organization classification of lymphoid neoplasms. Blood 2016;127:2375–90.

21. Reyes AJ, Ramcharan K, Aboh S, et al. Primary hepatic Burkitt's lymphoma as first manifestation of HIV-AIDS in a hepatitis B seropositive adult: when defences fail. BMJ Case Rep 2016;26:1–4.

22. Sekiguchi Y, Yoshikawa H, Shimada A, et al. Primary hepatic circumscribed Burkitt's lymphoma that developed after acute hepatitis B: report of a case with a review of the literature. J Clin Exp Hematop 2013;53:167–73.

23. Citak EC, Sari I, Demirci M, et al. Primary hepatic Burkitt lymphoma in a child and review of literature. J Pediatr Hematol Oncol 2011;33:e368–71.

24. Takamatsu T. Preferential infiltration of liver sinusoids in acute lymphoblastic leukemia. Rinsho Ketsueki 2001;42:1181–6.

25. Lin P, Jones D, Dorfman DM, et al. Precursor B-cell lymphoblastic lymphoma: a predominantly extranodal tumor with low propensity for leukemic involvement. Am J Surg Pathol 2000;24:1480–90.

26. Maitra A, McKenna RW, Weinberg AG, et al. Precursor B-cell lymphoblastic lymphoma. A study of nine cases lacking blood and bone marrow involvement and review of the literature. Am J Clin Pathol 2001; 115:868–75.

27. Litten JB, Rodríguez MM, Maniaci V. Acute lymphoblastic leukemia presenting in fulminant hepatic failure. Pediatr Blood Cancer 2006;47:842–5.

28. Wen KW, Gill RM. Immature B-cells are detected in a subset of adult and pediatric liver biopsies. Appl Immunohistochem Mol Morphol 2017, in press. PMID: 28968264.

29. Hasuike S, Hayashi K, Abe H, et al. Acute hepatic failure due to hepatic involvement by chronic lymphocytic leukemic cells in a patient with chronic hepatitis B. J Gastroenterol 2004;39:499–500.

30. Roquet ML, Zafrani ES, Farcet JP, et al. Histopathological lesions of the liver in hairy cell leukemia: a report of 14 cases. Hepatology 1985;5:496–500.

31. Sahar N, Schiby G, Davidson T, et al. Hairy cell leukemia presenting as multiple discrete hepatic lesions. World J Gastroenterol 2009;15:4453–6.

32. Gomyo H, Kagami Y, Kato H, et al. Primary hepatic follicular lymphoma : a case report and discussion of chemotherapy and favorable outcomes. J Clin Exp Hematop 2007;47:73–7.

33. Chan RC, Chu CM, Chow C, et al. A concurrent primary hepatic MALT lymphoma and hepatocellular carcinoma. Pathology 2015;47:178–81.

34. Mizuno S, Isaji S, Tabata M, et al. Hepatic mucosa-associated lymphoid tissue (MALT) lymphoma associated with hepatitis C. J Hepatol 2002;37: 872–3.

35. Ye MQ, Suriawinata A, Black C, et al. Primary hepatic marginal zone B-cell lymphoma of mucosa-associated lymphoid tissue type in a patient with primary biliary cirrhosis. Arch Pathol Lab Med 2000;124:604–8.

36. Prabhu RM, Medeiros LJ, Kumar D, et al. Primary hepatic low-grade B-cell lymphoma of mucosa-associated lymphoid tissue (MALT) associated with primary biliary cirrhosis. Mod Pathol 1998;11:404–10.

37. Koubaa Mahjoub W, Chaumette-Planckaert MT, Murga Penas EM, et al. Primary hepatic lymphoma of mucosa-associated lymphoid tissue type: a case report with cytogenetic study. Int J Surg Pathol 2008;16:301–7.

38. Doi H, Horiike N, Hiraoka A, et al. Primary hepatic marginal zone B cell lymphoma of mucosa-associated lymphoid tissue type: case report and review of the literature. Int J Hematol 2008;88: 418–23.

39. Isaacson PG, Banks PM, Best PV, et al. Primary low-grade hepatic B-cell lymphoma of mucosa-associated lymphoid tissue (MALT)-type. Am J Surg Pathol 1995;19:571–5.

40. Dong S, Chen L, Chen Y, et al. Primary hepatic extranodal marginal zone B-cell lymphoma of mucosa-associated lymphoid tissue type: a case report and literature review. Medicine (Baltimore) 2017;96:e6305.

41. Nart D, Ertan Y, Yilmaz F, et al. Primary hepatic marginal zone B-cell lymphoma of mucosa-associated lymphoid tissue type in a liver transplant patient with hepatitis B cirrhosis. Transplant Proc 2005;37:4408–12.

42. Swerdlow SH, Berger F, Pileri SA, et al. Lymphoplasmacytic lymphoma. In: Swerdlow SH, et al, editors. WHO classification of tumours of haematopoietic and lymphoid tissues. Lyon (France): IARC; 2008. p. 194–5.

43. Vitolo U, Ferreri AJ, Montoto S. Lymphoplasmacytic lymphoma-Waldenstrom's macroglobulinemia. Crit Rev Oncol Hematol 2008;67:172–85.

44. Stancu M, Jones D, Vega F, et al. Peripheral T-cell lymphoma arising in the liver. Am J Clin Pathol 2002;118:574–81.

45. Noronha V, Shafi NQ, Obando JA, et al. Primary non-Hodgkin's lymphoma of the liver. Crit Rev Oncol Hematol 2005;53:199–207.

46. Peng Y, Cai J, Yue C, et al. Primary hepatic Epstein-Barr virus-associated CD30-positive peripheral T-cell lymphoma of cytotoxic phenotype. Exp Mol Pathol 2016;100:207–11.

47. Siraj F, Dalal V, Khan AA, et al. Hepatosplenic T-cell lymphoma with coexistent hepatitis B infection: a rare clinicopathologic entity. Tumori 2016;102:S61–4.

48. Gaulard P, Jaffe ES, Krenacs L, et al. Hepatosplenic T-cell lymphoma. In: Swerdlow SH, et al, editors. WHO classification of tumours of haematopoietic and lymphoid tissues. Lyon: IARC; 2008. p. 292–3.

49. Belhadj K, Reyes F, Farcet JP, et al. Hepatosplenic gammadelta T-cell lymphoma is a rare clinicopathologic entity with poor outcome: report on a series of 21 patients. Blood 2003;102:4261–9.

50. Thai A, Prindiville T. Hepatosplenic T-cell lymphoma and inflammatory bowel disease. J Crohns Colitis 2010;4:511–22.

51. Falchook GS, Vega F, Dang NH, et al. Hepatosplenic gamma-delta T-cell lymphoma: clinicopathological features and treatment. Ann Oncol 2009;20:1080–5.

52. Wei SZ, Liu TH, Wang DT, et al. Hepatosplenic gammadelta T-cell lymphoma. World J Gastroenterol 2005;11:3729–34.

53. Veldt BJ, Meijers C, Zondervan PE, et al. Hepatosplenic gammadelta T cell lymphoma: a diagnostic pitfall. J Hepatol 2003;39:455–7.

54. Jonveaux P, Daniel MT, Martel V, et al. Isochromosome 7q and trisomy 8 are consistent primary, non-random chromosomal abnormalities associated with hepatosplenic T gamma/delta lymphoma. Leukemia 1996;10:1453–5.

55. Jain A, Nalesnik M, Reyes J, et al. Posttransplant lymphoproliferative disorders in liver transplantation: a 20-year experience. Ann Surg 2002;236:429–36.

56. Harris NL, Ferry JA, Swerdlow SH. Posttransplant lymphoproliferative disorders: summary of Society for hematopathology workshop. Semin Diagn Pathol 1997;14:8–14.

57. Swerdlow SH, Webber SA, Chadburn A, et al. Post-transplant lymphoproliferative disorders. In: Swerdlow SH, et al, editors. WHO classification of tumours of haematopoietic and lymphoid tissues. Lyon (France): IARC; 2008. p. 343–8.

58. Yokomori H, Kaneko F, Sato A, et al. Primary hepatic presentation of Hodgkin's lymphoma: a case report. Hepatol Res 2008;38:1054–7.

59. Vardareli E, Dündar E, Aslan V, et al. Acute liver failure due to Hodgkin's lymphoma. Med Princ Pract 2004;13:372–4.

60. Woolf KM, Wei MC, Link MP, et al. Nodular lymphocyte-predominant Hodgkin lymphoma presenting as fulminant hepatic failure in a pediatric patient: a case report with pathologic, immunophenotypic, and molecular findings. Appl Immunohistochem Mol Morphol 2008;16:196–201.

61. Willenbrock K, Kriener S, Oeschger S, et al. Nodular lymphoid lesion of the liver with simultaneous focal nodular hyperplasia and hemangioma: discrimination from primary hepatic MALT-type non-Hodgkin's lymphoma. Virchows Arch 2006;448:223–7.

62. Sharifi S, Murphy M, Loda M, et al. Nodular lymphoid lesion of the liver: an immune-mediated disorder mimicking low-grade malignant lymphoma. Am J Surg Pathol 1999;23:302–8.

Cholangiocarcinoma

Alyssa M. Krasinskas, MD

KEYWORDS

- Cholangiocarcinoma • Bile duct • Intrahepatic • Extrahepatic • IDH1 • IDH2

Key points

- Cholangiocarcinomas can be classified according to anatomic location, macroscopic growth pattern, microscopic features, and cell of origin.
- Intrahepatic cholangiocarcinomas have recently been divided into 2 subtypes based histologic features and cell of origin: small duct type/canals of Herring and large duct type/peribiliary glands.
- Intrahepatic cholangiocarcinomas of small duct type can express neural cell adhesion molecule, N-cadherin, and C-reactive protein, and can harbor mutations in *IDH1/2*.
- In intrahepatic cholangiocarcinomas, the main risk factor is chronic liver disease (viral hepatitis).
- Extrahepatic cholangiocarcinomas can express S100P.

ABSTRACT

This article focuses on cholangiocarcinoma, both intrahepatic and extrahepatic. The various classification schemes based on anatomic location, macroscopic growth pattern, microscopic features, and cell of origin are outlined. The clinicopathologic, immunohistochemical and molecular differences between intrahepatic cholangiocarcinoma and extrahepatic cholangiocarcinoma, as well as differences in the 2 subtypes of intrahepatic cholangiocarcinoma, are discussed. Finally, precursor lesions, prognosis, treatment, and promising new potential targeted therapies are reviewed.

OVERVIEW

Cholangiocarcinoma is the most common malignancy of the biliary tree. Gaining a complete understanding of this disease can be challenging for many reasons. Cholangiocarcinoma is a heterogenous disease with different definitions, different classification schemes, newly described subtypes, and an evolving knowledge of the molecular basis of this disease. By its most simple definition, cholangiocarcinoma is cancer of the bile ducts. However, although many people include cancers that involve both intrahepatic and extrahepatic bile ducts in their definition,[1–3] other sources only view cholangiocarcinoma as cancer of the intrahepatic bile ducts and perihilar bile ducts (the American Joint Committee on Cancer [AJCC]/International Union Against Cancer [UICC] does not specifically use the term cholangiocarcinoma for distal tumors)[4] or just the intrahepatic bile duct.[5] For the remaining of this discussion, cholangiocarcinoma is defined as a cancer that arises from either the intrahepatic or extrahepatic bile ducts, excluding the ampulla of Vater and gallbladder.

The incidence of cholangiocarcinoma is low in the United States, with reported rates ranging from 0.72 to 1.67 per 100,000.[1,6,7] The incidence varies widely worldwide and the highest incidence of the disease is in Asia (Northeast Thailand) with a rate of more than 80 per 100,000 population.[1] Interestingly, in the United States, the incidence of intrahepatic cholangiocarcinoma (ICC) from 1992 to 2000 showed a 4% annual increase,

---

Disclosure Statement: No disclosures.
Department of Pathology and Laboratory Medicine, Emory University Hospital, 1364 Clifton Road Northeast, Suite H180D, Atlanta, GA 30322, USA
E-mail address: akrasin@emory.edu

Surgical Pathology 11 (2018) 403–429
https://doi.org/10.1016/j.path.2018.02.005

whereas the incidence of extrahepatic cholangio-carcinoma (ECC) remained constant with annual percent changes of 1%.[8] The increasing incidence of ICC in the United States was also supported by another study that showed the rates of both hepatocellular carcinoma and ICC approximately doubled between 1976 and 2000.[9] These trends seem to also be occurring worldwide.[10,11]

Most of the risk factors for the development of cholangiocarcinoma are related to chronic inflammation and irritation (Box 1). Some well-established risk factors are similar for both ICC and ECC.[12,13] Because of the differences in the incidence rates between ICC and ECC, studies have shown some differences in risk factors as well. A population-based study in the United States showed liver cirrhosis, thyrotoxicosis, chronic pancreatitis, and possibly duodenal ulcer disease to be related to both ECC and ICC, and hepatitis C virus infection, obesity, chronic nonalcoholic liver disease, and smoking to be significantly more common in ICC; because of the rarity of liver fluke infections and hepatolithiasis in the United States, these entities were not found to be risk factors in this study.[13]

CLASSIFICATION SCHEMES

Owing to the heterogeneity of cholangiocarcinoma and multiple sites of origin in the biliary tree, many classification schemes have been developed and used in clinical practice, creating some confusion as to the best way to classify these lesions.[14] Cholangiocarcinomas can be classified according to anatomic location, macroscopic growth pattern, microscopic features, and cell of origin.

CLASSIFICATION BY ANATOMIC LOCATION

Cholangiocarcinomas can divided by location into 2 general categories: intrahepatic and extrahepatic. ICCs arise within the second-order bile duct branches and peripheral branches.[4,5,15] Although ECCs are further subdivided by location, the definition varies among different major publications. According to the AJCC/UICC and College of American Pathologists (CAP), ECCs are further divided into perihilar and distal bile duct tumors: Perihilar cholangiocarcinomas arise proximal to the cystic duct origin, distal to the second-order bile ducts, and often involve the hepatic duct bifurcation, whereas distal bile duct tumors arise between the cystic duct origin and the ampulla (AJCC/UICC, CAP).[3,4,16] According to the World Health Organization (WHO), hilar (extrahepatic) tumors arise at or near the junction of the right and left hepatic ducts, whereas perihilar intrahepatic tumors arise in the right and left hepatic ducts away from the junction; and tumors arising in the distal bile duct are not classified as cholangiocarcinoma.[5] According to guidelines published by the European Association for the Study of the Liver, cholangiocarcinoma should be subclassified as intrahepatic, perihilar, or distal, where intrahepatic cholangiocarcinoma arises within the liver parenchyma; use of the term Klatskin is discouraged and the term extrahepatic is felt to not be helpful.[1]

Although there are limitations to this classification scheme, and although more recent molecular and epidemiologic data support using different classification schemes for cholangiocarcinoma (discussed elsewhere in this article), classifying cholangiocarcinomas by anatomic location has been widely used in the literature. Many current treatment regimens are also based on this classification scheme and are

---

Box 1
Risk factors for cholangiocarcinoma

Risk factors for extrahepatic and intrahepatic cholangiocarcinoma

- Biliary diseases (primary sclerosing cholangitis; primary or secondary biliary cirrhosis)
- Biliary malformations/choledochal cysts
- Cholelithiasis/choledocholithiasis
- Cholecystitis/cholecystectomy
- Liver flukes (clonorchis sinensis should be italicized)
- Cirrhosis
- Alcoholic liver disease
- Type II diabetes
- Thyrotoxicosis
- Chronic pancreatitis

Risk factors for intrahepatic cholangiocarcinoma

- Hepatolithiasis
- Hepatitis C virus infection
- Chronic nonalcoholic liver disease
- Obesity
- Smoking

Fig. 1. Gross appearance of intra-hepatic cholangiocarcinoma (classification by macroscopic growth pattern). (*A*) Mass-forming tumor. Solid tumor with well-defined border and a rather homogenous grey-white cut surface. (*B*) Periductal infiltrating tumor with a mass forming component. In the top section, the tumor infiltrates around several small ductal structures and is associated with an area of atrophy containing cystically dilated ducts. In the bottom section, there is a solid, mass-forming component. (*C*) Intraductal growth with an invasive mass-forming component. Most of the tumor is expanding and filling a duct and there are foci where the tumor invades through the wall of the duct into the hepatic parenchyma.

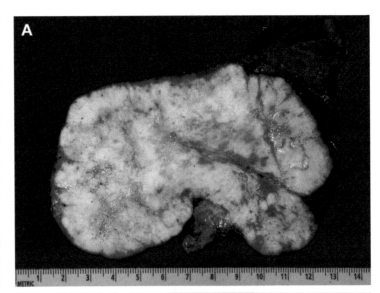

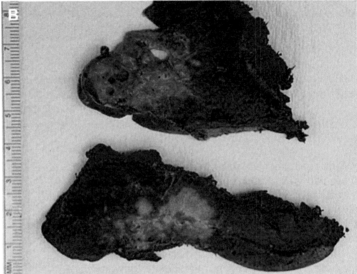

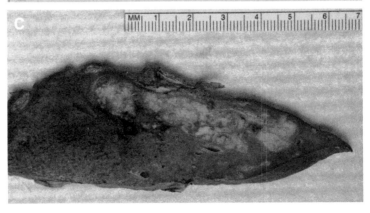

Table 1
Histologic classification of malignant epithelial tumors of the intrahepatic ducts

WHO 2010[5]	AJCC 7th Edition[18]	AJCC 8th Edition and CAP 2018[4,15]
Intrahepatic cholangiocarcinoma	Cholangiocarcinoma	Intrahepatic cholangiocarcinoma
Intraductal papillary neoplasm with an associated invasive carcinoma	Bile duct cystadenocarcinoma	Intraductal papillary neoplasm with an associated invasive carcinoma
Mucinous cystic neoplasm with an associated invasive carcinoma	Combined hepatocellular and cholangiocarcinoma	Mucinous cystic neoplasm with an associated invasive carcinoma
Combined hepatocellular-cholangiocarcinoma	High-grade neuroendocrine carcinoma, small cell or large cell type	Combined hepatocellular-cholangiocarcinoma
		Poorly differentiated neuroendocrine carcinoma, small cell or large cell type

Abbreviations: AJCC, American Joint Committee on Cancer; CAP, College of American Pathologists; WHO, World Health Organization.

discussed under "Treatment, Potential Targets and Prognosis."

CLASSIFICATION BY MACROSCOPIC GROWTH PATTERN

ICC can be further classified by macroscopic subtypes into mass forming, periductal infiltrating, or intraductal[17]; mixed growth patterns can occur (**Fig. 1**). The WHO recognizes these subtypes, but the AJCC/UICC and CAP only recognize the mass forming and periductal infiltrating types (or mixed mass-forming/periductal-infiltrating types); they do not recognize an intraductal growth pattern, again adding to the confusion of the classification of these tumors.

CLASSIFICATION BY MICROSCOPIC FEATURES

Histologically, cholangiocarcinomas are tubule or gland-forming adenocarcinomas. Traditionally, these adenocarcinomas are simply classified as well, moderately, or poorly differentiated. Rare variants[3,4] also exist, including squamous, adenosquamous, mucinous, signet ring cell, clear cell, undifferentiated, lymphoepithelial, mucoepidermoid, and sarcomatous. The WHO divides malignant epithelial tumors of the intrahepatic ducts into 4 categories, but this classification was modified in the AJCC 7th edition, and again in the AJCC 8th edition as well as the CAP 2018 cancer protocol (**Table 1**).[4,5,15,18] For malignant epithelial tumors of the extrahepatic ducts, the

WHO, AJCC 8th edition, and CAP 2018 cancer protocol all use the classification shown in **Box 2** (note, the term "adenocarcinoma" is used and not "extrahepatic cholangiocarcinoma").[3–5,16]

Box 2
Histologic classification of malignant epithelial tumors of the extrahepatic ducts

- Adenocarcinoma
  - Adenocarcinoma, biliary type
  - Adenocarcinoma, intestinal type
  - Adenocarcinoma, gastric foveolar type
  - Mucinous adenocarcinoma
  - Clear cell adenocarcinoma
  - Signet ring cell carcinoma
- Intraductal papillary neoplasm with an associated invasive carcinoma
- Mucinous cystic neoplasm with an associated invasive carcinoma
- Adenosquamous carcinoma
- Squamous cell carcinoma
- Poorly differentiated neuroendocrine carcinoma (small cell or large cell type)
- Mixed adenoneuroendocrine carcinoma
- Undifferentiated carcinoma

Fig. 2. Histologic appearance of intrahepatic cholangiocarcinoma (classification by microscopic features). (*A*) Large duct type (type 1). Tumor cells are columnar and form large glands dispersed within abundant desmoplastic stroma [H&E, original magnification ×40]. (*B*). Large duct type tumor cells are mucin producing and resemble classic pancreatic ductal adenocarcinoma [H&E, original magnification ×200].

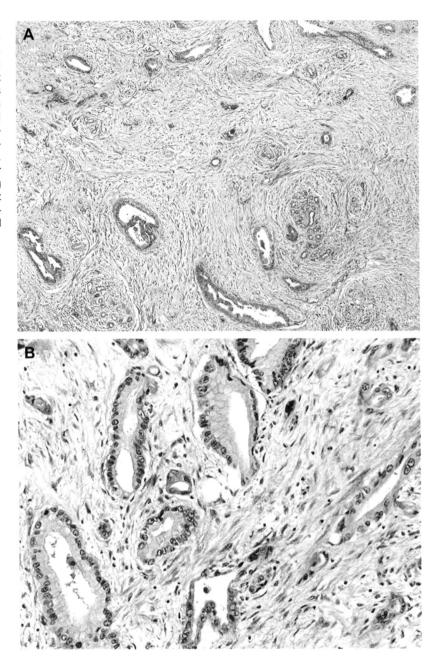

Morphologic similarities between cholangiocarcinomas arising in the extrahepatic ducts and those arising in the large intrahepatic ducts, and differences from cholangiocarcinomas arising from the peripheral bile ducts, had been observed in the past,[19] but only recently have these differences been studied more in depth. The newest classification based on histologic features basically divides ICCs into 2 groups, those with small duct or cholangiolar (cholangiolocellular) features, and those with large duct or bile duct features (**Fig. 2**). This classification has been shown to have clinicopathologic, molecular, and therapeutic significance.[20–23]

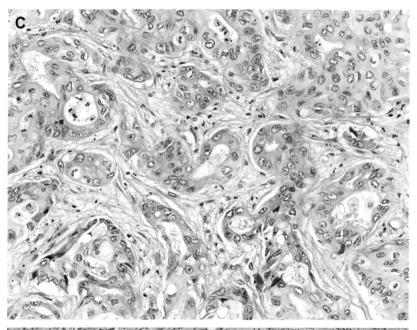

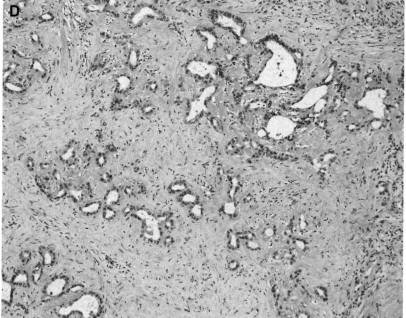

Fig. 2. (continued). (C) Small duct type (type 2). Tumor cells are cuboidal with scant eosinophilic cytoplasm and form small, anastomosing glands without mucin production [H&E, original magnification ×200]. (D). Small duct type tumors tend to be sclerotic, especially in the center of the tumor, rather than desmoplastic [H&E, original magnification ×100].

CLASSIFICATION BY CELL OF ORIGIN

Cholangiocarcinomas are known to arise from different cell types (different stem cell niches), including human hepatic stem cells residing in the canals of Hering and stem cells within peribiliary glands (biliary tree stem/progenitor cells).[24] Human hepatic stem cells can differentiate into hepatocytes and cholangiocytes, and hence can give rise to tumors with variable phenotypes. Biliary tree stem/progenitor cells within both intrahepatic and extrahepatic peribiliary glands give rise to mucin-producing tumors. Some authors have proposed classifying cholangiocarcinomas based on the presumed cell of origin, which correlates nicely with microscopic subtype.[24-26]

Key Points
CHOLANGIOCARCINOMA
CLASSIFICATION SCHEMES

Anatomic location
- Intrahepatic
- Extrahepatic

Macroscopic growth pattern
- Mass forming
- Periductal infiltrating
- Intraductal
- Mixed growth patterns

Microscopic features
- Extrahepatic: Adenocarcinoma and rare variants
- Intrahepatic: Small duct type versus large duct type

Cell of origin
- Stem cells residing in the canals of Hering
- Stem cells within peribiliary glands

INTRAHEPATIC CHOLANGIOCARCINOMA

Based on macroscopic growth pattern, most ICCs are mass-forming tumors. Grossly, these solid tumors typically have well-defined borders within the hepatic parenchyma and a gray or gray-white cut surface and firm texture (see **Fig. 1**A). Intrahepatic metastases or coalescing lesions can occur. ICCs of the periductal infiltrating type spread along the portal tracts and causes narrowing of the involved ducts (see **Fig. 1**B). ICCs with intraductal growth are characterized by a papillary or nodular lesion within a dilated duct (see **Fig. 1**C). As expected, ICCs can have mixed growth patterns, for example, mass forming and periductal infiltrating.

HISTOLOGIC SUBTYPES

Until recently, ICCs were classified as well, moderately, or poorly differentiated adenocarcinomas or as rare variants. Several publications support further subclassification based on histology into large duct (type 1) or small duct (type 2) types (see **Fig. 2**). Tumor cells of large duct (bile duct) type resemble bile duct cells: Tall columnar cells that usually contain mucin and usually form large glands within open luminal spaces often

associated with abundant desmoplastic stroma.[20–23,25] Tumor cells of small duct (cholangiolar) type resemble cholangiolar cells: Cuboidal cells with scant eosinophilic or amphophilic cytoplasm that often form small monotonous or anastomosing glands without mucin production.[20–23,25,27]

This histologic classification is associated with specific clinicopathologic, immunohistochemical, and molecular characteristics (**Table 2**). Small duct type ICC is associated with chronic liver disease/cirrhosis (especially viral hepatitis), whereas large duct type ICC is associated with chronic biliary disease, precursor lesions, and, especially outside of the United States, hepatolithiasis. Small duct type ICCs nearly always have a mass forming macroscopic growth pattern and often have scarlike central fibrosis, whereas large duct type ICCs have variable macroscopic growth patterns and are more associated with mucin production, cellular desmoplasia, poor differentiation, perineural invasion, and lymph node metastases.

IMMUNOHISTOCHEMICAL AND MOLECULAR CHARACTERISTICS

Cholangiocarcinomas, both ICC and ECC, are positive for CK7 and CK19, and negative for CDX2 and generally negative for CK20. Although these stains can help to rule out metastatic colorectal cancer, which is typically CK20[+], CDX2[+], and CK7[–], these stains cannot help to distinguish cholangiocarcinomas from pancreatic ductal adenocarcinoma and upper gastrointestinal tract cancers.

Several studies have shown that the 2 histologic subtypes of ICC have distinctly different immunohistochemical and molecular profiles. Large duct type ICCs are positive for S100P and TFF1 (**Fig. 3**A, B),[20,21,23,25] whereas small duct type ICCs tend to be positive for CD56 (neural cell adhesion molecule) and N-cadherin (see **Fig. 3**C, D),[20,21,25,27] and, more recently, C-reactive protein as well.[23,28] Because positivity rates range from 50% to 77% for neural cell adhesion molecule/N-cadherin (for small duct type)[20,21,27] and 56% to 79% for S100P/TFF1 (for large duct type),[20,21] there will be ICCs that are negative for both and can pose interpretive challenges. The addition of mucin production, as assessed by Alcian blue (pH 2.5), resulted in only 4% indeterminate cases in a study by Hayashi published in 2016[20]; however, another study found intracellular mucin in a significant proportion (45%) of ICCs with cholangiocellular differentiation.[23] Although not currently widely

Table 2
Histologic classification of ICC and association with clinicopathologic, immunohistochemical, and molecular features

	Large Duct Type (Type 1)	Small Duct Type (Type 2)
Location	Perihilar	Peripheral
Background condition	Chronic biliary disease, hepatolithiasis	Chronic liver disease, viral hepatitis, cirrhosis
Precursor lesion	+ (BilIN, IPNB, ITPN)	− (Occasionally ITPN)
Macroscopic growth pattern	Variable (PI, IG, +/− MF)	Mass forming
Shape of tumor cells	Columnar	Cuboidal to low columnar
Mucin production	++	+/−
Gland morphology	Large, widely spaced glands (similar to ECC); poorly differentiated	Small tubules, fused or anastomosing glands
Tumor fibrosis	Diffuse, desmoplastic	Central, sclerotic
Perinerual invasion	++	−
LVI/LN metastases	++	+/−
Tumor border	Infiltrative	Expansile or pushing, +/− infiltrative
Immunophenotype	S100P and TFF1	CD56 (NCAM), N-cadherin, CRP
Molecular alterations	*KRAS* mutations, *FGFR2* translocations	*IDH1/IDH2* mutations

Abbreviations: BilIN, biliary intraepithelial neoplasia; CRP, C-reactive protein; ECC, extrahepatic cholangiocarcinoma; ICC, intrahepatic cholangiocarcinoma; IG, intraductal growth; IPNB, intraductal papillary neoplasm of bile duct; ITPN, intraductal tubulopapillary neoplasm; LN, lymph node; LVI, lymphovascular invasion; MF, mass forming; NCAM, neural cell adhesion molecule; PI, periductal infiltrating; −, rare; +/−, uncommon; +, common.

used, immunophenotyping ICCs may become routine in the future as a method to triage cases for molecular testing and potential targeted therapy.

Significant advances in understanding the key genetic alterations in ICCs have been made recently. The most notable discovery was the detection of *IDH1* and *IDH2* missense mutations in ICCs.[29–35] These mutations were known to be present in low-grade gliomas, glioblastomas, and acute myeloid leukemias, but not in epithelial tumors. Importantly, the *IDH* mutant alleles present in ICC (*IDH1*[R132C] and *IDH2*[R172K/S]) are distinct from those found in glioma and acute myeloid leukemia (*IDH1*[R132H] and *IDH2*[R140Q]).[31,36] Several other genetic alterations have been reported in ICCs, including mutations in *KRAS*, *BRAF*, *TP53*, and inactivating mutations in chromatic remodeling genes *ARID1A*, *BAP1*, and *PBRM1*, as well as translocations involving *FGFR2*.[31,32,34,37–40] Interestingly, molecular alterations are also different between the 2 subtypes of ICCs. *IDH1/2* mutations and *FGFR2* translocations occur in 17% to 40% and 11%, respectively, of ICCs of the small duct type,[20,21,29] whereas *KRAS*

mutations occur in 20% to 29% of ICCs of the large duct type.[20,21,27,37,41] Many of the genetic alterations observed in ICCs are targetable and these potential therapeutic targets are discussed elsewhere in this article.

Key Points
INTRAHEPATIC CHOLANGIOCARCINOMA

- Often grossly appear as solid, firm tumors within the liver; can be multifocal

- Adenocarcinomas of 2 subtypes, small duct/cholangiolar type and large duct/bile duct type, that correlate with risk factors and immunohistochemistry/molecular features

- Neural cell adhesion molecule positive, N-cadherin[+], C-reactive protein positive (small duct type) or S100P[+], TFF1[+] (large duct type)

- *IDH1/2* mutations and *FGFR2* translocations (small duct type) or KRAS mutations (large duct type)

Fig. 3. Immunohistochemical features of intrahepatic cholangiocarcinoma (ICC). (*A, B*) S100P positivity in large duct type ICC (*A,* stain: hematoxylin and eosin [H&E, original magnification ×200]).

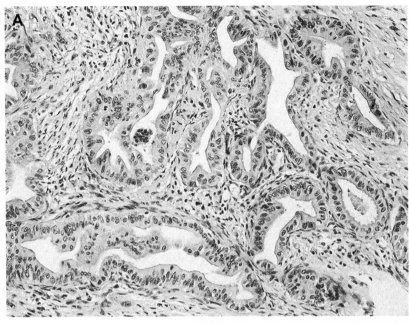

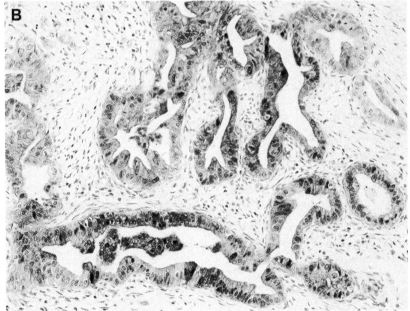

DIFFERENTIAL DIAGNOSIS

The presence of an adenocarcinoma in the liver should always raise the possibility of metastatic disease, particularly if the background parenchyma is not cirrhotic. If the adenocarcinoma is mucin producing or has large duct features, metastases from the pancreas and upper gastrointestinal tract need to be excluded.

Unfortunately, immunohistochemistry is not very helpful in distinguishing these types of tumors, and correlation with clinical history and imaging studies is required to exclude metastatic disease. If the adenocarcinoma is nonmucinous and has a more trabecular or nested appearance, metastatic breast cancer is a definite diagnostic consideration and, fortunately,

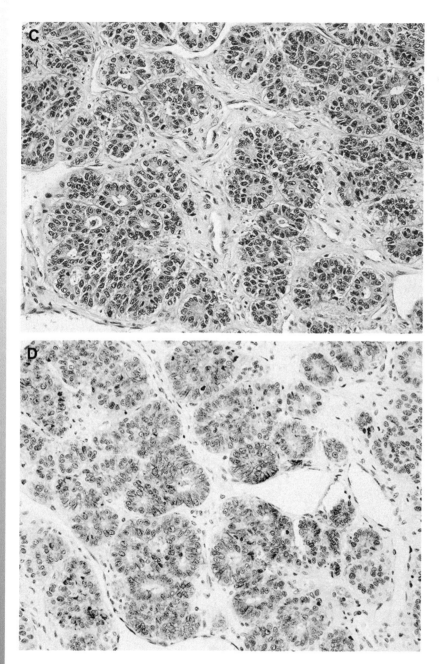

Fig. 3. (*continued*). (*C, D*) CD56 positivity in small duct type ICC (*C*, stain: H&E, original magnification ×200).

Immunohistochemical stains for breast cancer can be helpful (**Fig. 4**A, B).

In many institutions, MRI studies alone are used to diagnose hepatocellular carcinoma owing to the high specificity if the mass is mildly hyperintense precontrast, hyperenhances in the arterial phase, and hypoenhances in the portal venous and delayed phases (washout).[42] If the MRI findings are atypical or unequivocal, a liver biopsy is often performed. Biopsies of such lesions are hence expected to be challenging as well. Often, a straightforward diagnosis of either hepatocellular carcinoma or cholangiocarcinoma can be rendered. However, some tumors may show mixed or ambiguous features of hepatocellular and cholangiocarcinoma. Although

Fig. 4. Mimics of intrahepatic cholangio-carcinoma (ICC). (*A*) Metastatic breast cancer mimicking ICC (stain: hematoxylin and eosin, original magnification ×200). (*B*) Metastatic breast cancer is GATA3 positive (adjacent hepatocytes are negative) [GATA3, original magnification ×200]. (*C*) Segmental atrophy of the liver with bile ductular proliferation [H&E, original magnification ×100].

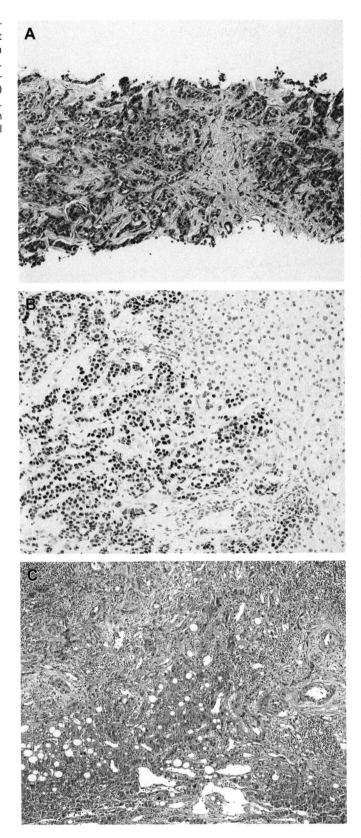

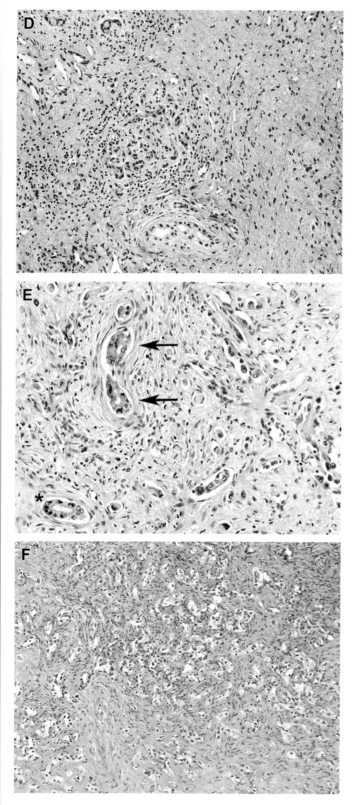

Fig. 4. (*continued*). (*D*) Segmental atrophy of the liver with bile ductules and marked elastosis [H&E, original magnification ×200]. (*E*) Epithelioid hemangioendothelioma mimicking a gland-forming malignancy with tumoral pseudoglands (*arrows*) and entrapped native ducts (*asterisks*) [H&E, original magnification ×100]. (*F*) Epithelioid hemangioendothelioma with epithelioid single cells and cell clusters within a sclerotic stroma [H&E, original magnification ×100].

a panel of immunohistochemical stains can help to confirm both hepatocytic (arginase-1, HepPar-1, pCEA, and CD10) and cholangiocytic (CK7 and CK19) differentiation within a single tumor, the diagnosis should rely on cytomorphologic features because there are pitfalls to the assessment of immunohistochemical stains in hepatic tumors. In situ hybridization for albumin is helpful to support hepatocellular differentiation, but ICCs can be positive.[43,44] Fibrolamellar carcinomas can be positive for CK7 and entrapped hepatocytes within a cholangiocarcinoma will be positive for hepatocellular markers such as arginase and HepPar-1.

Combined Hepatocellular Carcinoma and Cholangiocarcinoma

Rarely, mixed cholangiocarcinomas and hepatocellular carcinomas can occur; they comprise less than 1% of all primary liver cancers.[45] As noted, cholangiocarcinomas, as well as hepatocellular carcinomas, have been shown to arise from different stem cell niches. The most recent WHO classification of the digestive system introduced the concept that combined hepatocellular-cholangiocarcinomas also arise from hepatic progenitor cells.[45] According to the WHO 2010 classification, combined hepatocellular-cholangiocarcinomas are divided into a classical type and 3 subtypes with stem cell features: typical, intermediate, and cholangiolocellular subtypes. Although this classification was found to be reproducible, great histologic diversity and a complex mixture of histologic subtypes made the tumors challenging to classify, and no differences in survival were found.[46] In addition, a large study of cholangiocarcinomas showed that a substantial minority (39.2%) displayed histologic diversity, including focal hepatocytic differentiation and ductular areas (mixed tumors), and that these mixed tumors were similar to peripheral or small duct (cholangiolocellular) tumors.[26] Because mixed tumors seem to be heterogeneous and are challenging to classify, an international community of pathologists, radiologists, and clinicians have recommended consensus terminology. A primary liver carcinoma that is not classic HCC or ICC can be classified as (1) a combined hepatocellular-cholangiocarcinoma (a tumor with both hepatocytic and cholangiocytic features, either admixed or as separate areas within the same tumor), (2) intermediate cell carcinoma (composed only of "intermediate cells"), or (3) cholangiolocarcinoma.[47]

Other Histologic Mimics of Intrahepatic Cholangiocarcinoma

Other mimics of ICC include benign ductular reactions/proliferations, epithelioid hemangioendothelioma, and intraductal spread of metastases, especially on liver biopsies. Although small subcapsular biliary hamartomas or bile duct adenomas can mimic metastatic pancreatic ductal adenocarcinoma, these entities are usually so small that they do not mimic malignancy on imaging studies and usually pose a diagnostic challenge only when biopsied during surgery for pancreatic cancer. Atrophic hepatic parenchyma, in contrast, can mimic a mass (segmental atrophy) and contain abundant ductules that could cause concern for an ICC. Segmental atrophy of the liver is often subcapsular and, in addition to proliferating bile ductules without atypia, these lesions usually also contain thickened vessels, biliary cysts, and elastotic changes (see **Fig. 4**C, D).[48]

Epithelioid hemangioendothelioma of the liver is a rare malignancy that is often found incidentally, but can present with multiple hepatic lesions that can mimic ICC with intrahepatic metastases. Histologically, epithelioid cells are arranged as short strands, cohesive nests, and papillary-type clusters (tufts within vascular spaces; see **Fig. 4**E, F). Cytoplasmic vacuoles (small vascular lumens) and significant atypia with or without mitoses may be present. The malignant cells are surrounded by a myxoid or fibrotic stroma and may entrap normal structures, such as hepatocytes and bile ducts. Vascular invasion (large and small vessel) is common. If sampled on a liver biopsy, the epithelioid cells can mimic an epithelial malignancy, including ICC, as well as metastatic carcinoma, hepatocellular carcinoma, and angiosarcoma. Ancillary studies can confirm a diagnosis of epithelioid hemangioendothelioma. By immunohistochemistry, tumor cells are positive for endothelial markers, such as CD31 and ERG1, and a proportion of them are also positive for a newly described, highly sensitive and specific marker of epithelioid hemangioendothelioma, CAMTA1.[49] Caution is needed when performing a panel of stains, because an epithelioid hemangioendothelioma may be positive for pancytokeratin and CK7. These tumors harbor translocations that can be detected by fluorescence in situ hybridization (FISH): a WWTR1-CAMTA1 translocation in about 90% of cases or YAP1-TFE3 translocation in a subset of cases.[50–52]

The intraductal spread of metastases can mimic ICC, especially ICCs with an intraductal growth component. One study identified intrabiliary growth in 4.5% of metastatic colorectal cancers, but in only 0.8% of noncolorectal tumors.[53] Major ducts

△△ **Differential Diagnosis**
INTRAHEPATIC CHOLANGIOCARCINOMA

Entity	Helpful Distinguishing Features
Metastatic pancreatic adenocarcinoma	Clinical history Imaging studies No distinguishing histologic or immunohistochemical features
Metastatic breast cancer	Nonmucinous, trabecular or nested growth pattern GATA3[+], mammaglobin[+]
Combined hepatocellular-Cholangiocarcinoma	Hepatocellular differentiation Arginase[+], HepPar1[+], CK7/CK19[+]
Benign ductular reactions/proliferations	Bland histology without atypia Segmental atrophy is often subcapsular, contains thickened vessels, biliary cysts, and elastotic changes
Epithelioid hemangioendothelioma	Intravascular/sinusoidal growth and papillary tufting of epithelioid cells, cytoplasmic vacuoles, significant atypia CD31[+], ERG[+] Translocations: *WWTR1-CAMTA1* or *YAP1-TFE3*
Intraductal spread of metastases	Often from a colorectal cancer (CK20[+], CDX2[+])

were involved in 56%, minor ducts in 44%, and 5 (21%) cases were clinically challenging to distinguish from cholangiocarcinoma.[53] Hence, major duct involvement by metastatic colorectal carcinoma should be recognized.

GROSSING AND STAGING INTRAHEPATIC CHOLANGIOCARCINOMA

When grossing a solid hepatic tumor, an adequate sampling of both the periphery of the tumor, including the interface with the adjacent uninvolved hepatic parenchyma, and the center of the tumor, which may be fibrotic or sclerotic, is needed. Because some mass-forming tumors may be associated with intraductal or periductal infiltrating tumors, a sampling of adjacent large bile ducts and the bile duct margin is indicated.

Staging ICCs (carcinomas of the intrahepatic bile ducts) in the seventh edition of the AJCC staging manual[18] is primarily based on whether the tumor is solitary or multiple, or has vascular invasion or not (**Table 3**). The eighth edition of the AJCC classification (and the 2018 CAP cancer protocols)[4,15] use the same characteristics, but adds size criteria to the T stages (see **Table 3**). The new edition also modifies the T3 and T4 stages to align more with other gastrointestinal tumors (T3 tumors perforate the visceral peritoneum, whereas T4 tumors directly invade adjacent organs, including the colon, duodenum, stomach, common bile duct, portal lymph nodes, abdominal wall, and diaphragm). In addition, periductal invasion is no longer a part of the T classification because it is a growth pattern that has an unclear association with outcome. There is no change in the regional lymph node stage (stage is based on whether lymph node metastases are present [pN0] or absent [pN1]).

EXTRAHEPATIC CHOLANGIOCARCINOMA

Patients with ECCs, either perihilar or distal bile duct tumors, typically present with biliary obstructive symptoms, including jaundice. The clinical workup of a patient suspected of having ECC includes imaging studies, laboratory studies, and endoscopic cholangiography with biopsy and/or brush cytology with or without chromosomal abnormality detection by FISH.[54,55] For perihilar and distal bile duct tumors, if there is a dominant stricture in the perihilar biliary tree and positive cytology and/or polysomy on FISH analysis, a diagnosis of cholangiocarcinoma is rendered; a CA19-9 level of greater than 129 U/mL also supports a malignant diagnosis, but can be increased in patients with cholangitis.[56] In the absence of

Table 3
Staging the primary tumor (pT) of carcinomas of the intrahepatic bile ducts (Intrahepatic cholangiocarcinomas)

Primary Tumor (pT)			
AJCC 7th Edition[18]		**AJCC 8th Edition**[4]	
pTX	Cannot be assessed	pTX	Primary tumor cannot be assessed
pT0	No evidence of primary tumor	pT0	No evidence of primary tumor
pTis	Carcinoma in situ (intraductal tumor)	pTis	Carcinoma in situ (intraductal tumor)
pT1	Solitary tumor without vascular invasion	pT1	Solitary tumor without vascular invasion, ≤5 cm or >5 cm
		pT1a	Solitary tumor ≤5 cm without vascular invasion
		pT1b	Solitary tumor >5 cm without vascular invasion
pT2	Solitary tumor with vascular invasion or multiple tumors, with or without vascular invasion	pT2	Solitary tumor with intrahepatic vascular invasion, or multiple tumors, with or without vascular invasion
pT2a	Solitary tumor with vascular invasion		
pT2b	Multiple tumors, with or without vascular invasion		
pT3	Tumor perforating the visceral peritoneum or involving the local extrahepatic structures by direct invasion	pT3	Tumor perforating the visceral peritoneum
pT4	Tumor with periductal invasion	pT4	Tumor involving local extrahepatic structures by direct invasion

Abbreviation: AJCC, American Joint Committee on Cancer.

adenocarcinoma on biopsy or cytology and an absence of FISH abnormalities, a diagnosis of perihilar ECC can be rendered on imaging alone if there is a hilar mass on axial imaging with an associated biliary stricture and/or hypertrophy–atrophy complex (unilateral hepatic lobe hypertrophy with contralateral hepatic lobar atrophy).[56]

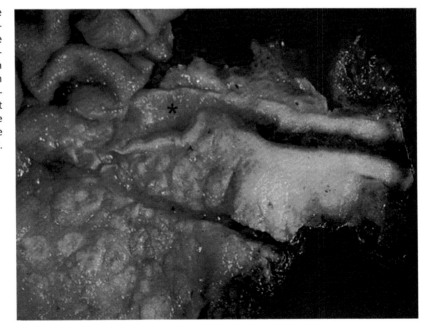

Fig. 5. Gross appearance of extrahepatic cholangiocarcinoma (ECC). The tumor spreads longitudinally along the common bile duct (*asterisks*) with circumferential thickening of the bile duct wall and a small masslike lesion within the pancreas (advanced ECC).

A pathologic diagnosis of ECC can be made on brush cytology or tissue biopsy. However, obtaining a definitive diagnosis of adenocarcinoma is difficult because of the challenges in accessing the biliary tree. Related both to the procedure and the inherent desmoplastic nature of these tumors, endoscopic retrograde cholangiopancreatography–guided brushings often provide only a limited number of cells, random biopsies may miss the lesion, and cholangioscopic-directed biopsies, although they may directly sample the lesion, are often limited by the small size of the sample. Hence, the sensitivity of conventional cytology ranges from 15% to 68%,[57–59] and the sensitivity for random and directed biopsies is only slightly better (range, 36%–81%).[57,60,61] With the application of FISH technology to biliary brush cytology, the sensitivity of brush cytology has been shown to improve from 20% to 43% when polysomy FISH was detected, along with high specificity of 99.6%.[54] Therefore, FISH is currently the most clinically relevant ancillary technique for cytology of bile duct strictures and has been incorporated into clinical diagnostic algorithms.[56]

Based on the macroscopic growth pattern, most ECCs are periductal-infiltrating tumors. Perihilar tumors can also be associated with an intraductal growth pattern. Mass lesions are uncommon in both perihilar and distal bile duct tumors, and if present, indicate advanced disease (**Fig. 5**). Histologically, most ECCs are well to moderately differentiated adenocarcinomas, often with mucin production and abundant fibrous stroma. Most ECCs are of a "pancreaticobiliary type" (**Fig. 6**) and hence perineural invasion is common and often extensive.

IMMUNOHISTOCHEMICAL AND MOLECULAR CHARACTERISTICS

As noted, ECCs are positive for CK7 and CK19, and there are currently no good markers to distinguish ECC form pancreatic ductal adenocarcinoma. There are several markers that show promise in distinguishing benign from malignant cells on bile duct brushings and biopsies. A panel of immunostains consisting of S100P, pVHL, and IMP3 can be helpful in distinguishing adenocarcinoma (S100P+/pVHL−/IMP+) from reactive epithelial atypia (S100P−/pVHL+/IMP3−).[62,63] Another study showed that the addition of maspin to S100P and VHL may also be helpful, because a maspin+/S100P+/pVHL− staining profile was seen in 75% of malignant biopsies but in none of the benign cases.[64]

There are currently no known genetic syndromes associated with cholangiocarcinoma. ECCs show overlap in driver gene mutations present in pancreatic ductal adenocarcinoma: *KRAS*, *p16/CDK2NA*, *TP53*, and *SMAD4*. *ERBB2/Her2Neu* gene amplification also occurs in about 20% to 30% of ECCs.[65] Studies have shown and emphasized the molecular differences between ICC and ECC, as highlighted in **Table 4**.[38]

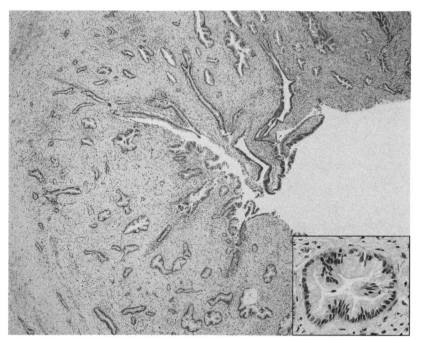

Fig. 6. Histology of extrahepatic cholangiocarcinoma (ECC). Pancreatobiliary-type glands infiltrate a bile duct. ECCs resemble both large duct type ICCs and classic pancreatic ductal adenocarcinoma (stain: hematoxylin and eosin [H×E, original magnification ×40]).

DIFFERENTIAL DIAGNOSIS

Although pancreatic ductal adenocarcinoma invading the bile duct is the main differential diagnosis of distal bile duct ECCs, a preoperative diagnosis of adenocarcinoma on bile duct sampling is often sufficient for clinical decision making. However, the distinction may be important postoperatively, especially if patients are interested in enrolling in clinical trials. Clinical trials are often strict about the pathologic diagnosis and patients who are otherwise eligible for a clinical trial for bile duct tumors would be excluded from participating if they were misdiagnosed as having pancreatic cancer, or vice versa. When the diagnosis is equivocal postoperatively, the gross appearance of the tumor in the Whipple resection is often the most helpful. As noted, helpful clues to a diagnosis of a distal bile duct ECC include circumferential growth along the bile duct without formation of a dominant mass. If the distinction remains difficult, a discussion with the clinical team might be helpful.

Other mimics of ECC include intraductal spread of metastatic tumors, especially from perihilar primaries (as discussed) and benign fibroinflammatory biliary strictures. Fibroinflammatory biliary stricture is a benign tumor-like process of the extrahepatic bile duct that mimics ECC clinically and radiographically.[66] Because preoperative tests are often inconclusive, surgery is the method of choice for both diagnosis and treatment. Histologically, the bile duct lesions exhibit varying degrees of fibrosis, mild to marked inflammation usually consisting of lymphocytes and plasma cells, and sometimes containing eosinophils and lymphoid follicles (**Fig. 7**). The mixed fibroinflammatory process may spread beyond the bile duct to involve adjacent structures. Some cases may represent examples of immunoglobulin G4–related sclerosing cholangitis.[66,67]

Table 4
Molecular differences between ICC and ECC

Genetic Alteration	ICC	ECC
TP53	+/−	+
KRAS	+/−	+
ERBB2 (HER2)	−	+/−
SMAD4	−	+/−
CDK2NA (p16)	−	+/−
FBXW7	−	+/−
IDH	+/−	−
ARID1A	+/−	−

All are gene mutations except for ERBB2, which includes mutations and amplification. −, rare; +/−, uncommon; +, common.
Abbreviations: ICC, intrahepatic cholangiocarcinoma; ECC, extrahepatic cholangiocarcinoma.

△△ Differential Diagnosis
EXTRAHEPATIC CHOLANGIOCARCINOMA

Entity	Helpful Distinguishing Features
Metastatic pancreatic adenocarcinoma	No distinguishing histologic or immunohistochemistry features Grossly, intrapancreatic or eccentric distal bile duct mass
Intraductal spread of metastases	Often from a colorectal cancer (CK20⁺, CDX2⁺)
Fibroinflammatory biliary stricture	Variable fibrosis and mild to marked inflammation Some represent IgG4-related sclerosing cholangitis

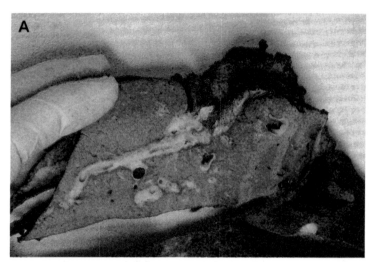

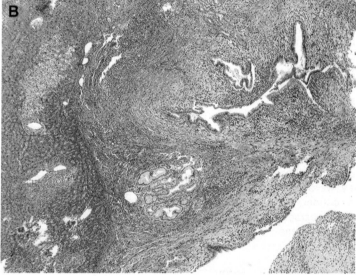

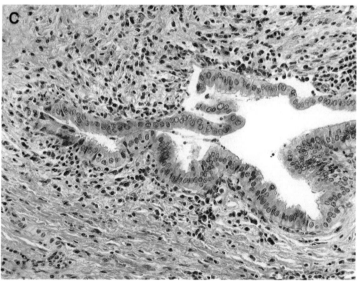

Fig. 7. Mimics of extrahepatic cholangiocarcinoma (ECC). Benign fibroinflammatory stricture. (*A*) Grossly, the fibrosis can mimic periductal infiltration by cholangiocarcinoma. (*B*) Histologically, fibrosis and chronic inflammation surround large ducts [H&E, original magnification ×40]. (*C*) The chronic inflammation is composed predominantly of lymphocytes and plasma cells [H×E, original magnification ×200].

GROSSING AND STAGING EXTRAHEPATIC CHOLANGIOCARCINOMA

When grossing tumors of the perihilar region and extrahepatic ducts, it is important to take perpendicular sections of the ducts to determine depth of invasion. Because most ECCs are periductal-infiltrating tumors, they can extend circumferentially along the ducts, requiring extensive sampling to determine tumor extent.

Because surgeons and radiologists may use the Bismuth-Corlette classification of perihilar tumors, it is worth mentioning here. Briefly, perihilar cholangiocarcinomas are divided into 4 classes based on the extent of involvement of the perihilar region: Type I tumors only involve the common hepatic duct (CHD), type II tumors involve the CHD and the confluence, type IIIa tumors involve the CHD, confluence and bifurcation of the right hepatic duct, type IIIb tumors involve the CHD, confluence and bifurcation of the left hepatic duct, and type IV tumors involve the CHD, confluence, and bifurcations of both the right and left hepatic ducts or cases with multifocal disease.[68]

The AJCC staging of perihilar primary tumors (pT) has not changed from the seventh to the eighth editions; however, the lymph node categories are now defined by the number of lymph nodes involved and not by location of the involved lymph nodes (**Table 5**).[4] However, significant changes have been made to the staging of distal bile duct tumors (**Table 6**). These changes were made because prior AJCC staging schemes showed poor ability to discriminate survival[69] and because the histologic assessment of the anatomic level of invasion was difficult. Detecting the anatomic barriers histologically is challenging because, even without distortion by tumor, the amount of smooth muscle within the wall of the distal bile duct varies along its length, as does the amount of fat versus pancreatic tissue surrounding the bile duct, and there is no serosa. When infiltrating carcinoma is present, its associated inflammatory cell response and desmoplastic reaction further blur these boundaries. In the eighth edition of the AJCC staging manual of distal bile duct tumors, T1, T2, and T3 tumors are defined by the depth of invasion as measured on the glass slide.[4] The depth is measured from the basement membrane of adjacent normal (nondistorted) epithelium to the point of deepest tumor invasion.[69,70] This examination requires properly oriented perpendicular sections and best estimates are acceptable when measuring the depth is challenging; longitudinal sections may be best at sampling deepest tumor invasion with adjacent epithelium. This staging scheme predicts prognosis (survival) better than the seventh AJCC edition.[69] The lymph node stages were modified in keeping with other malignancies, including pancreatic ductal adenocarcinomas and ampullary carcinomas.

PRECURSOR LESIONS

Precursor lesions to cholangiocarcinoma (nearly always perihilar and distal bile duct ECC) can be flat, cystic or tumoral. Biliary intraepithelial neoplasia (BilIN) is flat dysplasia that affects ducts of normal caliber and is similar in concept to pancreatic intraepithelial neoplasia (**Fig. 8A**).[71,72] Although initially divided into 3 grades, most have adopted a 2-tier grading scheme (low grade vs high grade) for BilIN after the 2015 Baltimore consensus meeting proposed a 2-tiered system for all precursor lesions of the pancreas.[73] As expected, BilIN is more common in patients with risk factors for cholangiocarcinoma (see **Box 1**). Mucinous cystic neoplasms with ovarian type stroma are known precursors to malignancy in the pancreas, even though the risk of malignancy is low.[74–76] Mucinous cystic neoplasms rarely

---

Table 5
Staging regional lymph nodes (pN) of carcinomas of the perihilar bile ducts (extrahepatic cholangiocarcinomas)

	AJCC 7th Edition[18]		AJCC 8th Edition[4]
pNX	Cannot be assessed	pNX	Regional lymph nodes cannot be assessed
pN0	No regional lymph node metastasis	pN0	No regional lymph node metastasis
pN1	Regional lymph node metastasis (including nodes along the cystic duct, common bile duct, hepatic artery, and portal vein)	pN1	One to 3 positive regional lymph nodes typically involving the hilar, cystic duct, common bile duct, hepatic artery, posterior pancreatoduodenal, and portal vein lymph nodes
pN2	Metastasis to periaortic, pericaval, superior mesentery artery, and/or celiac artery lymph nodes	pN2	Four or more positive lymph nodes from the sites described for N1

Abbreviation: AJCC, American Joint Committee on Cancer.

Table 6
Staging primary tumor (pT) and regional lymph nodes (pN) of carcinomas of the distal duct (extrahepatic cholangiocarcinomas)

AJCC 7th Edition[18]		AJCC 8th Edition[4]	
Primary tumor (pT)			
pTX	Cannot be assessed	pTX	Primary tumor cannot be assessed
pT0	No evidence of primary tumor	pT0	No regional lymph node metastasis
pTis	Carcinoma in situ	pTis	Carcinoma in situ/high-grade dysplasia
pT1	Tumor confined to the bile duct histologically	pT1	Tumor invades the bile duct wall with a depth <5 mm
pT2	Tumor invades beyond the wall of the bile duct	pT2	Tumor invades the bile duct wall with a depth of 5–12 mm
pT3	Tumor invades the gallbladder, pancreas, duodenum, or other adjacent organs without involvement of the celiac axis or the superior mesenteric artery	pT3	Tumor invades the bile duct wall with a depth >12 mm
pT4	Tumor involves the celiac axis or the superior mesenteric artery	pT4	Tumor involves the celiac axis, superior mesenteric artery, and/or common hepatic artery
Regional lymph nodes (pN)			
pNX	Cannot be assessed	pNX	Regional lymph nodes cannot be assessed
pN0	No regional lymph node metastasis	pN0	No regional lymph node metastasis
pN1	Regional lymph node metastasis	pN1	Metastasis in 1–3 regional lymph nodes
		pN2	Metastasis in ≥4 regional lymph nodes

Abbreviation: AJCC, American Joint Committee on Cancer.

occur in the liver and only a very small percent (6%) harbor small invasive adenocarcinomas.[75]

Tumoral intraepithelial neoplasia encompasses 2 related entities that fill and expand the bile duct with a solid mass or masslike lesion: Intraductal papillary neoplasm of the bile duct (IPNB) and intraductal tubular or tubulopapullary neoplasm (ITPN). IPNB (**Fig. 8**B, C) affects more men than women who are in their early 60s.[77] IPNB most commonly occurs in the hilar region and can be multifocal (papillomatosis). Other older terms for IPNB include bile duct adenoma, papillary neoplasm, and papillary adenocarcinoma. Histologically, IPNBs are similar to intraductal papillary mucinous neoplasms of the pancreas in that they form papillary structures that can be lined with different cell types, often biliary or intestinal, and rarely gastric or oncocytic; however, unlike intraductal papillary mucinous neoplasms, abundant mucin

production is uncommon. High-grade dysplasia is often present and extensive, and there is often an associated invasive component (in 74% of cases), which is usually of a pancreaticobiliary type.[78] Molecular alterations in *KRAS*, *TP53*, and loss of *CDKN2A/p16* were found in low-grade lesions, whereas loss of SMAD4 was found in advanced lesions; alterations of HER2, EGFR, and *GNAS* were rare.[77]

ITPNs (see **Fig. 8**D, E) are well-described in the pancreas[79] and can also occur in the bile ducts.[80] ITPN of the bile ducts affects women slightly more than men who are in their early 60s and they are most common in the intrahepatic bile ducts. Unlike IPNBs, ITPNs tend to be more solid grossly and have more tubular than papillary architecture histologically. Tumors composed of pure tubular structures can mimic intraductal growth of a neuroendocrine tumor or acinar cell carcinoma, but the

Fig. 8. Precursor lesions to cholangiocarcinoma. (*A*) Biliary intraepithelial neoplasia characterized by dysplastic biliary epithelium lining a normal-caliber duct [H&E, original magnification ×200]. (*B*) Grossly, this intraductal papillary neoplasm of the bile duct (IPNB) forms a mass within the common bile duct (*asterisks*). PD, pancreatic duct. (*C*) Histologically, this IPNB is filling the lumen of the bile duct with abundant papillary structures lined by mucin-producing cells with high-grade dysplasia (*inset*); abundant mucin production is lacking [H&E, original magnification ×40].

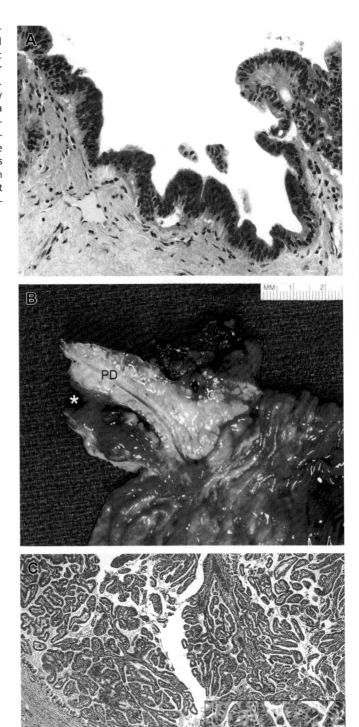

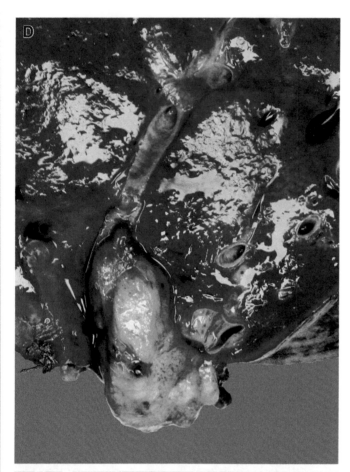

Fig. 8. (*continued*). (*D*) Grossly, this ITPN is forming a solid lesion within a proximal bile duct. (*E*) Histologically, the ITPN that is filling the lumen of the bile duct seems to be more compact and tubular rather than papillary; the tumor has abundant tightly packed tubules with high-grade cytologic dysplasia and without mucin production (*inset*). [H&E, original magnification ×40]

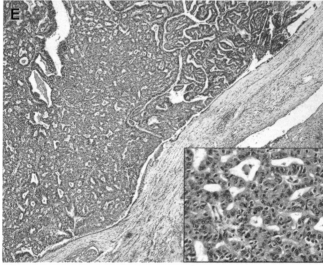

tumors are negative for neuroendocrine markers and trypsin. A solid growth pattern can be associated with comedo-type necrosis. Most ITPNs show at least focal high-grade dysplasia and up to 80% are associated with an invasive component, mainly conventional tubular adenocarcinoma.[80] Molecular alterations observed in many pancreatobiliary malignancies, including IPNB, are uncommon in ITPN; for example, alterations in *KRAS*, *TP53*, *PIK3CA*, *SMAD4*, and *GNAS* are rare.[80] The most common alteration was loss of *CDKN2A*/p16, which was found in 44% intraductal lesions and 33% invasive components.[80]

Key Points
PRECURSOR LESIONS

- BilIN is flat dysplasia that affects ducts of normal caliber

- Mucinous cystic neoplasm with ovarian type stroma portends a low risk of malignancy in the liver

- IPNB tends to arise in the hilar ducts and often harbors high-grade dysplasia/invasive carcinoma

- ITPN tends to involve intrahepatic ducts, has a solid appearance and often harbors high-grade dysplasia/invasive carcinoma

PROGNOSIS, TREATMENT, AND POTENTIAL TARGETS

Cholangiocarcinoma has a poor prognosis with a median survival of 24 months, primarily owing to lack of early detection and limited treatment options.[56] Surgery is the treatment of choice, but it can only be offered to patients with early stage disease. Factors impacting survival after surgery for ECC include margin status, lymph nodes metastases, vascular invasion, and, if applicable, function of the liver remnant.[81] For ICC, although margin status, number of tumors (single vs multiple), and vascular invasion are important determinants of prognosis, lymph node metastases have been shown to be the most important independent predictor of survival.[82]

Several guidelines exist for the treatment and management of patients with cholangiocarcinoma.[83] Most algorithms divide tumors by resectability. For unresectable tumors (usually locally advanced or with metastatic disease), the prognosis for untreated disease is a dismal median of 3.9 months.[84] Interestingly, liver transplantation may be an option for patients with inoperable perihilar ECC.[83,85] However, most patients with inoperable cholangiocarcinoma receive various combinations of chemotherapy and/or radiotherapy. The combination of gemcitabine and cisplatin chemotherapy is recommended as a standard first-line treatment for locally advanced and metastatic cholangiocarcinoma.[86,87] Although this drug combination improves overall survival compared with gemcitabine alone, the median overall survival is still only 1 year in metastatic disease.[86]

Locoregional therapies, such as transarterial chemoembolization, transarterial radioembolization, and radiofrequency ablation have been investigated for patients with ICC. Although the results are promising, conclusive studies are still needed before these are incorporated into existing guidelines.[2] Although the role of adjuvant radiation therapy is not well-defined in cholangiocarcinoma, radiation with concurrent chemotherapy has been recommended in margin-positive and node-positive ICC and perihilar ECC.[82,88]

As noted, genome-wide studies have revealed pertinent genes that are mutated or dysfunctional in cholangiocarcinoma, and some of these genes are targetable.[89,90] Although existing clinical trials using agents that target various molecular pathways demonstrate no or only very limited survival benefits, targeted therapy is beginning to show promise in the treatment of cholangiocarcinoma. Of particular interest are inhibitors of IDH1 and IDH2 in ICC and use of trastuzumab in HER2-positive ECC (distal cholangiocarcinoma).

REFERENCES

1. Bridgewater J, Galle PR, Khan SA, et al. Guidelines for the diagnosis and management of intrahepatic cholangiocarcinoma. J Hepatol 2014; 60(6):1268–89.

2. Banales JM, Cardinale V, Carpino G, et al. Expert consensus document: cholangiocarcinoma: current knowledge and future perspectives consensus statement from the European Network for the Study of Cholangiocarcinoma (ENS-CCA). Nat Rev Gastroenterol Hepatol 2016;13(5):261–80.

3. Kakar S, Shi C, Berlin J, et al. Protocol for the examination of specimens from patients with carcinoma of the distal extrahepatic bile ducts. 2017. Available at: http://www.cap.org/ShowProperty?nodePath=/UCM-Con/Contribution%20Folders/WebContent/pdf/cp-distal-extrahepatic-bileducts-17protocol-4000.pdf. Accessed November 12, 2017.

4. Amin MB, Edge SB, Greene FL, et al. AJCC cancer staging manual. 8th edition. New York: Springer; 2017.

5. Bosman FT, Carneiro F, Hruban RH, et al. WHO classification of tumours of the digestive system. 4th edition. Lyon (France): IARC; 2010.

6. Altekruse SF, Petrick JL, Rolin AI, et al. Geographic variation of intrahepatic cholangiocarcinoma, extrahepatic cholangiocarcinoma, and hepatocellular carcinoma in the United States. PLoS One 2015; 10(3):e0120574.

7. Tyson GL, Ilyas JA, Duan Z, et al. Secular trends in the incidence of cholangiocarcinoma in the USA and the impact of misclassification. Dig Dis Sci 2014;59(12):3103–10.

8. Welzel TM, McGlynn KA, Hsing AW, et al. Impact of classification of hilar cholangiocarcinomas (Klatskin tumors) on the incidence of intra- and extrahepatic cholangiocarcinoma in the United States. J Natl Cancer Inst 2006;98(12):873–5.

9. McGlynn KA, Tarone RE, El-Serag HB. A comparison of trends in the incidence of hepatocellular carcinoma and intrahepatic cholangiocarcinoma in the United States. Cancer Epidemiol Biomarkers Prev 2006;15(6):1198–203.

10. Alvaro D, Crocetti E, Ferretti S, et al, AISF Cholangiocarcinoma committee. Descriptive epidemiology of cholangiocarcinoma in Italy. Dig Liver Dis 2010; 42(7):490–5.

11. Wood R, Brewster DH, Fraser LA, et al. Do increases in mortality from intrahepatic cholangiocarcinoma reflect a genuine increase in risk? Insights from cancer registry data in Scotland. Eur J Cancer 2003; 39(14):2087–92.

12. Cardinale V, Semeraro R, Torrice A, et al. Intra-hepatic and extra-hepatic cholangiocarcinoma: new insight into epidemiology and risk factors. World J Gastrointest Oncol 2010;2(11):407–16.

13. Welzel TM, Graubard BI, El-Serag HB, et al. Risk factors for intrahepatic and extrahepatic cholangiocarcinoma in the United States: a population-based case-control study. Clin Gastroenterol Hepatol 2007;5(10):1221–8.

14. Cardinale V, Bragazzi MC, Carpino G, et al. Cholangiocarcinoma: increasing burden of classifications. Hepatobiliary Surg Nutr 2013;2(5):272–80.

15. Kakar S, Shi C, Adeyi OA, et al. Protocol for the examination of specimens from patients with carcinoma of the intrahepatic bile ducts. 2017. Available at: http://www.cap.org/ShowProperty?nodePath=/UCMCon/Contribution%20Folders/WebContent/pdf/cp-intrahepatic-bileducts-17protocol-4000.pdf. Accessed November 12, 2017.

16. Kakar S, Shi C, Fitzgibbons P, et al. Protocol for the examination of specimens from patients with carcinoma of the perihilar bile ducts. 2017. Available at: http://www.cap.org/ShowProperty?nodePath=/UCMCon/Contribution%20Folders/WebContent/pdf/cp-perihilar-bileducts-17protocol_4000.pdf. Accessed November 12, 2017.

17. Yamasaki S. Intrahepatic cholangiocarcinoma: macroscopic type and stage classification. J Hepatobiliary Pancreat Surg 2003;10(4):288–91.

18. Edge SB, Byrd DR, Compton CC, et al. AJCC cancer staging manual. 7th edition. New York: Springer; 2010.

19. Okuda K, Kubo Y, Okazaki N, et al. Clinical aspects of intrahepatic bile duct carcinoma including hilar carcinoma: a study of 57 autopsy-proven cases. Cancer 1977;39(1):232–46.

20. Hayashi A, Misumi K, Shibahara J, et al. Distinct clinicopathologic and genetic features of 2 histologic subtypes of intrahepatic cholangiocarcinoma. Am J Surg Pathol 2016;40(8):1021–30.

21. Liau JY, Tsai JH, Yuan RH, et al. Morphological subclassification of intrahepatic cholangiocarcinoma: etiological, clinicopathological, and molecular features. Mod Pathol 2014;27(8):1163–73.

22. Nakanuma Y, Sato Y, Harada K, et al. Pathological classification of intrahepatic cholangiocarcinoma based on a new concept. World J Hepatol 2010; 2(12):419–27.

23. Rhee H, Ko JE, Chung T, et al. Transcriptomic and histopathological analysis of cholangiolocellular differentiation trait in intrahepatic cholangiocarcinoma. Liver Int 2018;38(1):113–24.

24. Cardinale V, Carpino G, Reid L, et al. Multiple cells of origin in cholangiocarcinoma underlie biological, epidemiological and clinical heterogeneity. World J Gastrointest Oncol 2012;4(5):94–102.

25. Aishima S, Oda Y. Pathogenesis and classification of intrahepatic cholangiocarcinoma: different characters of perihilar large duct type versus peripheral small duct type. J Hepatobiliary Pancreat Sci 2015; 22(2):94–100.

26. Komuta M, Govaere O, Vandecaveye V, et al. Histological diversity in cholangiocellular carcinoma reflects the different cholangiocyte phenotypes. Hepatology 2012;55(6):1876–88.

27. Yu TH, Yuan RH, Chen YL, et al. Viral hepatitis is associated with intrahepatic cholangiocarcinoma with cholangiolar differentiation and N-cadherin expression. Mod Pathol 2011;24(6):810–9.

28. Yeh YC, Lei HJ, Chen MH, et al. C-Reactive protein (CRP) is a promising diagnostic immunohistochemical marker for intrahepatic cholangiocarcinoma and is associated with better prognosis. Am J Surg Pathol 2017;41(12):1630–41.

29. Borger DR, Tanabe KK, Fan KC, et al. Frequent mutation of isocitrate dehydrogenase (IDH)1 and IDH2 in cholangiocarcinoma identified through broad-based tumor genotyping. Oncologist 2012;17(1): 72–9.

30. Chan-On W, Nairismagi ML, Ong CK, et al. Exome sequencing identifies distinct mutational patterns in liver fluke-related and non-infection-related bile duct cancers. Nat Genet 2013;45(12):1474–8.

31. Farshidfar F, Zheng S, Gingras MC, et al. Integrative genomic analysis of cholangiocarcinoma identifies distinct IDH-mutant molecular profiles. Cell Rep 2017;18(11):2780–94.

32. Jiao Y, Pawlik TM, Anders RA, et al. Exome sequencing identifies frequent inactivating mutations in BAP1, ARID1A and PBRM1 in intrahepatic cholangiocarcinomas. Nat Genet 2013;45(12): 1470–3.

33. Kipp BR, Voss JS, Kerr SE, et al. Isocitrate dehydrogenase 1 and 2 mutations in cholangiocarcinoma. Hum Pathol 2012;43(10):1552–8.

34. Ross JS, Wang K, Gay L, et al. New routes to targeted therapy of intrahepatic cholangiocarcinomas revealed by next-generation sequencing. Oncologist 2014;19(3):235–42.

35. Wang P, Dong Q, Zhang C, et al. Mutations in isocitrate dehydrogenase 1 and 2 occur frequently in intrahepatic cholangiocarcinomas and share hypermethylation targets with glioblastomas. Oncogene 2013;32(25):3091–100.

36. Cancer Genome Atlas Research Network, Brat DJ, Verhaak RG, Aldape KD, et al. Comprehensive, integrative genomic analysis of diffuse lower-grade gliomas. N Engl J Med 2015;372(26):2481–98.

37. Borad MJ, Champion MD, Egan JB, et al. Integrated genomic characterization reveals novel, therapeutically relevant drug targets in FGFR and EGFR pathways in sporadic intrahepatic cholangiocarcinoma. PLoS Genet 2014;10(2):e1004135.

38. Churi CR, Shroff R, Wang Y, et al. Mutation profiling in cholangiocarcinoma: prognostic and therapeutic implications. PLoS One 2014;9(12):e115383.

39. Nakamura H, Arai Y, Totoki Y, et al. Genomic spectra of biliary tract cancer. Nat Genet 2015;47(9):1003–10.

40. Sia D, Losic B, Moeini A, et al. Massive parallel sequencing uncovers actionable FGFR2-PPHLN1 fusion and ARAF mutations in intrahepatic cholangiocarcinoma. Nat Commun 2015;6:6087.

41. Arai Y, Totoki Y, Hosoda F, et al. Fibroblast growth factor receptor 2 tyrosine kinase fusions define a unique molecular subtype of cholangiocarcinoma. Hepatology 2014;59(4):1427–34.

42. Tang A, Cruite I, Sirlin CB. Toward a standardized system for hepatocellular carcinoma diagnosis using computed tomography and MRI. Expert Rev Gastroenterol Hepatol 2013;7(3):269–79.

43. Coulouarn C, Cavard C, Rubbia-Brandt L, et al. Combined hepatocellular-cholangiocarcinomas exhibit progenitor features and activation of Wnt and TGFbeta signaling pathways. Carcinogenesis 2012;33(9):1791–6.

44. Ferrone CR, Ting DT, Shahid M, et al. The ability to diagnose intrahepatic cholangiocarcinoma definitively using novel branched DNA-enhanced albumin RNA in situ hybridization technology. Ann Surg Oncol 2016;23(1):290–6.

45. Theise ND, Nakashima O, Park YN, et al. Combined hepatocellular-cholangiocarcinoma. In: WHO classification of tumours of the digestive system. 4th edition. Lyon (France): IARC; 2010. p. 225–7.

46. Akiba J, Nakashima O, Hattori S, et al. Clinicopathologic analysis of combined hepatocellular-cholangiocarcinoma according to the latest WHO classification. Am J Surg Pathol 2013;37(4):496–505.

47. Brunt E, Aishima S, Clavien PA, et al. cHCC-CCA: consensus terminology for primary liver carcinomas with both hepatocytic and cholangiocytic differentiation. Hepatology 2018, [Epub ahead of print].

48. Singhi AD, Maklouf HR, Mehrotra AK, et al. Segmental atrophy of the liver: a distinctive pseudotumor of the liver with variable histologic appearances. Am J Surg Pathol 2011;35(3):364–71.

49. Doyle LA, Fletcher CD, Hornick JL. Nuclear expression of CAMTA1 distinguishes epithelioid hemangioendothelioma from histologic mimics. Am J Surg Pathol 2016;40(1):94–102.

50. Antonescu CR, Le Loarer F, Mosquera JM, et al. Novel YAP1-TFE3 fusion defines a distinct subset of epithelioid hemangioendothelioma. Genes Chromosomes Cancer 2013;52(8):775–84.

51. Errani C, Zhang L, Sung YS, et al. A novel WWTR1-CAMTA1 gene fusion is a consistent abnormality in epithelioid hemangioendothelioma of different anatomic sites. Genes Chromosomes Cancer 2011;50(8):644–53.

52. Flucke U, Vogels RJ, de Saint Aubain Somerhausen N, et al. Epithelioid Hemangioendothelioma: clinicopathologic, immunohistochemical, and molecular genetic analysis of 39 cases. Diagn Pathol 2014;9:131.

53. Estrella JS, Othman ML, Taggart MW, et al. Intrabiliary growth of liver metastases: clinicopathologic features, prevalence, and outcome. Am J Surg Pathol 2013;37(10):1571–9.

54. Fritcher EG, Kipp BR, Halling KC, et al. A multivariable model using advanced cytologic methods for the evaluation of indeterminate pancreatobiliary strictures. Gastroenterology 2009;136(7):2180–6.

55. DeHaan RD, Kipp BR, Smyrk TC, et al. An assessment of chromosomal alterations detected by fluorescence in situ hybridization and p16 expression in sporadic and primary sclerosing cholangitis-associated cholangiocarcinomas. Hum Pathol 2007;38(3):491–9.

56. Blechacz B, Komuta M, Roskams T, et al. Clinical diagnosis and staging of cholangiocarcinoma. Nat Rev Gastroenterol Hepatol 2011;8(9):512–22.

57. Rosch T, Hofrichter K, Frimberger E, et al. ERCP or EUS for tissue diagnosis of biliary strictures? A prospective comparative study. Gastrointest Endosc 2004;60(3):390–6.

58. Selvaggi SM. Biliary brushing cytology. Cytopathology 2004;15(2):74–9.

59. Weber A, Schmid RM, Prinz C. Diagnostic approaches for cholangiocarcinoma. World J Gastroenterol 2008;14(26):4131–6.

60. Hartman DJ, Slivka A, Giusto DA, et al. Tissue yield and diagnostic efficacy of fluoroscopic and cholangioscopic techniques to assess indeterminate biliary strictures. Clin Gastroenterol Hepatol 2012;10(9):1042–6.

61. Jahng AW, Chung D, Pham B, et al. Staining for intracytoplasmic lumina and CAM5.2 increases the detection rate for bile duct cancers. Endoscopy 2009;41(11):965–70.

62. Levy M, Lin F, Xu H, et al. S100P, von Hippel-Lindau gene product, and IMP3 serve as a useful immunohistochemical panel in the diagnosis of adenocarcinoma on endoscopic bile duct biopsy. Hum Pathol 2010;41(9):1210–9.

63. Schmidt MT, Himmelfarb EA, Shafi H, et al. Use of IMP3, S100P, and pVHL immunopanel to aid in the interpretation of bile duct biopsies with atypical histology or suspicious for malignancy. Appl Immunohistochem Mol Morphol 2012;20(5):478–87.

64. Chen L, Huang K, Himmelfarb EA, et al. Diagnostic value of maspin in distinguishing adenocarcinoma from benign biliary epithelium on endoscopic bile duct biopsy. Hum Pathol 2015;46(11):1647–54.

65. Galdy S, Lamarca A, McNamara MG, et al. HER2/HER3 pathway in biliary tract malignancies; systematic review and meta-analysis: a potential therapeutic target? Cancer Metastasis Rev 2017;36(1):141–57.

66. Gamblin TC, Krasinskas AM, Slivka AS, et al. Fibroinflammatory biliary stricture: a rare bile duct lesion masquerading as cholangiocarcinoma. J Gastrointest Surg 2009;13(4):713–21.

67. Rungsakulkij N, Sornmayura P, Tannaphai P. Isolated IgG4-related sclerosing cholangitis misdiagnosed as malignancy in an area with endemic cholangiocarcinoma: a case report. BMC Surg 2017;17(1):17.

68. Bismuth H, Corlette MB. Intrahepatic cholangioenteric anastomosis in carcinoma of the hilus of the liver. Surg Gynecol Obstet 1975;140(2):170–8.

69. Hong SM, Pawlik TM, Cho H, et al. Depth of tumor invasion better predicts prognosis than the current American Joint Committee on Cancer T classification for distal bile duct carcinoma. Surgery 2009;146(2):250–7.

70. Hong SM, Cho H, Moskaluk CA, et al. Measurement of the invasion depth of extrahepatic bile duct carcinoma: an alternative method overcoming the current T classification problems of the AJCC staging system. Am J Surg Pathol 2007;31(2):199–206.

71. Sato Y, Harada K, Sasaki M, et al. Histological characterization of biliary intraepithelial neoplasia with respect to pancreatic intraepithelial neoplasia. Int J Hepatol 2014;2014:678260.

72. Zen Y, Adsay NV, Bardadin K, et al. Biliary intraepithelial neoplasia: an international interobserver agreement study and proposal for diagnostic criteria. Mod Pathol 2007;20(6):701–9.

73. Basturk O, Hong SM, Wood LD, et al. A revised classification system and recommendations from the Baltimore consensus meeting for neoplastic precursor lesions in the pancreas. Am J Surg Pathol 2015;39(12):1730–41.

74. Crippa S, Salvia R, Warshaw AL, et al. Mucinous cystic neoplasm of the pancreas is not an aggressive entity: lessons from 163 resected patients. Ann Surg 2008;247(4):571–9.

75. Quigley B, Reid MD, Pehlivanoglu B, et al. Hepatobiliary mucinous cystic neoplasms with ovarian type stroma (So-Called "Hepatobiliary Cystadenoma/Cystadenocarcinoma"): clinicopathologic analysis of 36 cases illustrates rarity of carcinomatous change. Am J Surg Pathol 2018;42(1):95–102.

76. Yamao K, Yanagisawa A, Takahashi K, et al. Clinicopathological features and prognosis of mucinous cystic neoplasm with ovarian-type stroma: a multiinstitutional study of the Japan pancreas society. Pancreas 2011;40(1):67–71.

77. Schlitter AM, Born D, Bettstetter M, et al. Intraductal papillary neoplasms of the bile duct: stepwise progression to carcinoma involves common molecular pathways. Mod Pathol 2014;27(1):73–86.

78. Rocha FG, Lee H, Katabi N, et al. Intraductal papillary neoplasm of the bile duct: a biliary equivalent to intraductal papillary mucinous neoplasm of the pancreas? Hepatology 2012;56(4):1352–60.

79. Basturk O, Adsay V, Askan G, et al. Intraductal tubulopapillary neoplasm of the pancreas: a clinicopathologic and immunohistochemical analysis of 33 cases. Am J Surg Pathol 2017;41(3):313–25.

80. Schlitter AM, Jang KT, Kloppel G, et al. Intraductal tubulopapillary neoplasms of the bile ducts: clinicopathologic, immunohistochemical, and molecular analysis of 20 cases. Mod Pathol 2015;28(9):1249–64.

81. Zaydfudim VM, Rosen CB, Nagorney DM. Hilar cholangiocarcinoma. Surg Oncol Clin N Am 2014;23(2):247–63.

82. Weber SM, Ribero D, O'Reilly EM, et al. Intrahepatic cholangiocarcinoma: expert consensus statement. HPB (Oxford) 2015;17(8):669–80.

83. Cai Y, Cheng N, Ye H, et al. The current management of cholangiocarcinoma: a comparison of current guidelines. Biosci Trends 2016;10(2):92–102.

84. Park J, Kim MH, Kim KP, et al. Natural history and prognostic factors of advanced cholangiocarcinoma without surgery, chemotherapy, or radiotherapy: a large-scale observational study. Gut Liver 2009;3(4):298–305.

85. Razumilava N, Gores GJ. Classification, diagnosis, and management of cholangiocarcinoma. Clin Gastroenterol Hepatol 2013;11(1):13–21.e1, [quiz: e13–4].

86. Valle JW, Furuse J, Jitlal M, et al. Cisplatin and gemcitabine for advanced biliary tract cancer: a meta-analysis of two randomised trials. Ann Oncol 2014;25(2):391–8.

87. Valle J, Wasan H, Palmer DH, et al. Cisplatin plus gemcitabine versus gemcitabine for biliary tract cancer. N Engl J Med 2010;362(14):1273–81.

88. National Comprehensive Cancer Network. Hepatobiliary cancer (Version 4.2017). Available at: https://www.nccn.org/professionals/physician_gls/pdf/hepatobiliary.pdf. Accessed November 14, 2017.

89. Ahn DH, Bekaii-Saab T. Biliary cancer: intrahepatic cholangiocarcinoma vs. extrahepatic cholangiocarcinoma vs. gallbladder cancers: classification and therapeutic implications. J Gastrointest Oncol 2017; 8(2):293–301.

90. Geynisman DM, Catenacci DV. Toward personalized treatment of advanced biliary tract cancers. Discov Med 2012;14(74):41–57.

Acute, Chronic, and Humoral Rejection
Pathologic Features Under Current Immunosuppressive Regimes

Jamie Koo, MD[a], Hanlin L. Wang, MD, PhD[b],*

KEYWORDS

• Liver transplantation • Allograft rejection • Acute cellular rejection • T-cell–mediated rejection
• Chronic rejection • Antibody-mediated rejection • Humoral rejection

---

Key points

- Histopathologic assessment of allograft biopsies continues to serve an important role in the diagnosis of rejection to facilitate successful patient management.

- The diagnosis of acute and chronic antibody-mediated rejection requires integration of the results of histologic examination, donor-specific antibody testing and C4d immunostaining, and exclusion of other potential etiologies of allograft dysfunction.

- Antibody-mediated rejection should be suspected if histologic findings in an allograft biopsy cannot be adequately explained by an identifiable etiology.

ABSTRACT

Under current immunosuppressive regimes, T-cell–mediated acute and chronic rejection remain common and important posttransplant complications. The definition of humoral (antibody-mediated) rejection has been greatly expanded in recent years. The histopathologic assessment of allograft biopsies continues to serve an important role in the diagnosis of rejection and to facilitate patient management. The diagnosis of both acute and chronic antibody-mediated rejection requires integration of the results of donor-specific antibody testing and C4d immunostaining, as well as exclusion of other potential etiologies of allograft dysfunction. Chronic antibody-mediated rejection should also be included in the differential diagnosis for unexplained allograft fibrosis.

OVERVIEW

Since first performed by Dr Thomas E. Starzl and colleagues in 1963, liver transplantation has evolved to become the standard of care for patients with end-stage liver diseases, acute liver failure, liver-based metabolic disorders, and selected primary hepatic malignancies.[1,2] The range of posttransplant complications is broad, and includes surgical/technical complications, allograft rejection, infections, recurrent liver diseases, and acquired liver diseases, among others. Allograft rejection remains a major complication despite advances in immunosuppressive agents and regimens that have dramatically improved patient survival since the early days of liver transplantation. The histopathologic examination of allograft biopsies is an integral tool to the diagnosis of rejection, because many of the posttransplant

---

Disclosure Statement: The authors have nothing to disclose.
[a] Department of Pathology and Laboratory Medicine, Cedars-Sinai Medical Center, 8700 Beverly Boulevard, Room 8707, Los Angeles, CA 90048, USA; [b] Department of Pathology and Laboratory Medicine, David Geffen School of Medicine at UCLA, 10833 Le Conte Avenue, 27-061-C8 CHS, Los Angeles, CA 90095, USA
* Corresponding author.
E-mail address: hanlinwang@mednet.ucla.edu

complications cannot be easily differentiated from each other clinically, radiographically, or biochemically. In this article, current immunosuppressive agents and regimens are reviewed briefly, followed by a detailed discussion of the current diagnostic criteria for T-cell–mediated rejection (TCMR; acute cellular rejection), chronic rejection, and antibody-mediated rejection (AMR; humoral rejection). Relevant differential diagnoses and clinical aspects of these entities are also discussed briefly.

CURRENT STRATEGIES OF IMMUNOSUPPRESSION FOR LIVER TRANSPLANTATION

IMMUNOSUPPRESSIVE AGENTS

Corticosteroids are most commonly used during the induction phase immediately after transplantation and in the treatment of acute rejection.[3–5] They exert their antiinflammatory effects through multiple mechanisms, including decreased transcription of proinflammatory factors, inhibition of cell-mediated immunity and antibody production via decreased production of cytokines (interleukin [IL]-1, IL-2, IL-6, IL-8, tumor necrosis factor-α), and impairment of cell migration, phagocytosis, and respiratory burst mechanisms, and so on. Adverse side effects from long-term steroid use are numerous, including increased risk of opportunistic infections, metabolic derangements (such as hyperglycemia, hypertension, hyperlipidemia, weight gain, and osteoporosis), and in patients transplanted for active hepatitis C, the possibility for early and aggressive recurrence.

Calcineurin inhibitors (CNIs), including cyclosporine and tacrolimus (FK506, Prograf), are the most commonly used drugs for long-term maintenance immunosuppression. They exert their effects by binding to proteins that inhibit the phosphatase calcineurin, which in turn prevents transcription of the *IL-2* gene and, thus, T-cell proliferation. Tacrolimus is preferred over cyclosporine in the setting of liver transplantation, because it has been shown to be more potent and efficacious, with better graft survival rates and a fewer clinically significant side effects. The main complication from long-term CNI use is nephrotoxicity, which can lead to both acute and chronic renal insufficiency. Other significant side effects include hyperglycemia with development of diabetes mellitus, headaches, neurologic symptoms, and atherosclerotic cardiovascular disease.

The antimetabolites mycophenolic acid (MPA; CellCept) and azathioprine (Imuran) are second-line agents that are used in conjunction with CNIs for maintenance immunosuppression. Both exert their effects by inhibiting synthesis of purine nucleotides in T and B cells, thus, inhibiting lymphocyte proliferation. Over the past 20 years, the use of azathioprine has progressively decreased in the setting of liver transplantation and has now largely been replaced by MPA. The main side effects of MPA are dose-dependent leukopenia and gastrointestinal symptoms such as nausea, vomiting, and diarrhea, which usually respond to dose reduction or a switch to a different MPA formulation.

The mammalian target of rapamycin inhibitors sirolimus and everolimus are used less frequently for maintenance immunosuppression and are typically limited to patients who cannot tolerate CNIs, have renal dysfunction, or with high-risk hepatocellular carcinoma. They bind to the same protein (FKBP12) that binds tacrolimus but at a different site, which leads to inhibition of the kinase mammalian target of rapamycin, and thus inhibits T-cell activation and proliferation. Sirolimus has been associated with an increased risk of hepatic artery thrombosis, hyperlipidemia, hypertension, and cytopenia.

There are various polyclonal and monoclonal antibodies that either inhibit or deplete T cells, and can be used for steroid-free regimens or for treatment of steroid-resistant rejection. The polyclonal antibodies antithymocyte globulin and antilymphocyte globulin contain antibodies to multiple T-cell antigens, which leads to lymphocyte depletion via apoptosis and/or cell lysis. In general, they are well-tolerated, but can occasionally cause allergic reactions or a serum sickness-like illness. Monoclonal antibodies include those to CD3, IL-2 receptor, and CD52, but these are not widely used at this time.

STRATEGIES AND PROTOCOLS

Immunosuppression protocols can vary widely as a result of a combination of physician preference, primary disease necessitating transplantation, and an individual patient's side effect profile to particular medications. In the period immediately after transplantation, higher levels of immunosuppression are needed temporarily as the recipient's immune system is first exposed to various alloantigens from the donor liver. This immunosuppression is usually in the form of high-dose corticosteroids, up to 1000 mg at the time of transplantation, followed by a rapid taper over the first couple of weeks and maintenance on lower doses for the first 3 to 12 months after transplantation.[4–6] There has been growing interest in antibody-based steroid-free regimens, including the use of antithymocyte globulin or monoclonal antibodies, given the multiple adverse effects associated with steroid use. However, although the use of steroid-free induction regimens reduces the frequency of diabetes and hypertension and shows no statistically significant differences for infection, graft loss, and mortality in comparison with steroid-containing regimens, it is found to be associated with a higher rate of acute rejection based on a recent metaanalysis of 16 clinical trials that involved a total of 1347 participants.[7] Thus, corticosteroids will likely remain the mainstay of induction therapy at most transplant centers until more convincing data become available for steroid-free regimens.

In general, tacrolimus monotherapy is used for maintenance immunosuppression after liver transplantation and is started 1 to 3 days after transplantation. Drug levels are followed to ensure therapeutic efficacy and to minimize toxicity. The target trough levels are generally 10 to 15 ng/mL immediately after transplantation, 5 to 10 ng/mL in months 6 to 12, and 4 to 6 mg/mL thereafter.[5] Targeting of a lower trough level of tacrolimus or the addition of a second agent such as MPA can be beneficial in patients who have baseline renal insufficiency or who develop nephrotoxicity or other side effects while on tacrolimus.[4,5] It is unclear whether switching to monotherapy with sirolimus is beneficial in patients with preexisting renal disease.

IMMUNE TOLERANCE

As mentioned, long-term immunosuppression inevitably leads to a risk of various serious complications such as infections, metabolic disorders, direct drug toxicities, and even certain malignancies. Minimizing or even eliminating the use of immunosuppression without compromising graft function would, thus, be beneficial not only to minimize the morbidity associated with these complications, but also to improve quality of life and reduce medication costs.

Immunologically, the liver is uniquely tolerogenic compared with other organs. This allows for liver transplantation to be performed despite a positive crossmatch, with no substantial benefit from HLA matching. Less immunosuppression is needed as compared with other solid organ transplants, and chronic rejection occurs less frequently.[4,8] It has been observed that a certain proportion of liver transplant recipients, either as a result of noncompliance or as a deliberate decision to discontinue immunosuppression, develop spontaneous operational tolerance, and no longer seem to be at risk for the development of rejection. In an analysis of 7 major clinical trials on operational tolerance,

which included 265 adults and 20 children, tolerance was observed in 22.0% to 62.5% of patients after a mean follow-up duration of 1.0 to 7.3 years.[8] The mean time from transplantation to weaning ranged from 2 to 9 years. The rate of acute cellular rejection in these trials ranged widely, from 10% (pediatric cohort) to 76% (cohort with hepatitis C virus [HCV] infection). Based on the results of these trials, time after transplantation seems to be a key factor in the development of operational tolerance, with higher success rates seen in patients who are at least 3 years post transplantation. Weaning of immunosuppression also seemed to be more successful in older recipients (>60 years) and in those without autoimmune diseases. However, these results should be interpreted with some caution owing to the small size of the studies and the lack of uniform inclusion and exclusion criteria.

It has been recommended by the Banff Working Group on Liver Allograft Pathology that liver biopsy in conjunction with serum liver chemistry tests should play an integral role in the selection and monitoring of patients being considered or undergoing weaning of immunosuppression.[9] Briefly, a baseline (preweaning) biopsy that is considered conducive to the minimization of immunosuppression should show no or at the most minimal to focal mild portal mononuclear cell inflammation. There should be no or minimal interface necroinflammatory activity, no central perivenular inflammation, and no bile duct damage. If fibrosis is present, it should be mild overall, but rare portal-to-portal bridging and mild perivenular fibrosis are allowable. Those patients who have achieved sustained virologic response after HCV treatment can have more substantial fibrosis.[10] Patients transplanted for autoimmune hepatitis (AIH), primary biliary cholangitis (PBC), primary sclerosing cholangitis, or active HCV infection should be weaned only with caution or not at all according to the Banff recommendations.[9,10]

In the absence of other clinical parameters to suggest allograft injury, protocol biopsies with concurrent liver function tests are recommended at 1, 3, 5, and 10 years after major decreases in immunosuppression or after total withdrawal. These biopsies should be compared with the preweaning biopsy to assess whether there is increased portal inflammation, increased interface activity, new onset of endotheliitis, new onset of central perivenular inflammation, new onset of bile duct damage or loss that cannot be explained by a nonimmunologic etiology such as biliary stricture, a greater than 1-stage increase in fibrosis, or new onset of bridging fibrosis without an alternative explanation. Assessment of these histologic parameters would help to determine whether patients can be maintained on minimal or no immunosuppression.[9,10]

T-CELL–MEDIATED REJECTION (ACUTE CELLULAR REJECTION)

CLINICAL AND LABORATORY ASPECTS

TCMR is the currently preferred term for acute cellular rejection.[10] Although the reported incidence varies widely in the literature, the incidence of clinically significant TCMR is likely in the 20% to 40% range with current immunosuppression regimens.[11–13] This represents a dramatic decrease compared with the initial era of liver transplantation. TCMR typically occurs within the first 5 to 30 days after transplantation, but may occur as early as 2 days or as late as months to years after transplantation, and is usually the result of suboptimal immunosuppression.[13] Patients with TCMR can be asymptomatic, but many present with fever, abdominal pain, hepatomegaly, and fatigue. Serum liver chemistry tests generally lack specificity, but may show preferentially elevated serum alkaline phosphatase levels. Serum transaminase and bilirubin levels can also be significantly elevated. A definitive diagnosis of TCMR requires histologic confirmation in an allograft biopsy.

TYPICAL HISTOLOGIC FEATURES

The histologic features of typical TCMR are traditionally defined as a triad of (1) mixed portal inflammatory cell infiltrates, (2) bile duct damage, and (3) endotheliitis.[14] At least 2 of these 3 findings are required for the diagnosis, but the presence of unequivocal endotheliitis seems to be most diagnostic (Box 1). It is recommended that a minimum of 5 portal tracts and at least 2 sections at different levels be examined when evaluating a core biopsy for TCMR.[14]

Portal inflammatory cell infiltrates typically consist of a mixture of small and large (activated) lymphocytes. Other components include eosinophils, macrophages, plasma cells, and occasionally

neutrophils. Eosinophils are usually conspicuous, but still comprise a minority of the inflammatory cell infiltrates (Fig. 1A). Studies have shown that the presence of prominent portal eosinophils is a useful feature to suggest TCMR,[15,16] but its diagnostic usefulness should not be overvalued because eosinophils can also be seen in other conditions, such as drug-induced liver injury and viral hepatitis.[17] It should be noted that the commonly used immunosuppressive agents, such as tacrolimus and corticosteroids, do not cause eosinophilia in allografts.

Bile duct damage is characterized by infiltration of lymphocytes between duct epithelial cells and between the epithelial cells and basement membrane (Fig. 1B). The epithelial cells typically show features of injury characterized by nuclear overlapping, enlargement, pleomorphism, apoptosis, and cytoplasmic vacuolation and eosinophilia. In the setting of TCMR, bile ducts are usually cuffed by inflammatory cells, and may become obscured in cases with heavy portal inflammation. Ductular reaction is typically insignificant.

Endotheliitis is considered the most specific diagnostic feature of TCMR. It most commonly involves the portal veins, but may also involve the terminal hepatic venules (central veins) in some cases. It is characterized by subendothelial lymphocytic infiltrates that lift up and disrupt the overlying endothelial cells (Fig. 1C). Endotheliitis may also manifest as direct attachment of lymphocytes to the endothelium through cytoplasmic processes from the luminal side (Fig. 1D). The endothelial cells may be swollen and detached. Endotheliitis is usually focal but can be circumferential.

GRADING T-Cell–Mediated REJECTION

TCMR is graded for severity by either global assessment (Table 1) or the rejection activity index (Table 2) using the Banff schema.[10,14] The indeterminate category in the global assessment should be restricted to cases that only show mild portal and/or perivenular inflammatory cell infiltrates but lack evidence of bile duct damage, endotheliitis, or zone 3 confluent perivenular hepatocyte necrosis/dropout. The infiltrates should not be explainable by other conditions, such as recurrent liver disease. If the rejection activity index is used, a score of 1 to 2 roughly corresponds with indeterminate for TCMR, 3 to 4 with mild, 5 to 6 with moderate, and 7 to 9 with severe. Although the rejection activity index seems to offer a greater degree of precision, there have been no data to support that it is a better approach than global assessment.[14]

Box 1
Key histologic features of typical T-cell–mediated rejection

- Mixed portal inflammatory cell infiltrates

- Bile duct damage

- Portal vein endotheliitis

- Central perivenular inflammatory cell infiltrates with or without hepatocyte necrosis/dropout

Fig. 1. (*A*) T-cell–mediated rejection (TCMR) features mixed portal inflammatory cell infiltrates with prominent eosinophils (original magnification ×200). Endotheliitis involves the entire circumference of a portal vein (*left*). (*B*) TCMR showing mixed portal inflammatory cell infiltrates and bile duct damage. The bile duct (*arrow*) is obscured by dense infiltrates (original magnification ×400).

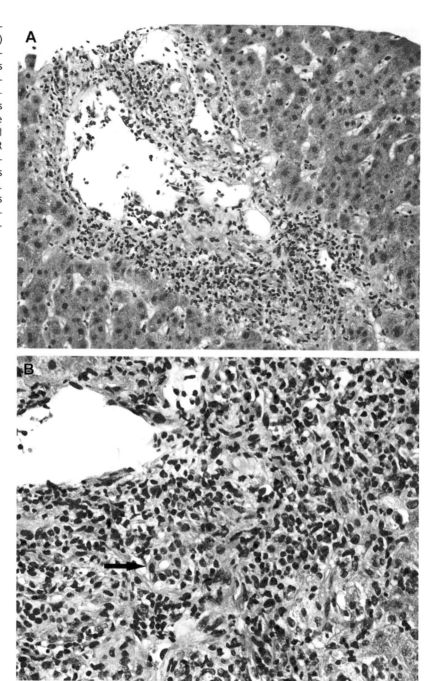

UNUSUAL FORMS OF T-Cell–Mediated REJECTION

Late-Onset Acute Rejection

Late-onset acute rejection occurs more than 6 months after transplantation.[10] The reported incidence varies from 7% to 40% in different studies, and it usually develops as a consequence of inadequate immunosuppression.[13,18]

The histologic features of late-onset acute rejection are essentially the same as those described for typical TCMR, but may show less prominent eosinophils, fewer activated lymphocytes, slightly more interface activity, less prominent bile duct damage, less intense endotheliitis, and slightly more lobular activity. Central perivenulitis may be seen in some cases and may be the only histologic finding (discussed elsewhere in this

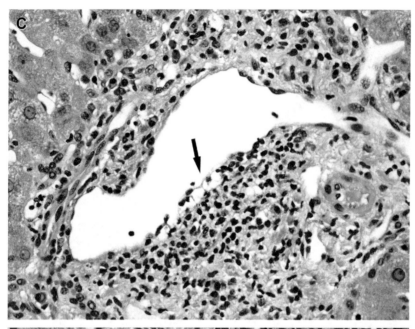

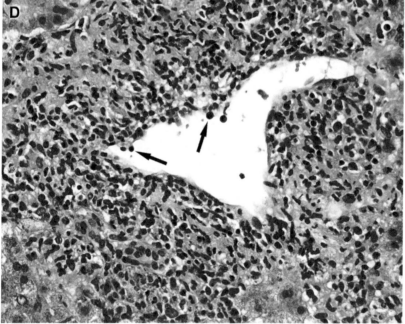

Fig. 1. (continued). (*C*) Endotheliitis focally involving a portal vein (*arrow*) characterized by subendothelial lymphocytic infiltrates that lift up and disrupt the overlying endothelium (original magnification ×400). (*D*) Endotheliitis also manifests as direct attachment of lymphocytes to the endothelium from the luminal side (*arrows*; original magnification ×400).

article). Patients with late-onset acute rejection may show a poorer response to increased immunosuppression. An increased risk to evolve to chronic rejection and graft loss has been observed.[18–21]

Central Perivenulitis

Central perivenulitis represents a spectrum of necroinflammatory changes involving the central veins and zone 3 hepatocytes. Histologically, it features endotheliitis of the central veins with subendothelial mononuclear cell infiltration (**Fig. 2**A). Frequently, there is also confluent perivenular hepatocyte necrosis/dropout. In some cases, zone 3 necrosis is prominent, but the inflammatory cell infiltrates are insignificant and the features of endotheliitis are not evident (**Fig. 2**B).

Table 1
Updated Banff schema for grading TCMR: global assessment

Grade	Criteria
Indeterminate	Portal and/or perivenular inflammatory infiltrate that is related to an alloreaction, but shows insufficient tissue damage to meet criteria for a diagnosis of mild acute rejection
Mild	Rejection-type infiltrate in a minority of the triads or perivenular areas, that is generally mild, and mostly confined within the portal spaces for portal-based rejection and an absence of confluent necrosis/ hepatocyte dropout for those presenting with isolated perivenular infiltrates
Moderate	Rejection-type infiltrate, expanding most or all of portal tracts and/or perivenular areas with confluent necrosis/ hepatocyte dropout limited to a minority of perivenular areas
Severe	As above for moderate, with spillover into periportal areas and/or moderate-to-severe perivenular inflammation that extends into the hepatic parenchyma and is associated with perivenular hepatocyte necrosis involving a majority of perivenular areas

Abbreviation: TCMR, T-cell–mediated rejection.

In the presence of typical portal changes of TCMR, central perivenulitis is generally regarded as a sign of TCMR.[10,22–28] For this reason, the updated Banff schema has incorporated central perivenulitis into the global assessment for TCMR grading (see **Table 1**).[10] However, isolated central perivenulitis not accompanied by portal changes of rejection may pose diagnostic challenges. In most cases, it is still believed to represent a form of rejection (either acute or chronic rejection), but other causes must be ruled out. These may include preservation/reperfusion injury, ischemic damage secondary to vascular thrombosis/stenosis, recurrent AIH, and drug toxicity.

Central perivenulitis may occur in the early posttransplant period, but is more commonly seen as a late event (after 3 months).[22] Compared with portal-based rejection, cases with central perivenulitis are less likely to respond to increased immunosuppression, and are more likely to develop subsequent episodes of acute rejection, chronic rejection, zone 3 fibrosis, and graft failure.[16,25–27,29]

Plasma Cell-Rich Rejection

Plasma cell-rich rejection is the currently preferred term for cases previously described as plasma cell hepatitis and de novo AIH.[10] It histologically resembles AIH, but occurs in patients whose original liver disease was not AIH. It is characterized by portal and lobular inflammatory cell infiltrates containing more than 30% plasma cells (**Fig. 3**). Interface activity is typically prominent and central perivenulitis may be present (**Box 2**). It is usually a late event, occurring several months or years after transplantation.[30,31] Although its pathogenesis is poorly understood,[30] it is now generally regarded as a special form of rejection resulting from both T-cell– and antibody-mediated mechanisms.[31–33] In addition to the presence of classical serum autoantibodies, some patients also have circulating donor-specific antibodies (DSA) to a liver/kidney cytosolic enzyme called glutathione S-transferase T1, which has been linked to the development of plasma cell-rich rejection when present in high titers.[34] It has also been shown that the development of plasma cell-rich rejection in the setting of recurrent HCV is a negative prognostic factor for graft and patient outcomes.[31,35]

Hepatitic Rejection

In addition to central perivenulitis, other features of lobular injury, such as lobular necroinflammation not restricted to perivenular or interface areas (**Fig. 4**A), lobular disarray, hepatocyte ballooning, sinusoidal lymphocytic infiltration (**Fig. 4**B), and sinusoidal endotheliitis, have also been observed in the setting of rejection.[36–39] These features are not considered in the current Banff schema, however. In a study of 28 cases with biopsy-confirmed moderate to severe TCMR,[39] Siddiqui and colleagues found that 7 also showed a sinusoidal lymphocytic infiltration pattern. All but 1 patients responded well to standard steroid boluses. None of them developed chronic rejection on follow-up. Six patients also showed a lobular necroinflammatory pattern. These patients had failed standard steroid boluses and 4 required thymoglobulin rescue. One

Table 2
Banff schema for grading TCMR: rejection activity index

Category	Criteria	Score
Portal inflammation	Mostly lymphocytic inflammation involving, but not noticeably expanding, a minority of the triads	1
	Expansion of most or all of the triads, by a mixed infiltrate containing lymphocytes with occasional blasts, neutrophils, and eosinophils. If eosinophils are conspicuous and accompanied by edema and microvascular endothelial cell hypertrophy is prominent, acute antibody-mediated rejection should be considered	2
	Marked expansion of most or all of the triads by a mixed infiltrate containing blasts and eosinophils with inflammatory spillover into the periportal parenchyma	3
Bile duct inflammation and damage	A minority of the ducts are cuffed and infiltrated by inflammatory cells and show only mild reactive changes such as increased nuclear:cytoplasmic ratio of the epithelial cells	1
	Most or all of the ducts infiltrated by inflammatory cells. More than an occasional duct shows degenerative changes such as nuclear pleomorphism, disordered polarity, and cytoplasmic vacuolization of the epithelium	2
	As above for 2, with most or all of the ducts showing degenerative changes or focal luminal disruption	3
Venous endothelial inflammation	Subendothelial lymphocytic infiltration involving some, but not a majority of the portal and/or hepatic venules	1
	Subendothelial infiltration involving most or all of the portal and/or hepatic venules with or without confluent hepatocyte necrosis/dropout involving a minority of perivenular regions	2
	As above for 2, with moderate or severe perivenular inflammation that extends into the perivenular parenchyma and is associated with perivenular hepatocyte necrosis involving a majority of perivenular regions	3

Abbreviation: TCMR, T-cell–mediated rejection.

patient developed chronic rejection on follow-up. These hepatitic features are generally thought to represent atypical forms of TCMR, but an antibody-mediated mechanism may also contribute.[36]

Idiopathic Posttransplant Hepatitis

Idiopathic posttransplant hepatitis refers to chronic hepatitis that cannot be attributed to a specific etiology and is thus a diagnosis of exclusion. It is characterized by mononuclear cell infiltrates in the portal tracts with varying degrees of interface and lobular activity, usually discovered more than 12 months after transplantation by protocol biopsies from asymptomatic patients with normal or near-normal liver tests.[23,40] By definition, bile duct damage, ductopenia, and endotheliitis are not present. A large proportion of these patients develop progressive fibrosis with time and may show bridging fibrosis or even cirrhosis by 10 years.[40,41] Studies have provided evidence to support the notion that most cases of so-called idiopathic

posttransplant hepatitis may represent a form of late-onset TCMR or chronic AMR in DSA-positive patients.[10,40,42]

DIFFERENTIAL DIAGNOSIS

In cases where the typical histologic features of TCMR are not fully present, other disease entities may enter into the differential diagnosis. This is particularly true if the biopsy shows hepatitic features, plasma cell-rich infiltrates, and/or central perivenulitis, and when the abnormalities are observed as a late event. In addition to recurrent HCV, AIH, and PBC, the possibility of unusual infections need to be borne in mind. These may include Epstein-Barr virus (EBV), hepatitis E, and human herpes virus 6, among others.

EBV hepatitis may show mixed inflammatory cell infiltrates, mild bile duct damage, and mild endotheliitis in the portal tracts, resulting in a histologic appearance similar to TCMR.[43] In contrast, the characteristic sinusoidal infiltrative pattern by lymphocytes seen in EBV hepatitis has also been described as an unusual feature of rejection as

Fig. 2. (*A*) Acute T-cell–mediated rejection (TCMR) with central perivenulitis showing prominent endotheliitis. Hepatocyte dropout and mild inflammatory cell infiltrates around the vein are also evident (original magnification ×400). (*B*) Central perivenulitis showing hepatocyte dropout and mild inflammatory cell infiltrates without endotheliitis (original magnification ×400). Features of ductopenic chronic rejection are also evident in this case.

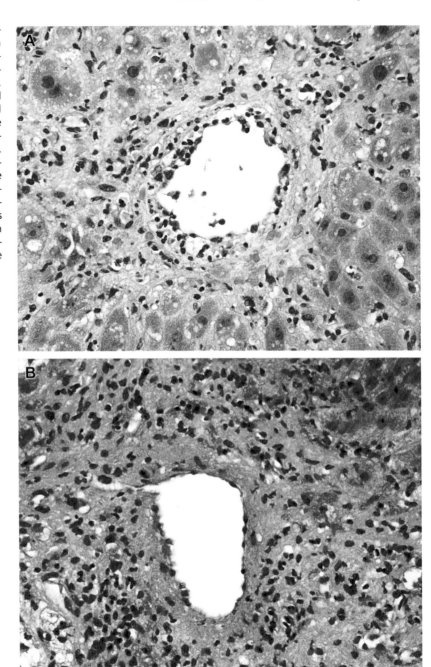

discussed above.[39] In situ hybridization to detect EBV early RNA can be valuable in this setting.

Hepatitis E has recently been recognized as a cause of chronic hepatitis in immunocompromised patients, including liver transplant recipients.[44–46] Chronic hepatitis E usually shows varying degrees of portal and lobular necroinflammation,[44,47] and may evolve rapidly to fibrosis and cirrhosis if not treated appropriately.[44–46] Although an uncommon occurrence, this condition may be easily

confused with late-onset rejection or idiopathic posttransplant hepatitis. Diagnosis requires a high index of suspicion.

Human herpes virus 6 infection or reactivation can be an early or late event after transplantation, and is another uncommon condition that may mimic TCMR. Histologically, human herpes virus 6 hepatitis features mild to moderate predominantly portal lymphocytic infiltrates. Minimal bile duct injury and focal mild portal vein

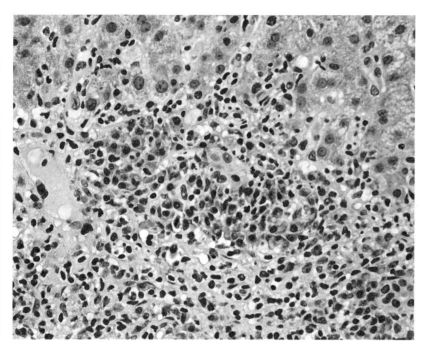

Fig. 3. Plasma cell-rich rejection showing lymphoplasmacytic infiltrates in a portal tract with interface activity rich in plasma cells (original magnification ×400). Central perivenulitis with prominent plasma cells is also evident in this case.

endotheliitis may be seen (**Fig. 5**A). In addition, spotty foci of lobular inflammation with apoptotic hepatocytes may be present (**Fig. 5**B), which is an unusual finding for TCMR. Confluent periportal necrosis may also be evident in some cases.[48] This diagnosis also requires a high index of suspicion and can be confirmed by polymerase chain reaction performed on serum or the biopsy tissue. Immunohistochemistry has been used to detect viral antigens on biopsy specimens,[49] but its diagnostic value has not been well-established.

TREATMENT AND PROGNOSIS

Mild TCMR may be treated with increased dosages of the immunosuppressive agents currently being used, whereas moderate to severe TCMR is typically treated with an additional steroid bolus followed by a slow taper over 10 to 14 days, which leads to successful resolution in 70% to 80% of cases by normalization of serum liver enzymes.[4–6] Histologic improvement after effective treatment begins with a decrease in inflammatory cell infiltrates, usually occurring within 24 hours. Complete recovery may take 7 to 10 days, and endotheliitis usually resolves before bile duct damage (**Fig. 6**).[13] A repeat biopsy is indicated for nonresponders, and may show ongoing or worsening rejection that warrants more vigorous immunosuppression or reveal an unrelated disease process that may be masked by concurrent rejection in the initial biopsy. Antithymocyte globulin is usually

---

Box 2
Banff criteria for the diagnosis of plasma cell-rich rejection

1. Portal and/or perivenular plasma cell–rich (estimated >30%) infiltrates with easily recognizable periportal/interface and/or perivenular necroinflammatory activity usually involving a majority of portal tracts and/or central veins. Most of these cases are graded at least moderate with a total RAI score of ≥ 5 because the V score is usually 3 because of aggressive perivenular activity, whereas the portal Inflammation score is usually ≥ 2.

2. Lymphocytic cholangitis is usually present and a desirable feature, but not absolutely required (inflammatory bile duct damage might be a relatively minor component, but Banff component score for bile duct injury is usually ≥ 1).

3. Original disease other than autoimmune hepatitis.

Must fulfill criteria 1 and 3; criterion 2 is desirable but not absolutely required.
Abbreviations: RAI, rejection activity index; V score, venous endothelial inflammation score (see **Table 2**).

Fig. 4. (*A*) Hepatitic rejection featuring lymphocytic infiltration of the lobules with frequent apoptotic hepatocytes (*arrows*; original magnification ×400). (*B*) Prominent sinusoidal lymphocytic infiltration can also be seen (original magnification ×400).

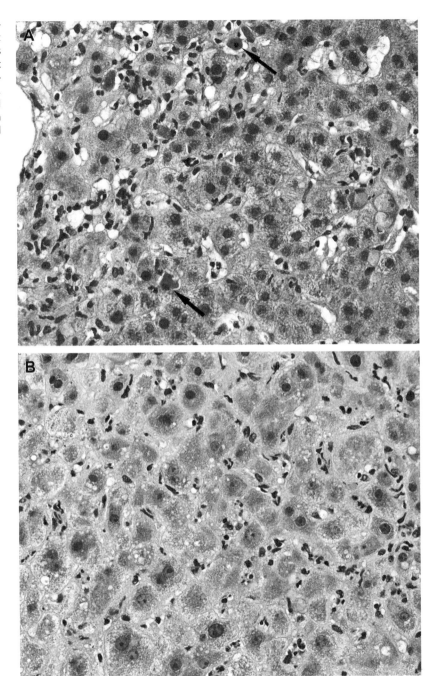

used as the first line to treat patients with steroid-resistant rejection.[5] After the rejection episode is treated successfully, the maintenance immunosuppressive therapy may need to be modified to either increase the target trough level or add another class of immunosuppressant. In patients with recurrent HCV, however, this addition will have to be carefully balanced with the risk of exacerbation of viral replication.

Unsuccessful treatment of acute rejection may lead to the development of chronic rejection, perivenular fibrosis, and graft loss. As discussed, patients with late-onset rejection and central perivenulitis tend to respond poorly to treatment and may carry a worse prognosis.

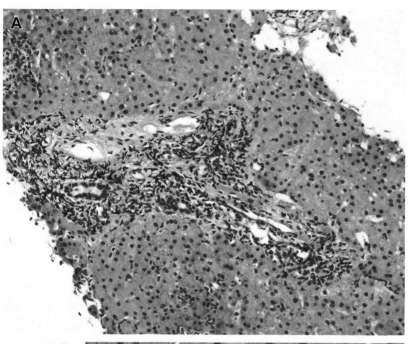

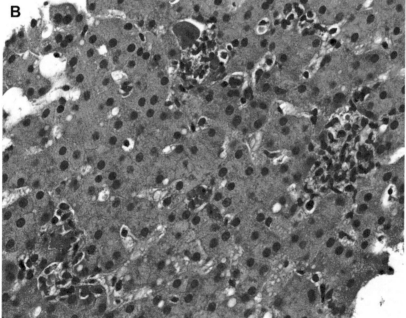

Fig. 5. (*A*) Human herpes virus 6 hepatitis in an allograft biopsy showing mild portal lymphocytic infiltrates that mimic acute T-cell–mediated rejection (original magnification ×200). (*B*) Spotty foci of lobular inflammation with frequent apoptotic hepatocytes are a clue to the proper diagnosis (original magnification ×400). The diagnosis was confirmed by polymerase chain reaction.

CHRONIC REJECTION

CLINICAL AND LABORATORY ASPECTS

Chronic rejection affects 2% to 5% of liver allografts, usually occurring more than 3 months after transplantation. It is typically preceded by episodes of TCMR, but may occur insidiously. Patients may present with progressive jaundice and a cholestatic pattern of abnormal serum liver chemistry tests with preferentially elevated serum alkaline phosphatase and γ-glutamyl transferase levels.[13,23]

HISTOLOGIC FEATURES

The 2 main histologic abnormalities that define chronic rejection are obliterative arteriopathy and progressive destruction of interlobular bile

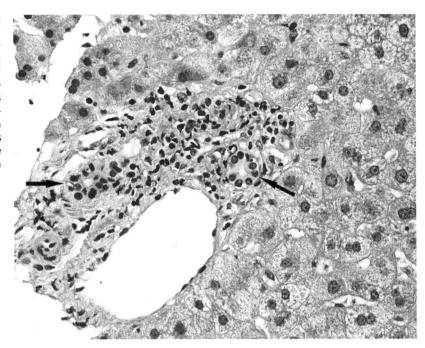

Fig. 6. Treated acute T-cell–mediated rejection showing mild inflammatory cell infiltrates in a portal tract with mild bile duct damage (*arrows*). No endotheliitis is seen (original magnification ×400). This is a follow-up biopsy 7 days after treatment from the same case shown in **Fig. 1A**.

ducts leading to ductopenia (**Box 3**). Obliterative arteriopathy is characterized by intimal thickening owing to accumulation of lipid-laden foamy macrophages that leads to progressive luminal narrowing and occlusion (**Fig. 7A**). Although this pathognomonic feature may be readily apparent in explanted failed allografts, it is seldom observed on a biopsy specimen because it primarily affects large- and medium-sized arteries at or near the hilum. A related finding that may be observed in biopsy specimens is the loss of small portal tract arterial branches, which may occur early before bile duct loss.[50] Biopsy specimens may also show evidence of ischemic injury, such as hepatocyte ballooning, necrosis/dropout, and cholestasis involving centrilobular areas. Sinusoidal accumulation of foamy macrophages may be evident. Perivenular fibrosis may develop, which can sometimes lead to central vein obliteration and even central-to-central or central-to-portal bridging fibrosis. In general, however, chronic rejection is not associated with significant portal or periportal fibrosis, and thus does not usually lead to cirrhosis.

Progressive bile duct loss is a hallmark of chronic rejection mediated by immunologic and ischemic mechanisms.[51] Because the small bile ducts in the portal tracts are the main antigenic targets, this abnormality can be recognized readily on biopsy specimens. It begins with degenerative or senescent changes of the ductal epithelium, characterized by nuclear enlargement, hyperchromasia and pleomorphism, unevenly spaced nuclei, and cytoplasmic eosinophilia (**Fig. 7B**).[52] A mild, predominantly lymphocytic infiltrate is usually present in the portal tracts at this phase, but there is less prominent lymphocytic infiltration of the duct epithelium when compared with that seen in acute rejection. By the time the bile ducts are completely gone, there may be no or only minimal inflammatory cells present (**Fig. 7C**). There is a general lack of ductular reaction, in marked contrast with most other biliary diseases that cause duct destruction and loss. In cases where both bile ducts and small arterial branches have vanished, the identification of portal tracts can be challenging. This may require a subjective interpretation based on the location, shape, and internal structure of small fibrotic areas that are presumed to represent portal tracts (**Fig. 7D**). Immunostains for cytokeratins, such as cytokeratin 7, may be helpful to confirm the

---

Box 3
Key histologic features of typical chronic rejection

- Obliterative arteriopathy
- Bile duct degeneration and loss

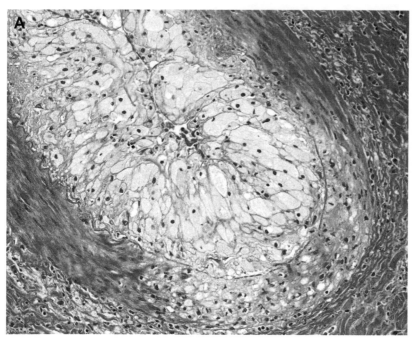

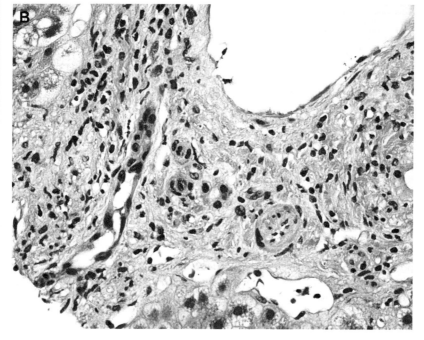

Fig. 7. (*A*) Obliterative arteriopathy in an explanted failed allograft owing to chronic rejection showing intimal thickening with lipid-laden foamy macrophages. The lumen is essentially completely occluded and the lesion focally involves the entire arterial wall (original magnification ×200). (*B*) Early chronic rejection featuring degenerative changes of the duct epithelium, characterized by cytoplasmic eosinophilia, unevenly spaced nuclei, and nuclear pleomorphism and hyperchromasia. The portal tract is usually infiltrated by inflammatory cells at this stage (original magnification ×400).

absence of bile ducts in difficult cases. Combined use with epithelial membrane antigen may further help to distinguish bile ducts from ductules in cases with ductular proliferation, because epithelial membrane antigen stains the brush border of interlobular bile ducts but not ductules, according to a recent study.[53]

STAGING CHRONIC REJECTION

Chronic rejection is divided into early and late stages according to the Banff schema (**Table 3**).[10,52] The distinction is clinically important because early chronic rejection is potentially reversible, whereas late stage rejection is

Fig. 7. (*continued*). (*C*) Chronic rejection showing bile duct loss. Note the presence of a hepatic artery (*arrow*). There is no inflammatory cell infiltrate in the portal tract in this case. No ductular reaction or portal fibrosis is evident (original magnification ×400). (*D*) Chronic rejection with loss of both bile duct and hepatic artery in this portal tract (original magnification ×400).

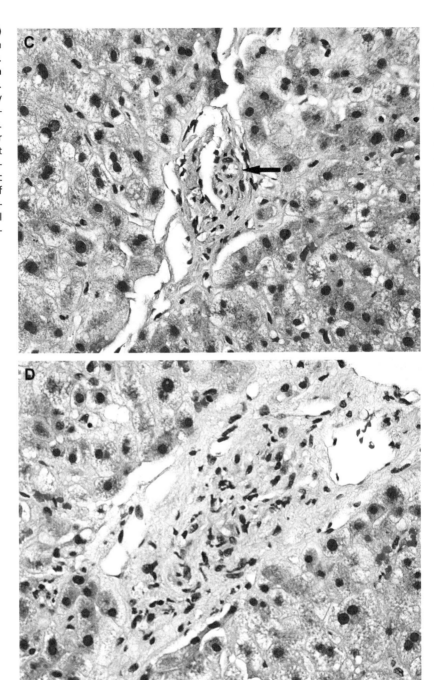

generally considered irreversible and usually requires retransplantation. To make an accurate assessment for the degree of ductopenia, 20 or more portal tracts should be assessed, which sometimes requires more than 1 biopsy over time.[54] However, there is evidence that ductopenic chronic rejection can be diagnosed reliably by experienced pathologists based on assessment of considerably fewer portal tracts.[55] It should be noted that up to 20% of portal tracts may physiologically lack bile ducts. Bile duct loss is thus considered present only when fewer than 80% of the portal tracts contain bile ducts.[52]

DIFFERENTIAL DIAGNOSIS

Bile duct degeneration, ductopenia, and centrilobular injury are not unique to chronic rejection and

Table 3
Banff schema for staging chronic rejection

Structure	Early Chronic Rejection[a]	Late Chronic Rejection[a]
Small bile ducts (<60 μm)	Degenerative changes involving a majority of ducts Bile duct loss in <50% of portal tracts	Loss in ≥50% of portal tracts Degenerative changes in remaining bile ducts
Portal tract hepatic arterioles	Occasional loss involving <25% of portal tracts	Loss involving >25% of portal tracts
Terminal hepatic venules and zone 3 hepatocytes	Perivenular mononuclear inflammation Lytic zone 3 necrosis and inflammation Mild perivenular fibrosis	Variable inflammation Focal obliteration Moderate to severe (bridging) fibrosis
Large perihilar hepatic artery branches[b]	Intimal inflammation Focal foam cell deposition without luminal compromise	Luminal narrowing by intimal foam cells Fibrointimal hyperplasia
Large perihilar bile ducts[b]	Inflammation damage and focal foam cell deposition	Mural fibrosis
Other	So-called transition hepatitis with spotty necrosis of hepatocytes	Sinusoidal foam cell accumulation Cholestasis

[a] At least 2 findings should be present.
[b] Usually seen in explanted failed allografts but not in biopsy specimens.

can also be seen in the setting of recurrent PBC, primary sclerosing cholangitis, ischemic cholangiopathy, drug-induced liver injury, and anastomotic biliary stricture, among others. As described, a salient feature of typical chronic rejection is the lack of ductular reaction, which is often not the case in other listed conditions. Additionally, chronic rejection typically shows no portal or periportal fibrosis, also in contrast with some of these conditions.

TREATMENT AND PROGNOSIS

If diagnosed early in its evolution, before the development of significant ductopenia, perivenular fibrosis, and obliterative arteriopathy, chronic rejection is potentially reversible with increases or changes in immunosuppression. Improved histology and resolution of liver function abnormalities can be seen in successfully treated patients. In contrast, advanced chronic rejection is usually unresponsive to increased immunosuppression and generally requires retransplantation. Thus, early detection and early therapeutic intervention provide the greatest chance for long-term preservation of allografts. However, although the histologic distinction between early and late chronic rejection can suggest the likelihood of reversibility, the severity of biopsy findings does not absolutely define

the transition between reversible and irreversible graft damage.[50,52] Correlation with clinical findings and serum biochemical markers is needed to determine the need for retransplantation.

ANTIBODY-MEDIATED REJECTION (HUMORAL REJECTION)

CLINICAL AND LABORATORY ASPECTS

AMR is mediated by either preformed or de novo DSAs that primarily target antigens on donor endothelial cells to cause graft dysfunction. The cascade includes fixation and activation of complement, activation of the clotting and fibrinolytic systems, impaired blood flow, and subsequent tissue damage.[13] AMR can be hyperacute, acute, or chronic according to the timing of occurrence.

Hyperacute AMR is exceedingly rare in modern transplantation medicine. It occurs in ABO-incompatible transplants within hours to days after an initial short period of normal reperfusion and bile production. It is characterized by a rapid increase in the serum liver enzyme and bilirubin levels, coagulopathy, thrombocytopenia, hypocomplementemia, and other signs of acute liver failure.[13] Acute AMR presents with varying degrees of graft dysfunction in ABO-compatible

Table 4
Banff criteria for the diagnosis of acute AMR

Definite for acute AMR (all 4 criteria required)	Scoring criteria
1. Histopathologic pattern of injury consistent with acute AMR, usually including the following: portal microvascular endothelial cell hypertrophy, portal capillary and inlet venule dilatation, monocytic, eosinophilic, and neutrophilic portal microvasculitis, portal edema, ductular reaction; cholestasis is usually present, but variable; edema and periportal hepatocyte necrosis are more common/prominent in ABO-incompatible allografts; variable active lymphocytic and/or necrotizing arteritis 2. Positive serum DSA 3. Diffuse (C4d score = 3) microvascular C4d deposition on frozen or formalin-fixed, paraffin-embedded tissue in ABO-compatible tissues or portal stromal C4d deposition in ABO-incompatible allografts 4. Reasonable exclusion of other insults that might cause a similar pattern of injury	h—(histopathology) score[a] 1. Portal microvascular endothelial cell enlargement (portal veins, capillaries, and inlet venules) involving a majority of portal tracts with sparse microvasculitis defined as 3–4 marginated and/or intraluminal monocytes, neutrophils, or eosinophils in the maximally involved capillary with generally mild dilation 2. Monocytic, eosinophilic, or neutrophilic microvasculitis/capillaritis, defined as $\geq$5–10 leukocytes marginated and/or intraluminal in the maximally involved capillary, prominent portal and/or sinusoidal microvascular endothelial cell enlargement involving a majority of portal tracts or sinusoids, with variable but noticeable portal capillary and inlet venule dilatation and variable portal edema 3. As above, with marked capillary dilatation, marked microvascular inflammation ($\geq$10 marginated and/or intraluminal leukocytes in the most severely affected vessels), at least focal microvascular disruption with fibrin deposition, and extravasation of red blood cells into the portal stroma and/or space of Disse (subsinusoidal space) C4d—(immune) score[b] 1. No C4d deposition in portal microvasculature 2. Minimal (<10% portal tracts) C4d deposition in >50% of the circumference of portal microvascular endothelia (portal veins and capillaries) 3. Focal (10%–50% portal tracts) C4d deposition in >50% of the circumference of portal microvascular endothelia (portal veins and capillaries), usually without extension into periportal sinusoids 4. Diffuse (>50% portal tracts) C4d deposition in >50% of the circumference of portal microvascular endothelia (portal veins and capillaries), often with extension into inlet venules or periportal sinusoids Most definite cases will have a C4d-score of 3, and a total score (with h-score) of 5 or 6

Suspicious for AMR (both criteria required)
1. DSA is positive
2. Nonzero h-score with C4d-score + h-score = 3 or 4
Indeterminate for AMR (requires 1 + 2 and 3 or 4)
1. C4d-score + h-score $\geq$2
2. DSA not available, equivocal, or negative
3. C4d staining not available, equivocal, or negative
4. Coexisting insult might be contributing to the injury

Abbreviations: AMR, antibody-mediated rejection; DSA, donor-specific antibody.
[a] Other features commonly seen but not necessarily associated with severity of rejection include ductular reaction and cholestasis.
[b] Immunohistochemistry on formalin-fixed, paraffin-embedded tissue.

transplants and is mediated by lymphocytotoxic antibodies against class I and class II major histocompatibility complex antigens. It also occurs in the setting of ABO-incompatible living donor transplantation treated with B-cell–directed immunosuppression. It is usually seen in the first several weeks after transplantation, but a late onset (>6 months) can occur. Chronic AMR in the setting of liver transplantation is an emerging concept that remains poorly defined. It seems to occur in patients who are suboptimally immunosuppressed with persistent DSAs, but usually with only mild to no signs of clinical or biochemical graft dysfunction.[10,56,57]

HISTOLOGIC FEATURES

The histologic findings of hyperacute AMR vary with the time of tissue examination after revascularization and may be modified by perioperative therapeutic interventions. It is typically characterized by patchy or massive hemorrhagic hepatic necrosis with fibrin thrombi in portal and central veins, sinusoidal congestion and fibrin deposition, endothelial cell swelling and neutrophil infiltration. Portal tracts may show edema, hemorrhage, ductular reaction, and neutrophilic infiltrates. Fibrinoid or neutrophilic arteritis may be seen.[10,13,58]

The histologic features of acute AMR are not as well-defined as those of TCMR. The recently published Banff criteria for the diagnosis of acute AMR (**Table 4**) emphasize the effects of microvascular injury.[10] These mainly include portal capillary and venular dilatation, endothelial cell hypertrophy and microvasculitis. Microvasculitis is characterized by the presence of marginated and/or intraluminal monocytes, eosinophils or neutrophils in dilated portal capillaries and the severity is scored by the number of inflammatory cells as 1 (3–4 cells), 2 (5–10), or 3 (>10). Varying degrees of portal edema, ductular reaction, centrilobular hepatocyte ballooning, spotty necrosis, and cholestasis may be present.

Chronic AMR lacks specific histologic features as outlined by the Banff Working Group document (**Box 4**). Most described findings that are potentially associated with chronic AMR are observed in protocol biopsies from patients who are clinically and biochemically doing well. The most common findings are low-grade portal and/or perivenular mononuclear cell inflammation and progressive portal, periportal, perisinusoidal, and/or perivenular fibrosis.[10,59]

There is increasing evidence to suggest that AMR may frequently overlap with typical TCMR. In that setting, the recipients tend to be less responsive to conventional immunosuppression and more likely to be steroid resistant, which increases the risk of progression to chronic rejection.[10,58] Some unusual forms of rejection discussed, such as plasma cell-rich rejection, central perivenulitis and idiopathic posttransplant hepatitis, may also serve as good examples of mixed TCMR and AMR.

C4D IMMUNOHISTOCHEMISTRY

The immunohistochemical detection of C4d, a marker of tissue-based complement activation, is now considered an integral component in the Banff criteria for the diagnosis of AMR (see **Box 4, Table 4**).[10] Linear or granular staining on endothelial cells lining the portal veins and capillaries, and less commonly the sinusoids, seems to be most useful to facilitate the diagnosis of

---

Box 4
Banff criteria for the diagnosis of chronic AMR

Probable chronic AMR (all 4 criteria required)

1. Histopathologic pattern of injury consistent with chronic AMR (both are required)

   a. Otherwise unexplained and at least mild mononuclear portal and/or perivenular inflammation with interface and/or perivenular necroinflammatory activity

   b. At least moderate portal/periportal, sinusoidal and/or perivenular fibrosis

2. Recent (eg, measured within 3 months of biopsy) circulating HLA DSA in serum samples

3. At least focal C4d-positive (>10% portal tract microvascular endothelia)

4. Reasonable exclusion of other insults that might cause a similar pattern of injury

Possible chronic AMR

1. As above, but C4d staining is minimal or absent

Abbreviations: AMR, antibody-mediated rejection; DSA, donor-specific antibody; HLA, human leukocyte antigen.

Fig. 8. (A) An allograft biopsy showing focal microvasculitis (*arrow*) suggestive of acute antibody-mediated rejection (AMR). However, ductular reaction with scattered neutrophils is also evident, suggestive of biliary obstruction (original magnification ×400). No evidence of biliary obstruction was demonstrated by radiographic studies, however. (B) Positive C4d immunostaining is evident in portal veins (*shorter arrow*) and capillaries (*longer arrows*) in nearly every portal tract in this biopsy (original magnification ×400). Donor-specific antibodies were also positive in this case, confirming the diagnosis of acute AMR.

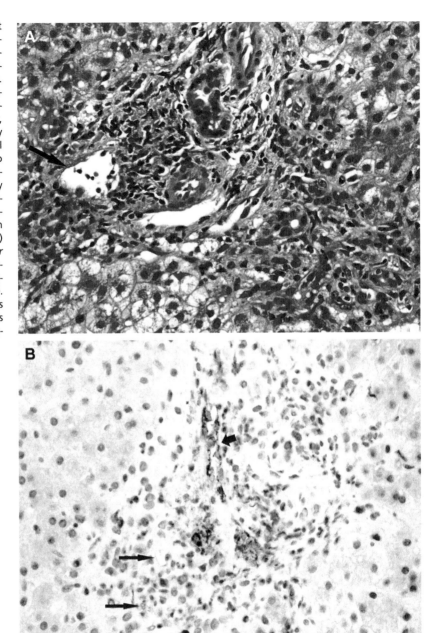

acute AMR. According to the Banff criteria, the staining on portal veins and capillaries should involve more than 50% of the luminal circumference of the vessels to be considered positive. Diffuse positivity, defined as greater than 50% portal tracts, seems to have the greatest diagnostic value. Positive C4d staining can also be detected in portal stroma, which may be more likely to be associated with acute AMR in ABO-incompatible transplants, TCMR, and chronic rejection.

It is clear that the diagnostic value of C4d immunostaining requires further investigation. There are occasional cases where C4d staining is convincingly positive and yet there are no DSAs. Positive C4d staining has been observed in allografts with recurrent HCV, AIH, and PBC, as well as cholangitis and biliary obstruction, albeit with less intensity and fewer frequencies.[13] In addition, high background C4d staining in hepatocytes and/or portal stroma can make interpretation of the staining challenging. Nevertheless, although positive C4d staining in isolation likely has little or no diagnostic value, especially if present focally, the detection of unequivocal diffusely positive C4d staining should raise the concern for AMR and should prompt DSA testing if not already performed.

DIFFERENTIAL DIAGNOSIS

Hyperacute AMR may need to be differentiated from primary nonfunction, vascular thrombosis, severe hypotension, and sepsis. The main differential diagnostic considerations for acute AMR include preservation injury, biliary obstruction, and fibrosing cholestatic hepatitis. However, the differential diagnosis for acute and chronic AMR can be difficult because of a lack of pathognomonic histologic features. The proposed features of microvascular injury for acute AMR, such as capillary dilatation, endothelial cell hypertrophy, and microvasculitis, can be easily overlooked, difficult to reproducibly recognize, and lack specificity. The lack of correlation of C4d immunostaining with DSA status in some cases also limits its usefulness as an ancillary tool in differential diagnosis.

The possibility of acute or chronic AMR should be considered if the histologic findings in an allograft biopsy cannot be explained adequately by an identifiable etiology. For example, if a biopsy shows features suggestive of biliary obstruction, such as portal edema and ductular reaction with neutrophils (**Fig. 8**A), but the diagnosis is ruled out by additional clinical and radiographic studies, C4d immunostaining can be performed (**Fig. 8**B). If positive, DSA testing should be recommended to further investigate the possibility of AMR. Cases showing features of TCMR that are refractory to treatment is another scenario where the possibility of overlapping AMR should be entertained.

Fibrosing cholestatic hepatitis demonstrates hepatocyte swelling with lobular disarray, cholestasis, ductular reaction, and periportal fibrosis,[60,61] and these features overlap somewhat with acute AMR. The presence of a high serum HCV load will lead to the correct diagnosis. Fortunately, with recent successful anti-HCV therapies, fibrosing cholestatic hepatitis has become a rare occurrence.[62]

TREATMENT AND PROGNOSIS

No standardized treatment protocols exist for acute AMR, but early intervention with plasmapheresis, intravenous immunoglobulin, and anti–B-cell agents (such as rituximab) are generally used for moderate to severe AMR. For chronic AMR, compliance with standard tacrolimus-based maintenance immunosuppression seems to be critical for its prevention and possibly treatment.[63] If unrecognized or undertreated, acute AMR may lead to early graft loss whereas chronic AMR results in progressive fibrosis, necessitating retransplantation.[64]

REFERENCES

1. Kohli R, Cortes M, Heaton ND, et al. Liver transplantation in children: state of the art and future perspectives. Arch Dis Child 2018;103(2):192–8.
2. Jadlowiec CC, Taner T. Liver transplantation: current status and challenges. World J Gastroenterol 2016; 22:4438–45.
3. Karam S, Wali RK. Current state of immunosuppression: past, present, and future. Crit Rev Eukaryot Gene Expr 2015;25:113–34.
4. Adams DH, Sanchez-Fueyo A, Samuel D. From immunosuppression to tolerance. J Hepatol 2015; 62(1 Suppl):S170–85.
5. Dhanasekaran R. Management of immunosuppression in liver transplantation. Clin Liver Dis 2017;21: 337–53.
6. Crippin JS. Approach to the liver transplant recipient: maintenance of allograft function. In: Liapis H, Wang HL, editors. Pathology of solid organ transplantation. Berlin: Springer; 2011. p. 212–22.
7. Fairfield C, Penninga L, Powell J, et al. Glucocorticosteroid-free versus glucocorticosteroid-containing immunosuppression for liver transplanted patients. Cochrane Database Syst Rev 2015;(12). CD007606.
8. Clavien PA, Muller X, de Oliveira ML, et al. Can immunosuppression be stopped after liver transplantation? Lancet Gastroenterol Hepatol 2017;2: 531–7.
9. Banff Working Group on Liver Allograft Pathology. Importance of liver biopsy findings in immunosuppression management: biopsy monitoring and working criteria for patients with operational tolerance. Liver Transpl 2012;18:1154–70.
10. Demetris AJ, Bellamy C, Hübscher SG, et al. 2016 Comprehensive update of the Banff Working Group on Liver Allograft Pathology: introduction of antibody-mediated rejection. Am J Transplant 2016;16:2816–35.
11. Shaked A, Ghobrial RM, Merion RM, et al. Incidence and severity of acute cellular rejection in recipients undergoing adult living donor or deceased donor liver transplantation. Am J Transplant 2009;9: 301–8.
12. Górnicka B, Ziarkiewicz-Wróblewska B, Bogdańska M, et al. Pathomorphological features of acute rejection in patients after orthotopic liver transplantation: own experience. Transplant Proc 2006;38:221–5.

13. Wang HL. Rejection. In: Liapis H, Wang HL, editors. Pathology of solid organ transplantation. Berlin: Springer; 2011. p. 244–62.

14. Anonymous. Banff schema for grading liver allograft rejection: an international consensus document. Hepatology 1997;25:658–63.

15. Kishi Y, Sugawara Y, Tamura S, et al. Histologic eosinophilia as an aid to diagnose acute cellular rejection after living donor liver transplantation. Clin Transplant 2007;21:214–8.

16. Demirhan B, Bilezikçi B, Haberal AN, et al. Hepatic parenchymal changes and histologic eosinophilia as predictors of subsequent acute liver allograft rejection. Liver Transpl 2008;14:214–9.

17. Tarantino G, Cabibi D, Cammà C, et al. Liver eosinophilic infiltrate is a significant finding in patients with chronic hepatitis C. J Viral Hepat 2008;15:523–30.

18. Nacif LS, Pinheiro RS, Pécora RA, et al. Late acute rejection in liver transplant: a systematic review. Arq Bras Cir Dig 2015;28:212–5.

19. Ramji A, Yoshida EM, Bain VG, et al. Late acute rejection after liver transplantation: the Western Canada experience. Liver Transpl 2002;8:945–51.

20. Uemura T, Ikegami T, Sanchez EQ, et al. Late acute rejection after liver transplantation impacts patient survival. Clin Transplant 2008;22:316–23.

21. Thurairajah PH, Carbone M, Bridgestock H, et al. Late acute liver allograft rejection; a study of its natural history and graft survival in the current era. Transplantation 2013;95:955–9.

22. Hübscher SG. Central perivenulitis: a common and potentially important finding in late posttransplant liver biopsies. Liver Transpl 2008;14:596–600.

23. Demetris AJ, Adeyi O, Bellamy CO, et al. Liver biopsy interpretation for causes of late liver allograft dysfunction. Hepatology 2006;44:489–501.

24. Khettry U, Backer A, Ayata G, et al. Centrilobular histopathologic changes in liver transplant biopsies. Hum Pathol 2002;33:270–6.

25. Hassoun Z, Shah V, Lohse CM, et al. Centrilobular necrosis after orthotopic liver transplantation: association with acute cellular rejection and impact on outcome. Liver Transpl 2004;10:480–7.

26. Abraham SC, Freese DK, Ishitani MB, et al. Significance of central perivenulitis in pediatric liver transplantation. Am J Surg Pathol 2008;32:1479–88.

27. Krasinskas AM, Demetris AJ, Poterucha JJ, et al. The prevalence and natural history of untreated isolated central perivenulitis in adult allograft livers. Liver Transpl 2008;14:625–32.

28. Demetris AJ. Central venulitis in liver allografts: considerations of differential diagnosis. Hepatology 2001;33:1329–30.

29. Lovell MO, Speeg KV, Halff GA, et al. Acute hepatic allograft rejection: a comparison of patients with and without centrilobular alterations during first rejection episode. Liver Transpl 2004;10:369–73.

30. Kerkar N, Yanni G. 'De novo' and 'recurrent' autoimmune hepatitis after liver transplantation: a comprehensive review. J Autoimmun 2016;66:17–24.

31. Fiel MI, Agarwal K, Stanca C, et al. Posttransplant plasma cell hepatitis (de novo autoimmune hepatitis) is a variant of rejection and may lead to a negative outcome in patients with hepatitis C virus. Liver Transpl 2008;14:861–71.

32. Fiel MI, Schiano TD. Plasma cell hepatitis (de-novo autoimmune hepatitis) developing post liver transplantation. Curr Opin Organ Transplant 2012;17: 287–92.

33. Wozniak LJ, Hickey MJ, Venick RS, et al. Donor-specific HLA antibodies are associated with late allograft dysfunction after pediatric liver transplantation. Transplantation 2015;99:1416–22.

34. Salcedo M, Rodriguez-Mahou M, Rodriguez-Sainz C, et al. Risk factors for developing de novo autoimmune hepatitis associated with anti-glutathione S-transferase T1 antibodies after liver transplantation. Liver Transpl 2009;15:530–9.

35. Khettry U, Huang WY, Simpson MA, et al. Patterns of recurrent hepatitis C after liver transplantation in a recent cohort of patients. Hum Pathol 2007;38:443–52.

36. Sawada T, Shimizu A, Kubota K, et al. Lobular damage caused by cellular and humoral immunity in liver allograft rejection. Clin Transplant 2005;19:110–4.

37. Quaglia AF, Del Vecchio Blanco G, Greaves R, et al. Development of ductopaenic liver allograft rejection includes a "hepatitic" phase prior to duct loss. J Hepatol 2000;33:773–80.

38. Shi Y, Dong K, Zhang YG, et al. Sinusoidal endotheliitis as a histological parameter for diagnosing acute liver allograft rejection. World J Gastroenterol 2017; 23:792–9.

39. Siddiqui I, Selzner N, Hafezi-Bakhtiari S, et al. Infiltrative (sinusoidal) and hepatitic patterns of injury in acute cellular rejection in liver allograft with clinical implications. Mod Pathol 2015;28:1275–81.

40. Kelly D, Verkade HJ, Rajanayagam J, et al. Late graft hepatitis and fibrosis in pediatric liver allograft recipients: current concepts and future developments. Liver Transpl 2016;22:1593–602.

41. Syn WK, Nightingale P, Gunson B, et al. Natural history of unexplained chronic hepatitis after liver transplantation. Liver Transpl 2007;13:984–9.

42. Miyagawa-Hayashino A, Yoshizawa A, Uchida Y, et al. Progressive graft fibrosis and donor-specific human leukocyte antigen antibodies in pediatric late liver allografts. Liver Transpl 2012;18:1333–42.

43. Suh N, Liapis H, Misdraji J, et al. Epstein-Barr virus hepatitis: diagnostic value of in situ hybridization, polymerase chain reaction, and immunohistochemistry on liver biopsy from immunocompetent patients. Am J Surg Pathol 2007;31:1403–9.

44. Mazzola A, Tran Minh M, Charlotte F, et al. Chronic hepatitis E viral infection after liver transplantation:

a regression of fibrosis after antiviral therapy. Transplantation 2017;101:2083–7.

45. Unzueta A, Rakela J. Hepatitis E infection in liver transplant recipients. Liver Transpl 2014;20:15–24.

46. Wang Y, Metselaar HJ, Peppelenbosch MP, et al. Chronic hepatitis E in solid-organ transplantation: the key implications of immunosuppressants. Curr Opin Infect Dis 2014;27:303–8.

47. Kamar N, Selves J, Mansuy JM, et al. Hepatitis E virus and chronic hepatitis in organ-transplant recipients. N Engl J Med 2008;358:811–7.

48. Buyse S, Roque-Afonso AM, Vaghefi P, et al. Acute hepatitis with periportal confluent necrosis associated with human herpesvirus 6 infection in liver transplant patients. Am J Clin Pathol 2013;140: 403–9.

49. Hill JA, Myerson D, Sedlak RH, et al. Hepatitis due to human herpesvirus 6B after hematopoietic cell transplantation and a review of the literature. Transpl Infect Dis 2014;16:477–83.

50. Neil DA, Hubscher SG. Histologic and biochemical changes during the evolution of chronic rejection of liver allografts. Hepatology 2002;35: 639–51.

51. Nakanuma Y, Tsuneyama K, Harada K. Pathology and pathogenesis of intrahepatic bile duct loss. J Hepatobiliary Pancreat Surg 2001;8:303–15.

52. Demetris A, Adams D, Bellamy C, et al. Update of the International Banff Schema for liver allograft rejection: working recommendations for the histopathologic staging and reporting of chronic rejection. An International panel. Hepatology 2000;31: 792–9.

53. Herman HK, Abramowsky CR, Caltharp S, et al. Identification of bile duct paucity in Alagille syndrome: using CK7 and EMA immunohistochemistry as a reliable panel for accurate diagnosis. Pediatr Dev Pathol 2016;19:47–50.

54. International Working Party. Terminology for hepatic allograft rejection. Hepatology 1995;22:648–54.

55. Demetris AJ, Seaberg EC, Batts KP, et al. Chronic liver allograft rejection: a National Institute of Diabetes and Digestive and Kidney Diseases Inter-institutional study analyzing the reliability of current criteria and proposal of an expanded definition. National Institute of Diabetes and Digestive and Kidney Diseases Liver Transplantation Database. Am J Surg Pathol 1998;22:28–39.

56. Del Bello A, Congy-Jolivet N, Muscari F, et al. Prevalence, incidence and risk factors for donor-specific anti-HLA antibodies in maintenance liver transplant patients. Am J Transplant 2014;14:867–75.

57. O'Leary JG, Cai J, Freeman R, et al. Proposed diagnostic criteria for chronic antibody-mediated rejection in liver allografts. Am J Transplant 2016;16: 603–14.

58. Hübscher SG. Antibody-mediated rejection in the liver allograft. Curr Opin Organ Transplant 2012;17: 280–6.

59. Kim PT, Demetris AJ, O'Leary JG. Prevention and treatment of liver allograft antibody-mediated rejection and the role of the 'two-hit hypothesis'. Curr Opin Organ Transplant 2016;21:209–18.

60. Verna EC, Abdelmessih R, Salomao MA, et al. Cholestatic hepatitis C following liver transplantation: an outcome-based histological definition, clinical predictors, and prognosis. Liver Transpl 2013; 19:78–88.

61. Salomao M, Verna EC, Lefkowitch JH, et al. Histopathologic distinction between fibrosing cholestatic hepatitis C and biliary obstruction. Am J Surg Pathol 2013;37:1837–44.

62. Vukotic R, Conti F, Fagiuoli S, et al. Long-term outcomes of direct acting antivirals in post-transplant advanced hepatitis C virus recurrence and fibrosing cholestatic hepatitis. J Viral Hepat 2017;24:858–64.

63. O'Leary JG, Samaniego M, Barrio MC, et al. The influence of immunosuppressive agents on the risk of de novo donor-specific HLA antibody production in solid organ transplant recipients. Transplantation 2016;100:39–53.

64. Hogen R, DiNorcia J, Dhanireddy K. Antibody-mediated rejection: what is the clinical relevance? Curr Opin Organ Transplant 2017;22:97–104.

Frozen Sections of the Liver

Meredith E. Pittman, MD, MSCI*, Rhonda K. Yantiss, MD

KEYWORDS

- Liver biopsy • Frozen section • Donor evaluation • Metastatic carcinoma

Key points

- Subcapsular benign biliary proliferations display an even distribution of glands in variably cellular collagenous stroma without significant nuclear atypica or infiltration of adjacent hepatic parenchyma.
- Metastatic adenocarcinoma is characterized by haphazardly arranged glands, fibroinflammatory stroma, nuclear hyperchromasia, size variability, and infiltration of normal hepatic structures, including sinusoids and portal tracts.
- Knowledge of the clinical history is often critical to the correct classification of tumors that features epithelioid cells with eosinophilic cytoplasm.
- Steatosis, fibrosis, inflammation, and necrosis should be documented and quantified when evaluating the suitability of donor liver for transplantation.

ABSTRACT

Intraoperative consultation requires skills in gross examination and histologic diagnosis, as well as an ability to perform rapid interpretations under time constraints. The aim of this review is to provide surgical pathologists with a framework for dealing with hepatic specimens in the frozen section area by covering common clinical scenarios and histologic findings. Differential diagnoses are considered in relation to primary hepatic neoplasia and metastatic diseases. Benign mimics of malignancy and other pitfalls in frozen section diagnosis of lesional tissue are covered. Finally, assessment of donor liver biopsy for organ transplant evaluation is discussed.

OVERVIEW

Despite advances in cross-sectional imaging techniques, intraoperative frozen sections still play an important role in the immediate management of surgical patients. Most frozen sections performed on the liver are intended to evaluate margins for tumors in partial resection specimens or to assess for hepatic metastases in oncology patients undergoing potentially curative resection of a primary tumor, although frozen sections are also used to determine the suitability of potential donor livers. The purpose of this review is to provide the practicing pathologist with an overview of common issues encountered during frozen section of liver samples, which are organized according to the clinical scenarios in which they are likely to be encountered.

SURGICAL RESECTION OF ADENOCARCINOMA

COLORECTAL CANCER METASTASES

Hepatic metastases are far more common than primary tumors among noncirrhotic patients.[1] Although hepatic metastases were historically treated in a palliative manner, patients with some types of cancer, particularly colorectal cancer, may benefit from surgical resection of isolated hepatic metastases.[2–4] In fact, targeted chemotherapeutic agents in combination with ablative techniques and high-resolution

Disclosure Statement: The authors have no financial relationships to disclose.
Department of Pathology and Laboratory Medicine, Weill Cornell Medicine, 525 East 68th Street, Starr 10, New York, NY 10065, USA
* Corresponding author.
E-mail address: mep9071@med.cornell.edu

Surgical Pathology 11 (2018) 453–466
https://doi.org/10.1016/j.path.2018.02.012

imaging have improved surgical management to the point that 5-year survival rates approach 60% among selected patients.[5]

Intraoperative consultation begins with careful gross inspection and identification of vascular and biliary margins, if present. The cauterized parenchymal margin is readily identified and should be assessed for the possibility of visible tumor before the application of ink. Palpation facilitates localization of the mass, and perpendicular sections demonstrating the relationship between the tumor and resection margin can be used to determine the adequacy of resection (**Fig. 1**A). Most surgeons are satisfied with a gross assessment of the distance between the tumor and margin, provided that distance is greater than 0.5 cm. Frozen sections performed on close margins are best assessed with thin perpendicular sections documenting the tumor and margin the same section. Negative resection margins are associated with improved survival.[6,7]

INTRAHEPATIC CHOLANGIOCARCINOMA

Although intrahepatic cholangiocarcinoma is the second most common primary liver tumor, it remains a rare malignancy. Currently, surgical resection is the only treatment modality that offers curative intent for this malignancy, yet the postoperative 5-year survival remains less than 50%.[8] As was described for colorectal metastatic disease, resection specimens for intrahepatic cholangiocarcinoma should first be palpated, inked, and sectioned perpendicular to the margin so that the mass can be demonstrated in relation to the inked margin (**Fig. 1**B). Because intrahepatic cholangiocarcinoma may have an infiltrating growth pattern along sinusoids and portal tracts, care should be

taken to identify irregular glands or cytologically atypical cells at the parenchymal, vascular, and biliary margins, where applicable. The histologic appearance of intrahepatic cholangiocarcinoma is discussed in more detail in the section on primary hepatic tumors.

Distinguishing Adenocarcinoma from Primary Hepatic Bile Duct Lesions

Surgeons may request intraoperative consults to evaluate small (<1 cm) nodules that are discovered at laparotomy, particularly when resecting primary adenocarcinomas of the pancreas, extrahepatic bile ducts, gallbladder, esophagus, and stomach. In this situation, the classification of hepatic lesions directly affects immediate patient management. If the hepatic nodule is classified as metastatic carcinoma, then the operative procedure is aborted, whereas a benign diagnosis is usually followed by surgical resection of the primary tumor. The differential diagnosis of metastatic adenocarcinoma includes 3 benign entities: bile duct hamartoma, bile duct adenoma, and ductular reactions that develop as a result of an obstructing mass in the head of the pancreas (**Table1**).

Clues to a diagnosis of adenocarcinoma are best appreciated at low magnification. Adenocarcinomas are expansile nodules composed of irregularly distributed, angulated glands embedded in fibroinflammatory (desmoplastic) stroma (**Fig. 2**A, B). They tend to overrun preexisting benign elements, including portal tracts, and display an irregular interface with adjacent hepatic parenchyma (**Fig. 2**C, D). Glands vary in size and shape. They may contain mucin, but are usually unassociated with luminal bile, reflecting a lack of communication with the biliary tract. Malignant glands contain

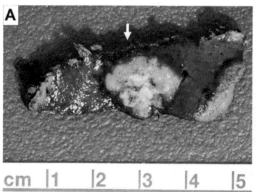 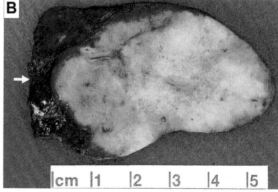

Fig. 1. (*A*) The parenchymal margin is inked (*arrow*) and the specimen is sectioned to evaluate the distance from the tumor to the inked margin. Colorectal carcinoma metastases are white, lobulated, and show variable necrosis. (*B*) An intrahepatic cholangiocarcinoma is close to the inked resection margin (*arrow*); it has a firm, homogeneous white cut surface.

Table 1
Features that distinguish between benign bile duct proliferations and metastatic adenocarcinoma

Feature	Bile Duct Hamartoma	Bile Duct Adenoma	Biliary Ductular Reaction	Metastatic Adenocarcinoma
Anatomic location	Subcapsular	Subcapsular	Variable	Variable
Size	<1 cm	<1 cm	Variable	Variable
Tumor centricity	Solitary or multiple	Solitary or multiple	Usually multiple	Usually multiple
Quality of stroma	Densely collagenous	Cellular	Edematous	Desmoplastic
Appearance	Circumscribed	Circumscribed	Ill-defined	Ill-defined
Intralesional portal tracts	Common	Common	Common	Present at lesional edge
Organization of epithelium	Uniformly spaced, variably dilated tubules	Uniformly spaced, small round tubules	Irregularly spaced, variably dilated tubules	Irregular aggregates of variably sized glands
Luminal mucin	Absent	May be present	Absent	Present
Bile	May be present	Absent	May be present	Absent
Cytologic atypia	Absent	Minimal	Minimal	Present
Mitotic figures	Absent	Absent	Absent	Present

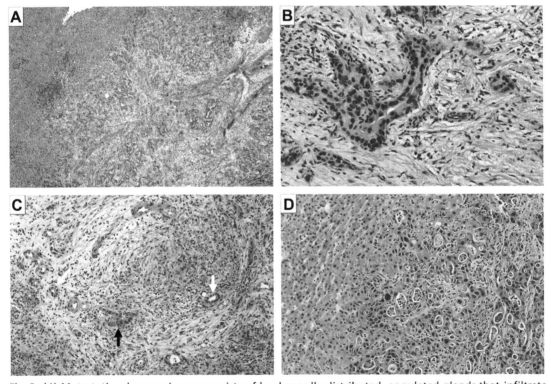

Fig. 2. (*A*) Metastatic adenocarcinoma consists of haphazardly distributed, angulated glands that infiltrate adjacent hepatic parenchyma (stain: hematoxylin and eosin [H&E]; original magnification ×40). (*B*) Tumor cells show nuclear enlargement, hyperchromasia, and variability; irregularly shaped glands are embedded in dense fibrotic stroma (stain: H&E, original magnification ×400). (*C*) Metastatic adenocarcinoma can infiltrate normal hepatic structures, including portal tracts and sinusoids. Nonneoplastic glands (*white arrows*) are in close proximity to arteries and contain uniform nuclei, whereas a malignant gland (*black arrow*) is angulated and contains large, atypical nuclei (stain: H&E; original magnification ×100). (*D*) Metastatic adenocarcinoma infiltrates hepatic parenchyma, which is not a feature of benign mimics (stain: H&E; original magnification ×100).

highly variable and enlarged nuclei that are often at least 4 times the size of nonneoplastic ductal epithelial cells. Foamy, vacuolated cytoplasm, necrosis, and mitotic activity are also features of malignancy.

> ### Key Features
> #### ADENOCARCINOMA
>
> 1. Adenocarcinomas appear as expansile nodules with ill-defined borders and irregularly distributed glands in fibroinflammatory stroma.
> 2. Cancers contain haphazardly arranged glands, some of which may be incompletely formed, that infiltrate between hepatocytes.
> 3. Tumor cells show nuclear variability and nucleomegaly; tumor cell nuclei may be 4 times that of a benign biliary epithelial cell.

BILE DUCT HAMARTOMA

Bile duct hamartomas (von Meyenburg complex) are developmental anomalies associated with ductal plate malformations. They are often multiple and can be mistaken for metastatic seeding by a primary malignancy.[9] Bile duct hamartomas contain lobules of ectatic, angulated, and branched ductules that are evenly distributed in densely collagenous stroma (**Fig. 3**A). Epithelial cells are flat and monomorphic with bland, basally oriented nuclei and attenuated, eosinophilic cytoplasm; mitotic figures are conspicuously absent (**Fig. 3**B). Bile duct hamartomas communicate with nonlesional bile ducts and, thus, often contain inspissated bile that can be a helpful diagnostic clue (**Fig. 3**C). Dense regular collagen separates lesional epithelium from adjacent hepatic parenchyma (**Fig. 3**D).

Metastatic adenocarcinomas occasionally contain dilated glands that superficially resemble bile duct hamartomas. However, such cases generally show a greater degree of architectural complexity with fused, anastomosing glands and fibroinflammatory or desmoplastic stroma (**Fig. 3**E). Cancer cells show a greater degree of cytologic atypia with cell-to-cell variability, conspicuous nucleoli, and luminal mucin (**Fig. 3**F). They also contain more voluminous cytoplasm, which can be mucinous.

BILE DUCT ADENOMA (PERIBILIARY GLAND HAMARTOMA)

Bile duct adenomas are wedge-shaped or circumscribed yellow nodules that are usually solitary and located just under the capsule (**Fig. 4**A). They are more cellular than bile duct hamartomas and often contain a central, uninvolved portal tract without infiltration by lesional elements (**Fig. 4**B). Small, minimally dilated ductules are evenly distributed in variably inflamed fibrotic stroma, which is often associated with a peripheral cuff of lymphocyte-predominant inflammation (**Fig. 4**C). Lesional cells are cuboidal and contain eosinophilic cytoplasm with round, uniform nuclei and small, but conspicuous nucleoli (**Fig. 4**D). Mild nuclear enlargement may be present, but mitotic figures and cellular necrosis are lacking. Bile duct adenomas do not communicate with the biliary system and do not contain bile, but luminal mucin is often present. Similar to bile duct hamartomas, bile duct adenomas are distinct from the adjacent hepatic parenchyma; comingling of lesional epithelium and hepatocytes is not a feature.

Metastatic adenocarcinomas can appear as round or wedge-shaped nodules containing small glands that simulate bile duct adenoma. However, glands usually show a greater degree of architectural variability and may show fused growth or papillary infoldings, neither of which are typical of bile duct adenoma (**Fig. 4**E). They also infiltrate between hepatocyte cords at the advancing edge of the lesion and invade entrapped portal tracts (**Fig. 4**F).

BENIGN DUCTULAR REACTIONS ASSOCIATED WITH BILE DUCT OBSTRUCTION AND CHOLECYSTITIS

Obstructing cancers in the head of the pancreas, ampulla, or distal common bile duct can produce inflammatory changes with benign proliferating ducts in the liver, some of which may be large enough to be grossly apparent. Generally, these lesions contain a disproportionate amount of inflamed or edematous stroma than would be expected in a focus of metastatic adenocarcinoma. They may have an infiltrative appearance at low magnification owing to the presence of abundant inflammation, but proliferating ductules maintain a lobular architecture or appear as scattered linear arrays (**Fig. 5**A). They contain small, uniform nuclei with round contours, evenly dispersed chromatin, and small nucleoli (**Fig. 5**B).

Patients with cholecystitis can develop inflammatory changes in the adjacent liver that form an ill-defined mass or show increased radiolabeled tracer uptake on imaging.[10] Histologic sections of this inflammatory pseudotumor typically show xanthogranulomatous inflammation with

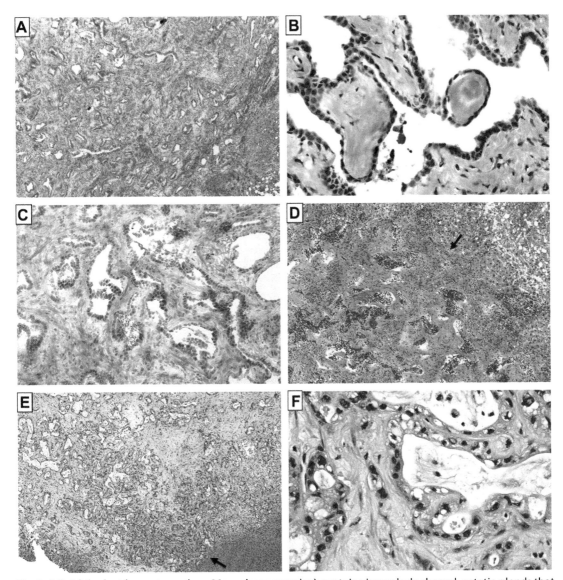

Fig. 3. (*A*) A bile duct hamartoma (von Meyenberg complex) contains irregularly shaped, ectatic glands that are evenly distributed in a dense, collagenous stroma (stain: hematoxylin and eosin [H&E]; original magnification ×40). (*B*) They contain cuboidal cells with eosinophilic cytoplasm and round, regular nuclei (stain H&E; original magnification ×200). (*C*) Bile duct hamartomas communicate with the biliary system and often contain bile (stain: H&E; original magnification ×100). (*D*) Artifactually "telescoped" glands seem to be hypercellular, although the even distribution of branched glands in dense collagenous stroma, and clear demarcation from hepatic parenchyma (*black arrow*) suggest a benign diagnosis (stain: H&E; original magnification ×40). (*E*) Metastatic adenocarcinoma can show gland dilation that simulates bile duct hamartoma. This nodule, however, contains a haphazard mixture of small and large glands embedded in cellular stroma and infiltrating adjacent hepatic parenchyma (*black arrow*; stain: H&E; original magnification ×40). (*F*) Cytologic features are more atypical than should be seen in a bile duct hamartoma: nuclear variability, nuclear overlap, and foamy cytoplasm (stain: H&E; original magnification ×200).

proliferative spindle cells, macrophages, and multinucleated giant cells associated with bile pigment and accompanying entrapped ducts (**Fig. 5**C). Although the presence of ducts in the setting of a mass rightly raises concern for adenocarcinoma, accessory biliary ducts, or ducts of Luschka, grow along the gallbladder fossa, and represent a normal variant of gallbladder

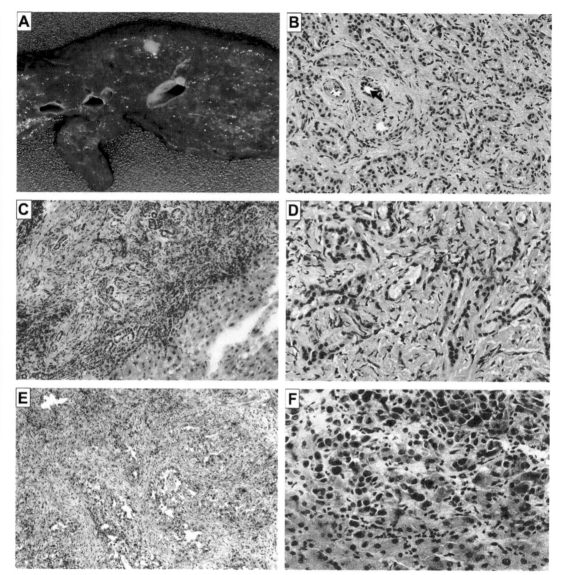

Fig. 4. (*A*) Bile duct adenomas are solitary, well-circumscribed, and white to pale yellow lesions. (*B*) They consist of small glands that proliferate around a normal portal tract (*black arrow*). The glands are singly dispersed or fused, and the background stroma is slightly more cellular than that of a bile duct hamartoma (stain: hematoxylin and eosin [H&E]; original magnification ×200). (*C*) Chronic inflammation is often prominent at the periphery of the lesion, which is clearly demarcated from the adjacent hepatic parenchyma (stain: H&E; original magnification ×100). (*D*) Cells are flat to cuboidal with eosinophilic cytoplasm and round nuclei; luminal mucin may be present, but inspissated bile is not seen (stain: H&E; original magnification ×200). (*E*) Adenocarcinoma may contain small glands that mimic bile duct adenoma, but they usually show complex glandular structures with papillary projections and cribriform growth. Nucleomegaly and hyperchromasia are evident at low magnification (stain: H&E; original magnification ×100). (*F*) Malignant cells insinuate between hepatocytes; this feature is never seen in bile duct adenomas.

anatomy.[11] Clues to the benign nature of these ducts include a linear arrangement or lobular configuration of the ducts with concentric fibroblasts that highlight the underlying architecture (**Fig. 5**D). Ductal epithelial cells are cuboidal to columnar with eosinophilic cytoplasm and small, uniform nuclei. Reactive epithelial atypia may be present secondary to inflammation, but nuclear abnormalities are mild and unassociated with mitotic activity or necrosis.

SURGICAL RESECTION OF PRIMARY HEPATIC TUMORS

> ### Key Points
> #### HEPATOCELLULAR NEOPLASIA
>
> 1. Hepatocellular neoplasms lack normal architectural features, often showing loss of identifiable portal tracts and central veins with expanded hepatocellular plates and indistinct sinusoids.
>
> 2. Hepatocellular neoplasms often contain increased fat, bile, or Mallory's hyaline compared with nonlesional liver.
>
> 3. Distinguishing adenoma from carcinoma is unnecessary at the time of frozen section because both types of lesion will be similarly treated at the time of the procedure.

> ### Key Points
> #### METASTATIC MIMICS OF HEPATOCELLULAR NEOPLASIA
>
> 1. Several types of metastatic tumors can contain cells with oncocytic cytoplasm that mimic primary hepatocellular neoplasms.
>
> 2. Metastases are the most common malignant tumors of the liver; knowledge of the clinical history is key, especially among patients without chronic liver disease.
>
> 3. Common pink cell tumors that mimic hepatocellular carcinoma include renal cell carcinoma, adrenal cortical carcinoma, (neuro)endocrine tumors, malignant melanoma, and gastrointestinal stromal tumors.

DISTINGUISHING HEPATOCELLULAR CARCINOMA FROM OTHER HEPATOCELLULAR LESIONS

Surgeons infrequently request intraoperative consultation to assess resection specimens for primary hepatocellular tumors because sophisticated imaging facilitates a preoperative diagnosis in many cases.[12] When evaluating resection specimens, the hepatic parenchymal margin is of primary concern; it should be examined and inked before sectioning the lesion perpendicular to the margin. Most tumors associated with a background of cirrhosis are hepatocellular carcinomas. They tend to be bulging brown or yellow-green nodules that are sharply circumscribed from the adjacent parenchyma (Fig. 6A). Focal nodular hyperplasia is yellow-brown, and large lesions often have a central fibrotic scar. These usually develop in patients without underlying liver disease (Fig. 6B). Hepatocellular adenomas can be nearly the same color as the background liver, yellow or red-tinged, and are somewhat distinct from the nonlesional liver (Fig. 6C). If a frozen section evaluation of the parenchymal margin is requested, a perpendicular section through the inked parenchymal margin including both nonneoplastic and tumor tissue, when possible, should be frozen and assessed.

All hepatocellular neoplasms display variable architectural abnormalities, including disorganized hepatocellular growth, thickened cords, and loss of portal tracts (Fig. 6D). Often there will be a shift in cellular composition between tumor and normal: the background liver does not have steatosis but the adenoma does, the carcinoma has abundant Mallory's hyaline but the adjacent nonneoplastic liver does not, and so forth (Fig. 6E). The distinction between well-differentiated hepatocellular carcinoma and hepatocellular adenoma can be difficult, if not impossible, to determine at the time of frozen section. In these cases, a diagnosis of well-differentiated hepatocellular neoplasm is sufficient, because both tumor types require surgical excision. Both hepatocellular adenoma and focal nodular hyperplasia occur in noncirrhotic livers. Broad fibrous bands that mimic cirrhotic septa and/or biliary ductal proliferation without a portal tract are clues to the diagnosis of focal nodular hyperplasia (Fig. 6F).

Intrahepatic Cholangiocarcinoma

Frozen sections are usually performed on hepatic specimens to assess the surgical resection margins. Assessment of the portal vein, hepatic artery, and bile duct with appropriate shave margins is critical to evaluation because intrahepatic cholangiocarcinoma commonly infiltrates along these structures. These tumors are firm and light yellow or white with a fibrotic surface. Histologic features include irregularly distributed and angulated glands or sheets of cells surrounded by dense, pink, collagenous stroma. The cytologic features are variable; cells may have abundant eosinophilic, cleared, or foamy cytoplasm with pleomorphic nuclei. Mucin may or may not be apparent. Bile production is not a feature of intrahepatic cholangiocarcinoma, unless it colonizes a preexisting bile duct hamartoma.

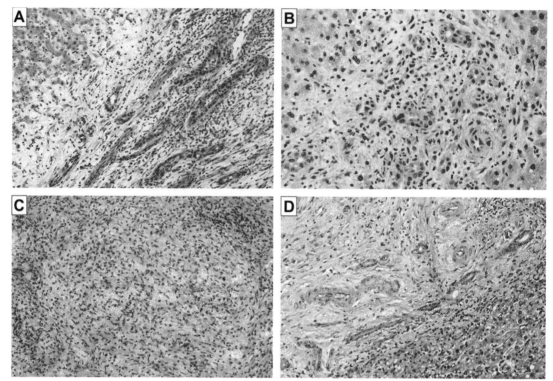

Fig. 5. (A) Bile duct obstruction can cause upstream biliary proliferations that mimic adenocarcinoma. Proliferating ductules surround portal veins and hepatic arteries, often in combination with neutrophils, lymphocytes, and edematous collagenous stroma (stain: hematoxylin and eosin [H&E]; original magnification ×100). (B) Ductules contain round, uniform nuclei with minimal-to-mild atypia (stain: H&E; original magnification ×200). (C) Postinflammatory changes secondary to cholangitis or prior surgery also mimic carcinoma, particularly in the gallbladder fossa. Xanthogranulomatous inflammation features sheets of cells with pink or foamy macrophages with ovoid nuclei and extracellular bile (stain: H&E; original magnification ×100). (D) Benign ducts (of Luschka) are normally located between the liver and gallbladder and may be prominent in some cases. Clues to a benign diagnosis include their linear or lobular distribution within fibrous tissue, minimal cytologic abnormalities, and lack of infiltration of hepatic parenchyma (stain: H&E; original magnification ×100).

Cavernous Hemangioma

Benign cavernous hemangiomas may be resected if they are large or if a patient is symptomatic. Gross examination reveals a red, spongy, ill-defined lesion with variable fibrosis. A frozen section is generally not required unless the lesion is a subcapsular sclerosed hemangioma. Thought to represent a hemangioma that has atrophied and been replaced by primarily fibrotic tissue, sclerosed hemangiomas may retain a histologic suggestion of glandular lumina because of residual vascular spaces (**Fig. 7**A). These lesions are benign and carry no risk of malignant degeneration for the patient.

Epithelioid Hemangioendothelioma

Epithelioid hemangioendotheliomas are firm and white infiltrative lesions that grossly resemble intrahepatic cholangiocarcinoma. Histologically,

the tumor comprises multiple cell types in a myxoid or hyalinized stroma. The leading edge of the tumor tends to be the most cellular: epithelioid cells with clear or eosinophilic cytoplasm and spindle-shaped dendritic cells grow within existing liver sinusoids. Vacuolated cells mimic signet ring cells, but lack cytoplasmic mucin. Vacuoles represent cytoplasmic lumina that may contain eosinophilic globules or fragmented red blood cells. If evaluation of the margin is requested for frozen section, special care should be taken to observe portal tracts and sinusoids for the presence of malignant cells percolating through these structures to the parenchymal margin.

DISTINGUISHING HEPATOCELLULAR CARCINOMA FROM METASTASES

There are several nonhepatocellular neoplasms to keep in mind when confronted with a solid tumor

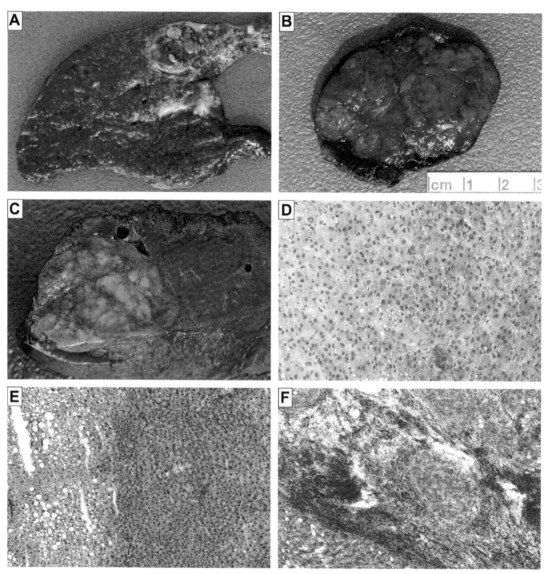

Fig. 6. (*A*) Hepatocellular carcinomas are typically associated with chronic liver disease and cirrhosis; they are bulging, well-circumscribed yellow, brown, or green nodules. (*B*) Focal nodular hyperplasia, which develops in a noncirrhotic liver, is somewhat lobulated with yellow-brown coloration and central fibrosis. (*C*) Hepatocellular adenomas are brown, yellow, or red, and may not have a sharply defined border with nonneoplastic parenchyma. They do not develop in association with cirrhosis and, thus, one should be cautious rendering this diagnosis anytime cirrhosis is present. (*D*) All hepatocellular neoplasms show variably disorganized hepatocyte plates with loss of portal structures and identifiable sinusoids. Bile can be present (stain: hematoxylin and eosin [H&E]; original magnification ×200). (*E*) When asked to evaluate the parenchymal margin it is helpful to first identify nonlesional liver with portal tracts and central veins, and then look for areas that are different. For example, nonlesional steatotic liver (*left*) is distinct from the adjacent adenoma that does not contain fat (stain: H&E; original magnification ×40). (*F*) Focal nodular hyperplasia contains broad fibrous septa that harbor a ductular proliferation, thereby mimicking cirrhosis. The septa lack portal vein branches (stain: H&E; original magnification ×40).

composed of cells with eosinophilic cytoplasm. Multiple tumors are more likely to represent metastatic disease. Be wary of diagnosing hepatocellular carcinoma in a patient who does not have chronic liver disease.

Gastrointestinal Endocrine Tumors

Patients with limited metastatic disease from primary pancreatic or small bowel (neuro)endocrine tumors may be resected, although such cases rarely pose diagnostic challenges at the

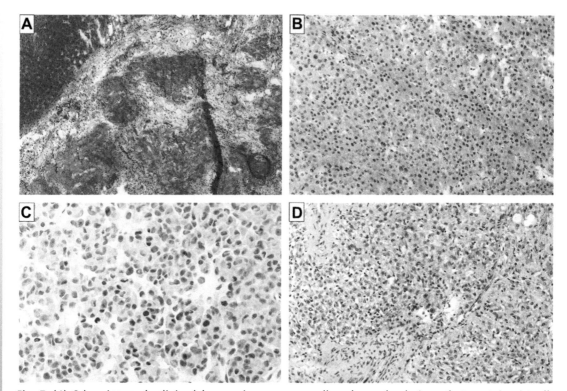

Fig. 7. (*A*) Sclerosing or hyalinized hemangiomas are usually subcapsular lesions that contain virtually acellular dense collagenous stroma. Vascular spaces may be present, but have flat endothelial lining without atypia (stain: hematoxylin and eosin [H&E]; original magnification ×40). (*B*) Adrenal cortical carcinoma is an eosinophilic tumor that can mimic hepatocellular carcinoma (stain: H&E; original magnification ×100). (*C*) Gastrointestinal stromal tumors that metastasize to the liver may have epithelioid morphology. They tend to display less nuclear pleomorphism than hepatocellular carcinoma (stain: H&E; original magnification ×200). (*D*) Hepatic angiomyolipoma can again mimic primary hepatocellular tumors. Many cases contain fat as well as dystrophic muscular vessels surrounded by spindled or epithelioid cells with eosinophilic cytoplasm.

time of frozen section.[13] Low-grade tumors display a tubular, nested, or sheetlike growth pattern and contain cells with scant eosinophilic to amphophilic cytoplasm, monomorphic nuclei, stippled chromatin, and inconspicuous nucleoli. Higher grade lesions may have more abundant eosinophilic cytoplasm and nuclear pleomorphism, mimicking a primary hepatocellular neoplasm.

Renal Cell Carcinoma

Renal cell carcinoma typically metastasizes to lung, lymph nodes, and bone, but up to 20% of patients develop hepatic metastases, which may be solitary.[14,15] Because liver metastases are often identified several years after the original diagnosis, renal cell carcinoma may not be initially suspected as the cause of a liver mass. The majority of renal cell carcinomas that metastasize to the liver show clear cell cytologic features and prominent vascularity. Metastases from papillary and

chromophobe renal cell carcinoma are more difficult to identify on frozen section because their cells may contain abundant eosinophilic cytoplasm and round nuclei that mimic a hepatocellular primary.

Adrenal Cortical Carcinoma

Like renal cell carcinoma, adrenal cortical carcinoma may consist of polygonal cells with clear to eosinophilic cytoplasm and round nuclei (**Fig. 7**B). In the absence of a clinical history, a diagnosis of metastatic adrenal cortical carcinoma requires immunohistochemical confirmation.

Malignant Melanoma

Uveal malignant melanoma commonly metastasizes to the liver, and the primary presentation may be that of a hepatic mass.[16] Tumors can be pigmented or amelanotic, epithelioid or spindled, but most contain characteristic single prominent nucleoli (see **Fig. 4**C). Hepatic metastases from cutaneous melanoma is less common but does occur.[4]

Gastrointestinal Stromal Tumor

The liver is a common site for metastasis from gastrointestinal stromal tumors. Hepatic involvement may be synchronous, in which case patients are treated with chemotherapy followed by surgical resection of primary and metastatic disease, or metachronous, usually occurring within 2 years of primary tumor resection.[17,18] Like malignant melanoma, these neoplasms can have a spindled or epithelioid morphology. If predominantly epithelioid, the cells commonly have abundant eosinophilic cytoplasm and can mimic hepatocellular lesions; clinical history is critical at the time of frozen section (**Fig. 7**C).

Angiomyolipoma

Angiomyolipoma is a rare tumor that can arise in the liver and mimic a primary hepatocellular neoplasm. It contains sheets of epithelioid cells with eosinophilic cytoplasm and thick-walled dystrophic blood vessels (**Fig. 7**D). The clue to the nonhepatocellular nature of this tumor is the presence of lipoma-like fatty growth, or, in the absence of a fat cell component, the presence of spindle cells that have a smooth muscle phenotype. On frozen section, nuclear pleomorphism and hyperchromasia may provide a clue that the lesion is not a hepatocellular adenoma. Although the vast majority of hepatic angiomyolipoma act in a benign manner, these tumors may rupture or cause abdominal discomfort. Surgical resection is indicated for symptoms or growth on imaging and is generally curative.[19]

DONOR LIVER EVALUATION

The decision to use an available organ for transplant depends on many clinical factors, one of which may be histologic evaluation of the donor liver.[20,21] Four features should be noted and quantified on frozen section review of a donor liver biopsy: steatosis, fibrosis, inflammation, and necrosis. A donor liver with more than 25% to 30% macrovesicular steatosis has an increased risk of primary graft dysfunction in the immediate posttransplant interval, and livers with greater than 60% macrovesicular steatosis have an increased risk of graft failure overall.[20,22,23] Transplant surgeons often have a high index of suspicion for fatty liver disease before sending a biopsy for frozen section evaluation because of the pale and/or yellow color of the organ. True macrovesicular steatosis in a frozen liver core appears as clear cytoplasmic globules that distort the hepatocytes and displace nuclei (**Fig. 8**A). Because steatotic hepatocytes are swollen, it is possible to overestimate the amount of steatosis in a liver core.[24] It is helpful to note which zones of the liver are involved to better estimate percentage of steatosis. If fat accumulation is confined to zone 3 (perivenular), then the amount of steatosis is 30% or less; panlobular involvement from central vein to portal tract reflects at least 60% steatosis. Potential mimics include bubbles that form as a frozen artifact, especially when tissue cores are transported in saline rather than procurement medium (**Fig. 8**B). Artifacts can be distinguished from steatosis because fat globules distort and displace hepatocyte nuclei.

> ## Key Points
> ### DONOR LIVER EVALUATION
>
> 1. Steatosis of less than 30% is acceptable for transplantation; mimics include frozen artifact and necrosis.
>
> 2. Inflammation should be grade 2 or less (moderate portal/interface hepatitis is acceptable) and fibrosis should be stage 2 or less (some periportal fibrosis is acceptable) for extended criteria donors.
>
> 3. Hepatocellular necrosis correlates with warm ischemia time, and more than 10% necrosis (generally found in zone 3) corresponds with graft dysfunction.

Fibrosis is the second important element to quantify in the liver biopsy, especially when expanded criteria donors are used.[25] The presence of fibrous septa, or more advanced fibrosis (Batts and Ludwig system stage 2/4 or greater), is a risk factor for poor patient outcome after transplant.[26] Although frozen section is not the optimal method to evaluate for minimal to mild fibrosis, careful evaluation of the architecture, including spacing of portal tracts and central veins, the presence of bridging septa, and entrapped hepatocytes in the periportal area allow one to rule out increased fibrosis (**Fig. 8**C). Inflammation (hepatitis) can also be present in extended criteria donors, and the grade of portal and lobular inflammation should be reported (**Fig. 8**D). Grafts with an inflammatory grade of 3 or 4 are generally excluded from transplantation because of poor graft survival.[26,27]

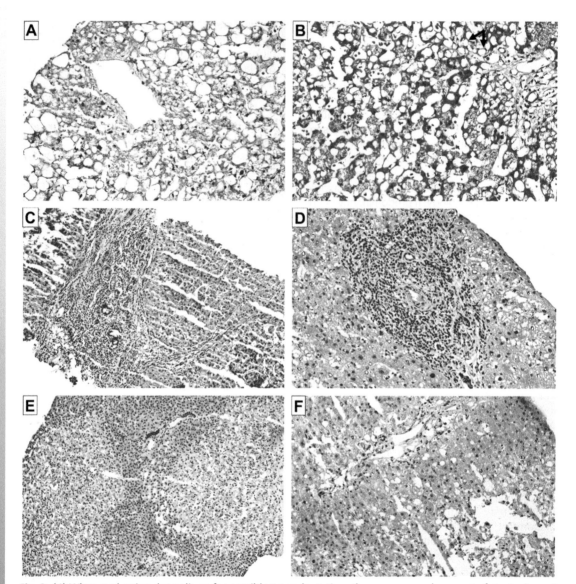

Fig. 8. (*A*) When evaluating donor livers for possible transplantation, the presence and amount of steatosis must be noted. Macrovesicular fat distorts hepatocellular plates and displaces hepatocyte nuclei (stain: hematoxylin and eosin [H&E]; original magnification ×100). (*B*) Frozen artifacts can result in massive dilation of sinusoids that mimics steatosis. Longitudinally sectioned dilated sinusoids are a helpful clue. There is very little steatosis is present in this sample, which is recognized by the presence of displaced nuclei (*black arrows*; stain: H&E; original magnification ×100). (*C*) Extended criteria donor livers often have some degree of chronic hepatitis and, in these cases, the amounts of periportal and perisinusoidal fibrosis should be staged. Bridging fibrosis is a contraindication for transplantation (stain: H&E; original magnification ×100). (*D*) Grade of inflammation should also be assessed. This portal tract is inflamed, but interface hepatitis is lacking and the liver may be used for transplantation (stain: H&E; original magnification ×200). (*E*) Hepatocellular necrosis occurs secondary to warm ischemia begins in zone 3. Hepatocytes may be pale or darkly eosinophilic with pyknotic or absent nuclei. Prominent endothelial cells and Kupffer cells can mimic viable hepatocytes in necrotic areas, resulting in an underestimation of the extent of injury (stain: H&E; original magnification ×100). (*F*) Hepatocellular drop out may leave empty spaces that mimic fat, or extensive necrosis may result in tissue tears during sectioning that may be misinterpreted as a cutting artifact rather than necrosis. In this patient, all of the centrilobular region was clearly necrotic on permanent section (stain: H&E; original magnification ×200). (*Courtesy of* Dr Rao Watson, University of Wisconsin, Department of Pathology.)

Finally, the extent of hepatocellular necrosis also predicts graft function. Extended warm ischemia time, the interval where the organ has decreased blood flow but remains at a physiologic temperature, is associated with noninflammatory hepatocellular necrosis. This interval may be increased in certain donors, including those who experience cardiac death. Although acidophil bodies may be seen throughout the lobule, the necrosis from warm ischemia is usually most prominent around the central veins (zone 3). Greater than 10% hepatocyte necrosis is considered undesirable because of potential graft dysfunction (**Fig. 8**E).[28] A pitfall in recognizing necrosis is that it may be interpreted as mild steatosis or frozen artifact. Hepatocellular dropout can form spaces that simulate centrilobular fat globules (**Fig. 8**F). Although cold ischemic time, which begins when the procured organ is placed in a cooling solution and ends when the organ is reperfused in the recipient, is also associated with graft dysfunction, the primary injury seems to be related to biliary damage rather than hepatocellular death.[25,29]

SUMMARY

Intraoperative consultation on specimens from the liver are useful for diagnosing metastatic disease, confirming negative margins, and evaluating a donor liver for transplantation. Metastases are the most common malignancies of the noncirrhotic liver, but benign biliary proliferations may mimic seeding of the liver by metastatic disease. Hepatocellular carcinoma is primarily a disease of the cirrhotic liver, but other primary liver tumors, including epithelioid hemangioendothelioma and focal nodular hyperplasia, arise in the noncirrhotic liver. Gross examination of primary liver tumors is key to the diagnosis of these lesions. Finally, frozen section evaluation of donor liver biopsies for steatosis, fibrosis, necrosis, and inflammation assists in optimal allocation of available organs for transplantation.

REFERENCES

1. Suriawinata AA. Miscellaneous liver tumors and tumor-like lesions. In: Saxena R, editor. Practical hepatic pathology: a diagnostic approach. 2nd edition. Philadelphia: Elsevier; 2018. p. 583–601. Available at: https://www.clinicalkey.com/#!/content/book/3-s2.0-B9780323428736000366?scrollTo=%23hl0001378.
2. Chatelain D, Shildknecht H, Trouillet N, et al. Intraoperative consultation in digestive surgery. A consecutive series of 800 frozen sections. J Visc Surg 2012; 149(2):e134–42.
3. Frankel TL, D'Angelica MI. Hepatic resection for colorectal metastases. J Surg Oncol 2014;109(1): 2–7.
4. Page AJ, Weiss MJ, Pawlik TM. Surgical management of noncolorectal cancer liver metastases. Cancer 2014;120(20):3111–21.
5. Rees M, Tekkis PP, Welsh FKS, et al. Evaluation of long-term survival after hepatic resection for metastatic colorectal cancer: a multifactorial model of 929 patients. Ann Surg 2008;247(1):125–35.
6. Poultsides GA, Schulick RD, Pawlik TM. Hepatic resection for colorectal metastases: the impact of surgical margin status on outcome. HPB (Oxford) 2010;12(1):43–9.
7. Bhutiani N, Philips P, Martin RCG, et al. Impact of surgical margin clearance for resection of secondary hepatic malignancies. J Surg Oncol 2016; 113(3):289–95.
8. Banales JM, Cardinale V, Carpino G, et al. Expert consensus document: cholangiocarcinoma: current knowledge and future perspectives consensus statement from the European Network for the Study of Cholangiocarcinoma (ENS-CCA). Nat Rev Gastroenterol Hepatol 2016;13(5):261–80.
9. Fritz S, Hackert T, Blaker H, et al. Multiple von Meyenburg complexes mimicking diffuse liver metastases from esophageal squamous cell carcinoma. World J Gastroenterol 2006;12(26): 4250–2.
10. Spinelli A, Schumacher G, Pascher A, et al. Extended surgical resection for xanthogranulomatous cholecystitis mimicking advanced gallbladder carcinoma: a case report and review of literature. World J Gastroenterol 2006;12(14): 2293–6.
11. Singhi AD, Adsay NV, Swierczynski SL, et al. Hyperplastic Luschka ducts: a mimic of adenocarcinoma in the gallbladder fossa. Am J Surg Pathol 2011; 35(6):883–90.
12. Anis M, Irshad A. Imaging of hepatocellular carcinoma: practical guide to differential diagnosis. Clin Liver Dis 2011;15(2):335–52, vii–x.
13. Glazer ES, Tseng JF, Al-Refaie W, et al. Long-term survival after surgical management of neuroendocrine hepatic metastases. HPB (Oxford) 2010; 12(6):427–33.
14. Ruys AT, Tanis PJ, Nagtegaal ID, et al. Surgical treatment of renal cell cancer liver metastases: a population-based study. Ann Surg Oncol 2011; 18(7):1932–8.
15. Hamada S, Ito K, Kuroda K, et al. Clinical characteristics and prognosis of patients with renal cell carcinoma and liver metastasis. Mol Clin Oncol 2015; 3(1):63–8.
16. Eskelin S, Pyrhönen S, Summanen P, et al. Screening for metastatic malignant melanoma of the uvea revisited. Cancer 1999;85(5):1151–9.

17. Gomez D, Al-Mukthar A, Menon KV, et al. Aggressive surgical resection for the management of hepatic metastases from gastrointestinal stromal tumours: a single centre experience. HPB (Oxford) 2007;9(1):64–70.

18. Turley RS, Peng PD, Reddy SK, et al. Hepatic resection for metastatic gastrointestinal stromal tumors in the tyrosine kinase inhibitor era. Cancer 2012; 118(14):3571–8.

19. Klompenhouwer AJ, Verver D, Janki S, et al. Management of hepatic angiomyolipoma: a systematic review. Liver Int 2017;37(9):1272–80.

20. Strasberg SM, Howard TK, Molmenti EP, et al. Selecting the donor liver: risk factors for poor function after orthotopic liver transplantation. Hepatology 1994;20(4 Pt 1):829–38.

21. Ploeg RJ, D'Alessandro AM, Knechtle SJ, et al. Risk factors for primary dysfunction after liver transplantation–a multivariate analysis. Transplantation 1993;55(4):807–13.

22. Adani GL, Baccarani U, Sainz-Barriga M, et al. The role of hepatic biopsy to detect macrovacuolar steatosis during liver procurement. Transplant Proc 2006;38(5):1404–6.

23. de Graaf EL, Kench J, Dilworth P, et al. Grade of deceased donor liver macrovesicular steatosis impacts graft and recipient outcomes more than the donor risk index. J Gastroenterol Hepatol 2012; 27(3):540–6.

24. D'Alessandro E, Calabrese F, Gringeri E, et al. Frozen-section diagnosis in donor livers: error rate estimation of steatosis degree. Transplant Proc 2010;42(6):2226–8.

25. Feng S, Lai JC. Expanded criteria donors. Clin Liver Dis 2014;18(3):633–49.

26. Ydreborg M, Westin J, Lagging M, et al. Impact of donor histology on survival following liver transplantation for chronic hepatitis C virus infection: a Scandinavian single-center experience. Scand J Gastroenterol 2012;47(6):710–7.

27. Rayhill SC, Wu YM, Katz DA, et al. Older donor livers show early severe histological activity, fibrosis, and graft failure after liver transplantation for hepatitis C. Transplantation 2007;84(3): 331–9.

28. Reich DJ, Hong JC. Current status of donation after cardiac death liver transplantation. Curr Opin Organ Transplant 2010;15(3):316–21.

29. Taner CB, Bulatao IG, Keaveny AP, et al. Use of liver grafts from donation after cardiac death donors for recipients with hepatitis C virus. Liver Transpl 2011;17(6):641–9.

Printed and bound by CPI Group (UK) Ltd, Croydon, CR0 4YY

03/10/2024

01040298-0015